evolve

W9-BTN-205

To access your Student Resources, visit:

http://evolve.elsevier.com/KeeMarshall/clinical/

Evolve® Student Resources for Kee/Marshall: *Clinical Calculations With Applications to General and Specialty Areas, Sixth Edition,* offer the following features:

Student Resources

- **WebLinks**
  An exciting resource that lets you link to hundreds of websites carefully chosen to supplement the content of your textbook. The WebLinks are regulary updated with new ones added as they develop.

CLINICAL
CALCULATIONS

With Applications to General and Specialty Areas

Sixth Edition

CLINICAL CALCULATIONS

With Applications to General and Specialty Areas

Joyce LeFever Kee, RN, MS
Associate Professor Emerita
College of Health Sciences
Department of Nursing
University of Delaware
Newark, Delaware

Sally M. Marshall, RN, MSN
Nursing Service
Department of Veterans Affairs
Regional Office and Medical Center
Wilmington, Delaware

SAUNDERS

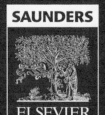

ELSEVIER

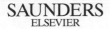

SAUNDERS
ELSEVIER

11830 Westline Industrial Drive
St. Louis, Missouri 63146

CLINICAL CALCULATIONS WITH APPLICATIONS TO GENERAL   ISBN: 978-1-4160-4740-7
AND SPECIALTY AREAS, SIXTH EDITION
Copyright © 2009, 2004, 2000, 1996, 1992, 1988 by Mosby, Inc., an affiliate of Elsevier Inc.

Notice

Knowledge and best practice in this field are constantly changing. As new research and experience broaden our knowledge, changes in practice, treatment, and drug therapy may become necessary or appropriate. Readers are advised to check the most current information provided (i) on procedures featured or (ii) by the manufacturer of each product to be administered, to verify the recommended dose or formula, the method and duration of administration, and contraindications. It is the responsibility of practitioners, relying on their own experience and knowledge of the patient, to make diagnoses, to determine dosages and the best treatment for each individual patient, and to take all appropriate safety precautions. To the fullest extent of the law, neither the Publisher nor the Authors assumes any liability for any injury and/or damage to persons or property arising out of or related to any use of the material contained in this book.

Library of Congress Control Number 978-1-4160-4740-7

Senior Editor: Yvonne Alexopoulos
Senior Developmental Editor: Danielle M. Frazier
Publishing Services Manager: John Rogers
Senior Project Manager: Helen Hudlin
Designer: Maggie Reid

Printed in Canada

Last digit is the print number: 9 8 7 6 5 4 3 2

**Working together to grow
libraries in developing countries**

www.elsevier.com | www.bookaid.org | www.sabre.org

ELSEVIER   BOOK AID
International   Sabre Foundation

To my grandchildren, Christopher, Brenda, Jessica, and Kimberly

Joyce Kee

————•————

To my mother and to my children, Drew and Sarah

Sally Marshall

————•————

To our nursing colleagues

Reviewers

Marjorie Campbell, RN, MSN
Nursing Faculty
University of New Mexico
Gallup, NM

Jennifer Clark, MSN, ARNP-BC
Assistant Professor
Florida Hospital College
Orlando, FL

Rebekah Delafield, RN, ADN
Nursing Instructor
San Jancinto College
Houston, TX

Dori Gilman, RN, BS, MSN
Instructor of Nursing
North Country Community College
Saranac Lake, NY

Kathleen K. Gudgel, RN, MSN
Instructor of Nursing
School of Health Sciences
Pennsylvania College of Technology
Williamsport, PA

Carla Hilton, MSN, RN
Instructor of Nursing
Covenant School of Nursing
Lubbock, TX

Ruth Lebet, RN, MSN, CCNS, CCRN
Clinical Nurse Specialist, PICU
Alfred I duPont Hospital for Children/Nemours
Wilmington, DE

Maria McCabe, RN, MS
Industrial Assistant in Nursing
SUNY Ulster Community College
Stone Ridge, NY

Diane M. Shannon, RNC, MSN
Certified School Nurse
Previously Perinatal Clinical Nurse Specialist
Thomas Jefferson University Hospital
Philadelphia, PA

Tamara Shields, RN, MS, CFNP
Instructor of Nursing
St. Elizabeth School of Nursing
Lafayette, IN

Jo Voss, RN, PhDc, CNS
Assistant Professor
College of Nursing
South Dakota State University
Rapid City, SD

Frances Warrick, MS, RN
Program Coordinator, Vocational Nursing
El Centro College
Dallas, TX

Preface to the Instructor

Clinical Calculations With Applications to General and Specialty Areas arose from the need to bridge the learning gap between education and practice. We believe that this bridge is needed for the student to understand the wide range of clinical calculations used in nursing practice. This book provides a comprehensive application of calculations in nursing practice.

Clinical Calculations has been expanded in this sixth edition on topics in several areas to show the interrelationship between calculation and drug administration. The use of the latest methods, techniques, and equipments are included: unit dose dispensing system, electronic medication administration record (eMAR), computerized prescriber order system (CPOS), various methods of calculating drug doses with the use of Body Mass Index (BMI), Ideal Body Weight (IBW) with Adjusted Body Weight (ABW), insulin pump, insulin inhalant, patient-controlled analgesia pumps, multi-channel infusion pumps, IV filters, and many more. This text also provides the six (6) methods for calculating drug dosages—basic formula, ratio and proportion, fractional equation, dimensional analysis, body weight, and body surface area.

Clinical Calculations is unique in that it has problems not only for the general patient areas but also for the specialty units—pediatrics, critical care, pediatric critical care, labor and delivery, and community. This text is useful for nurses at all levels of nursing education who are learning for the first time how to calculate dosage problems and for beginning practitioners in specialty areas. It also can be used in nursing refresher coursers, inservice programs, hospital units, home health care, and other places of nursing practice.

This book is divided into five parts. Part I is the basic math review, written concisely for nursing students to review Roman numerals, fractions, decimals, percentages, and ratio and proportion. A post-math review test follows. The post-math test can be taken first, and, if the student has a score of 90% of higher, the basic review section can be omitted. Part II covers metric, apothecary, and household systems used in drug calculations; conversion of units; reading drug labels, drug orders, eMAR, computerized prescriber order systems, and abbreviations; and methods of calculations. We suggest that you assign Parts I and II, which cover delivery of medication, prior to the class. Part III covers calculation of drug and fluid dosages for oral, injectable, and intravenous administration. Clinical drug calculations for specialty areas are found in Part IV. This part includes pediatrics, critical care for adults and children, labor and delivery, and community. Part V contains the Post-Test for students to test their competency in mastering oral, injectable, intravenous, and pediatric drug calculations. A passing grade is 88%.

Appendix A includes guidelines for administrations of medications (oral, injectable, and intravenous), and Appendix B contains nomograms.

Each chapter has a content list, objectives, introduction, and numerous practice problems. The practice problems are related to clinical drug problems that are currently used in clinical settings. Illustrations such as tablets, capsules, medicine cup, syringes, ampules, vials, intravenous bag and bottle, IV tubing, electronic IV devices, intramuscular injection sites, central venous sites, and many others are provided throughout the text.

Calculators may be used in solving dosage problems. Many institutions have calculators available. The nurse should work the problem without a calculator and then check the answer with a calculator.

FEATURES OF THE SIXTH EDITION

- Problems using the newest drug labels are provided in most chapters.
- Six methods for calculating drug dosages have been divided into two chapters. Chapter 5 gives four methods—basic formula, ratio and proportion, fractional equations, and dimensional analysis. Chapter 6 contains two individual methods for calculating drug doses—body weight and body surface area.
- Additional dimensional analysis has been added to the examples of drug dosing and to the answers to practice problems in most of the chapters.
- Additional drug problems have been added throughout.
- More emphasis is placed on the metric system than on the apothecary system.
- Several chapters have nomograms for adults and children.
- Explanation on the unit dose dispensing system, computer-based drug administration, computerized prescriber order system, bar code medication administration, MAR, electronic medication administration record (eMAR), and automation of medication dispensing administration are provided.
- Incorporation of guidelines for safe practice and the medication administration set by The Joint Commission (TJC) and the Institute for Safe Medicine Practices (ISMP) are included.
- Explanation of the four groups of inhaled medications include: MDI inhalers with and without spacers, dry powder inhalers, and the nebulizers.
- Calculations by BMI, IBW, and ABW for obese and debilitated persons are presented.
- Body Surface Area (BSA or m^2) using the square root method is included.
- Use of fingertip units for cream applications is illustrated.
- Explanations are provided for the use of the insulin pump, insulin pen injectors, insulin inhalant, and the patient-controlled analgesic pump.
- Illustrations of new types of syringes, safety needle shield, various insulin and tuberculin syringes, and needleless syringes are provided.
- Illustrations of pumps are provided, including insulin, enteral infusion, and various intravenous infusion pumps (single and multi-channel, patient-controlled analgesia, and syringe).
- Coverage of direct intravenous injection (IV push or IV bolus) is provided with practice problems in Chapter 9.
- Updated methods and information for critical care, pediatrics, and OB calculations are presented.

ANCILLARIES

Instructor Resources for Clinical Calculations With Applications to General and Specialty Areas, Sixth Edition, is specifically geared toward this edition and includes the following:

- Teaching strategies
- Three different course outlines for teaching calculation of drug dosage: (1) as a separate course, (2) as part of a pharmacology course, or (3) as integrated into the nursing curriculum and covered in the skill laboratory and clinical courses
- A Basic Math Test for the instructor to administer to the students early in the course to evaluate basic math skills
- A Test Bank with over 300 drug calculation problems covering general and specialty areas

To use this great resource online visit the **Evolve** website at http:// evolve.elsevier.com/KeeMarshall/clinical/

TEACH for Clinical Calculations With Applications to General and Specialty Areas, Sixth Edition is an online resource designed to help instructors reduce their lesson preparation time, give them new and creative ideas to promote student learning, and help them to make full use of the rich array of resources in the Kee/Marshall teaching package.

TEACH consists of customizable Lesson Plans and Lecture Outlines that are based on the learning objectives from the text. Provided for each book chapter, the lesson plans are divided into 50-minute lessons. These lesson plans include features such as teaching focus summaries, lesson preparation checklists, pretests and background assessment questions, critical thinking questions, and class activities. The lecture outlines are also available for each book chapter and include PowerPoint slides to provide visual presentation and summary of the main chapter points. Lecture notes for each slide highlight key topics and provide thought-provoking questions for discussion to help create an interactive classroom environment.

TEACH is available online through the **Evolve** website at http:// evolve.elsevier.com/KeeMarshall/clinical/

Dosages and Solutions Computerized Test Bank (Version II) is a generic testbank that contains over 700 questions on general mathematics, converting within the same system of measurements, between different systems of measurement, oral dosages, parenteral dosages, flow rates, pediatric dosages, IV calculations, and more.

CTB is available online through the Evolve website at http://evolve. elsevier.com/KeeMarshall/clinical/

Drug Calculations Student CD-ROM (Version III) is a completely updated, user-friendly, interactive student tutorial with a brand new organization and design for easier navigation. It includes an extensive menu of various topic areas within drug calculations such as oral, parenteral, pediatric, and intravenous calculations to name a few. It includes exercises where students can fill in syringes to answer problems. Covering the ratio and proportion, basic formula, and dimensional analysis methods, this CD contains 565 practice problems including a comprehensive post-test. It is packaged with every copy of the text.

Preface to the Student

Clinical Calculations With Applications to General and Specialty Areas, Sixth Edition, can be used as a self-instructional mathematics and dosage calculation review tool.

Part I, *Basic Math Review,* is a review of math concepts usually taught in middle school. Some of you may need to review Part I as a refresher of basic math and then take the comprehensive math test at the end of the chapter. Others may choose to take the math test first. If your score on this test is 90% or higher, you should proceed to Part II; if your score is less than 90%, you should review Part I.

Part II, *Systems, Conversion, and Methods of Drug Calculation,* should be studied before the class on oral, injectable, and intravenous calculations, which is covered in Part III. In Part II you will learn the various systems of drug administration, conversion within the various systems, charting (MAR and eMAR), drug orders, abbreviations, methods of drug calculation, and alternative methods for drug administration. You can study Part II on your own. Chapter 5, "Methods of Calculation," gives the four methods commonly used to calculate drug dosages. You or the instructor should select one of the four methods to calculate drug dosages. Use that method in all practice problems starting in Chapter 5. This approach will improve your proficiency in the calculation of drug dosages.

Part III, *Calculations for Oral, Injectable, and Intravenous Drugs,* is usually discussed in class and during a clinical practicum. Before class, you should review the three chapters in Part III. Questions may be addressed and answered during class time. During the class or clinical practicum, you may practice drug calculations and the drawing up of drug doses in a syringe.

Part IV, *Calculations for Specialty Areas,* is usually presented when the topics are discussed in class. You should review the content in these chapters— "Pediatrics," "Critical Care," "Pediatric Critical Care," "Labor and Delivery," and "Community"—before the scheduled class. According to the requirements of your specific nursing program, this content may or may not be covered.

Part V has 60 post-test questions for the students to determine their competency in mastering oral, injectable, intravenous, and pediatric drug calculations.

Take a look at the following features so that you may familiarize yourself with this text and maximize its value:

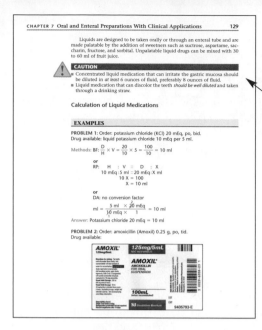

> *Caution* boxes alert you to potential problems related to various medications and their administration.

> *Notes* emphasize important points for students as they learn material in each chapter.

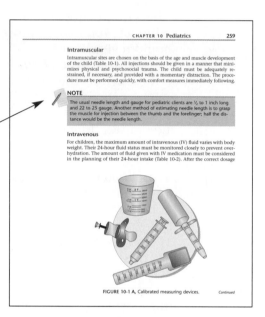

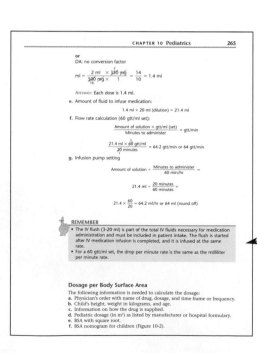

> *Remember* boxes identify pertinent concepts that students should commit to memory.

Drug Calculations Student CD-ROM (Version III). Completely updated, this user friendly, interactive student tutorial has a brand new organization and design for easier navigation. It includes an extensive menu of various topic areas within drug calculations such as oral, parenteral, pediatric, and intravenous calculations to name a few. It includes exercises where students can fill in syringes to answer problems. Covering the ratio and proportion, formula, and dimensional analysis methods, this CD contains 565 practice problems including a comprehensive post-test. Packaged with every copy of the text.

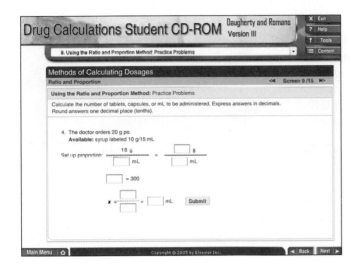

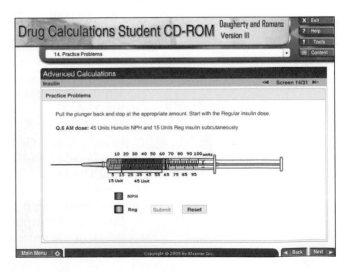

Here is an outline of the table of contents for the *Drug Calculations Student CD-ROM (Version III)*

I.   Mathematics Review
   A. Fractions
   B. Decimals
   C. Ratios
   D. Proportions
   E. Percents

II. Introducing Drug Measures
   A. Systems of Measurement
   B. Measuring Dosages

III. Safety in Medication Administration
   A. The "Six" Rights
   B. Pyxis
   C. Bar Code
   D. MAR and eMAR
   E. Parts of a Drug Label
   F. Reading Drug Labels
   G. Reading Syringes

IV. Methods of Calculating Dosages
   A. Basic Formula
   B. Ratio and Proportion
   C. Dimensional Analysis

V.   Basic Calculations
   A. Oral Dosages
   B. Parenteral Dosages
   C. Reconstitution of Powdered Drugs
   D. Intake and Output (I & O)
   E. Tube Feedings

VI. Pediatric Calculations
   A. Pediatric Dosages per Body Weight
   B. Pediatric Dosages per Body Surface Area (BSA)

VII. Intravenous Calculations
   A. Understanding IV Flow Rates
   B. Mixing IVs
   C. Intravenous Push (IVP)

VIII. Advanced Calculations
   A. Critical Medications
   B. Titrating Medications
   C. Insulin
   D. Heparin
   E. Patient Controlled Analgesia (PCA)

IX. Comprehensive Post-Test
   A. Oral Dosages
   B. Parenteral Dosages
   C. Reconstitution of Powdered Drugs
   D. Intake and Output (I & O)
   E. Pediatric Calculations
   F. Mixing IV's

Look for this icon at the end of the chapters. It will refer you to the *Drug Calculations Student CD-ROM (Version III)* for additional practice problems and content information.

Acknowledgments

We wish to extend our sincere appreciation to the individuals who have helped with this Sixth Edition: Ruth Lebet, RN, MSN, CCNS, CCRN, Clinical Nurse Specialist, PICU, Alfred I. duPont Hospital for Children/Nemours, Wilmington, Delaware; Diane Shannon, RNC, MSN, Certified School Nurse, previously Perinatal Clinical Nurse Specialist, Thomas Jefferson University Hospital, Philadelphia, Pennsylvania; Drew Marshall for his typing assistance, particularly with the references; and to our husbands, Edward Kee and Robert Marshall, for their support. We also thank Don Passidomo, Head Librarian at the Veterans Administration Medical Center, for his research assistance.

Joyce LeFever Kee
Sally M. Marshall

Contents

BASIC MATH REVIEW

OBJECTIVES

- Convert Roman numerals to Arabic numerals.
- Multiply and divide fractions and decimals.
- Solve ratio and proportion problems.
- Change percentages to decimals, fractions, and ratio and proportion.
- Demonstrate an understanding of Roman numerals, fractions, decimals, ratio and proportion, and percentage by passing the math test.

OUTLINE

NUMBER SYSTEMS
    Arabic System
    Roman System
    Conversion of Systems

FRACTIONS
    Proper, Improper, and Mixed
       Fractions
    Multiplying Fractions
    Dividing Fractions
    Decimal Fractions

DECIMALS
    Multiplying Decimals
    Dividing Decimals

RATIO AND PROPORTION
PERCENTAGE
POST-MATH TEST
    Roman and Arabic Numerals
    Fractions
    Decimals
    Ratio and Proportion
    Percentage

The basic math review assists nurses in converting Roman and Arabic numerals, multiplying and dividing fractions and decimals, and solving ratio and proportion problems and percentage problems. Nurses need to master basic math skills to solve drug problems used in the administration of medication.

A math test, found on pages 13 to 16, follows the basic math review. The test may be taken first, and, if a score of 90% or greater is achieved, the math review, or Part I, can be omitted. If the test score is less than 90%, the student should do the basic math review section. Some students may choose to start with Part I and then take the test.

Answers to the Practice Problems are at the end of Part I, before the Post-Math Test.

NUMBER SYSTEMS

Two systems of numbers currently used are Arabic and Roman. Both systems are used in drug administration.

Arabic System

The Arabic system is expressed in numbers: 0, 1, 2, 3, 4, 5, 6, 7, 8, 9. These can be written as whole numbers or with fractions and decimals. This system is commonly used today.

Roman System

Numbers used in the Roman system are designated by selected capital letters, e.g., I, V, X. Roman numbers can be changed to Arabic numbers.

Conversion of Systems

Roman Number	Arabic Number
I	1
V	5
X	10
L	50
C	100

The apothecary system of measurement uses Roman numerals for writing drug dosages. The Roman numerals are written in lower case letters, e.g., i, v, x, xii. The lower case letters can be topped by a horizontal line, e.g., ī, v̄, x̄, x̄īi.

Roman numerals can appear together, such as xv and ix. Reading multiple Roman numerals requires the use of addition and subtraction.

METHOD A

If the first Roman numeral is greater than the following numeral(s), then **ADD.**

EXAMPLES

$$\overline{viii} = 5 + 3 = 8$$
$$\overline{xv} = 10 + 5 = 15$$

METHOD B

If the first Roman numeral is less than the following numeral(s), then **SUBTRACT.** Subtract the first numeral from the second (i.e., the smaller from the larger).

EXAMPLES

$$\overline{iv} = 5 - 1 = 4$$
$$\overline{ix} = 10 - 1 = 9$$

Some Roman numerals require both addition and subtraction to ascertain their value. Read from left to right.

EXAMPLES

$$\overline{xix} = 10 + 9 \, (10 - 1) = 19$$
$$\overline{xxxiv} = 30 \, (10 + 10 + 10) + 4 \, (5 - 1) = 34$$

PRACTICE PROBLEMS: I Roman Numerals

Answers can be found on page 11.

1. $\overline{xvi}$

_____

2. $\overline{xii}$

_____

3. $\overline{xxiv}$

_____

4. $\overline{xxxix}$

_____

5. XLV

_____

6. XC

_____

FRACTIONS

Fractions are expressed as part(s) of a whole or part(s) of a unit. A fraction is composed of two basic numbers: a *numerator* (the top number) and a *denominator* (the bottom number). The denominator indicates the total number of parts.

EXAMPLES

Fraction: $\dfrac{3}{4}$ numerator (3 of 4 parts)
denominator (4 of 4 parts, or 4 total parts)

The value of a fraction depends mainly on the denominator. When the denominator increases, for example, from $\frac{1}{10}$ to $\frac{1}{20}$, the value of the fraction decreases, because it takes more parts to make a whole.

EXAMPLES

Which fraction has the greater value: $\frac{1}{4}$ or $\frac{1}{6}$? The denominators are 4 and 6.

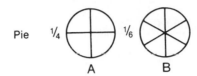

The larger value is $\frac{1}{4}$, because four parts make the whole, whereas for $\frac{1}{6}$, it takes six parts to make a whole. Therefore $\frac{1}{6}$ has the smaller value.

Proper, Improper, and Mixed Fractions

In a *proper fraction* (simple fraction), the numerator is less than the denominator, e.g., $\frac{1}{2}$, $\frac{2}{3}$, $\frac{3}{4}$, $\frac{2}{6}$. When possible, the fraction should be reduced to its lowest terms, e.g., $\frac{2}{6} = \frac{1}{3}$ (2 goes into 2 and 6).

In an *improper fraction*, the numerator is greater than the denominator, e.g., $\frac{4}{2}$, $\frac{8}{5}$, $\frac{14}{4}$. Reduce improper fractions to whole numbers or mixed numbers, e.g., $\frac{4}{2} = 2$ ($\frac{4}{2}$ means the same as $4 \div 2$); $\frac{8}{5} = 1\frac{3}{5}$ ($8 \div 5$, 5 goes into 8 one time with 3 left over, or $\frac{3}{5}$); and $\frac{14}{4} = 3\frac{2}{4} = 3\frac{1}{2}$ ($14 \div 4$, 4 goes into 14 three times with 2 left over, or $\frac{2}{4}$, which can then be reduced to $\frac{1}{2}$).

A *mixed number* is a whole number and a fraction, e.g., $1\frac{3}{5}$, $3\frac{1}{2}$. Mixed numbers can be changed to improper fractions by multiplying the denominator by the whole number, then adding the numerator, e.g., $1\frac{3}{5} = \frac{8}{5}$ ($5 \times 1 = 5 + 3 = 8$).

The apothecary system uses fractions to indicate drug dosages. Fractions may be added, subtracted, multiplied, or divided. Multiplying fractions and dividing fractions are the two common methods used in solving dosage problems.

Multiplying Fractions

To multiply fractions, multiply the numerators and then the denominators. Reduce the fraction, if possible, to lowest terms.

EXAMPLES

PROBLEM 1: $\dfrac{1}{3} \times \dfrac{3}{5} = \dfrac{\overset{1}{\cancel{3}}}{\underset{5}{\cancel{15}}} = \dfrac{1}{5}$

The answer is $\frac{3}{15}$, which can be reduced to $\frac{1}{5}$. The number that goes into both 3 and 15 is 3. Therefore 3 goes into 3 one time, and 3 goes into 15 five times.

PROBLEM 2: $\dfrac{1}{3} \times 6 = \dfrac{6}{3} = 2$

A whole number can also be written as that number over one $(\tfrac{6}{1})$. Six is divided by 3 $(6 \div 3)$; 3 goes into 6 two times.

Dividing Fractions

To divide fractions, invert the *second fraction*, or divisor, and then multiply.

EXAMPLES

PROBLEM 1: $\dfrac{3}{4} \div \dfrac{3}{8}$ (divisor) $= \dfrac{\overset{1}{\cancel{3}}}{\underset{1}{\cancel{4}}} \times \dfrac{\overset{2}{\cancel{8}}}{\underset{1}{\cancel{3}}} = \dfrac{2}{1} = 2$

When dividing, invert the divisor ⅜ to ⅞₃ and multiply. To reduce the fraction to lowest terms, 3 goes into both 3s one time, and 4 goes into 4 and 8 one time and two times, respectively.

PROBLEM 2: $\dfrac{1}{6} \div \dfrac{4}{18} = \dfrac{1}{\underset{1}{\cancel{6}}} \times \dfrac{\overset{3}{\cancel{18}}}{4} = \dfrac{3}{4}$

Six and 18 are reduced, or canceled, to 1 and 3.

Decimal Fractions

Fractions can be changed to decimals. Divide the numerator by the denominator, e.g., ¾ = 4)3.00 with quotient 0.75. Therefore ¾ is the same as 0.75.

PRACTICE PROBLEMS: II Fractions

Answers can be found on pages 11 and 12.

1. **a.** Which has the greatest value: ½₀, ¹⁄₁₀₀, or ¹⁄₁₅₀? _____

    b. Which has the lowest value: ½₀, ¹⁄₁₀₀, or ¹⁄₁₅₀? _____

2. Reduce improper fractions to whole or mixed numbers.

    a. ¹²⁄₄ =   **c.** ²²⁄₃ =

    _____   _____

    b. ²⁰⁄₅ =   **d.** ³²⁄₆ =

    _____   _____

3. Multiply fractions to whole number(s) or lowest fraction or decimal.

    a. ⅔ × ⅛ =   **c.** ⁵⁰⁰⁄₃₅₀ × 5 =

    _____   _____

b. $2\frac{2}{5} \times 3\frac{3}{4} =$
   $\frac{12}{5} \times \frac{15}{4} =$

d. $\frac{400,000}{200,000} \times 3 =$

---

4. Divide fractions to whole number(s) or lowest fraction or decimal.

   a. $\frac{2}{3} \div 6 =$

   d. $\frac{1}{150}/\frac{1}{100} = (\frac{1}{150} \div \frac{1}{100}) =$

   ---

   b. $\frac{1}{4} \div \frac{1}{5} =$

   e. $\frac{1}{200} \div \frac{1}{300} =$

   ---

   c. $\frac{1}{6} \div \frac{1}{8} =$

   f. $9\frac{3}{5} \div 4 =$
      $\frac{48}{5} \div \frac{4}{1} =$

   ---

5. Change each fraction to a decimal.

   a. $\frac{1}{4} =$

   b. $\frac{1}{10} =$

   c. $\frac{2}{5} =$

DECIMALS

Decimals consist of (1) whole numbers (numbers to the left of decimal point) and (2) decimal fractions (numbers to the right of decimal point). The number 2468.8642 is an example of the division of units for a whole number with a decimal fraction.

Whole Numbers					Decimal Fractions			
2	4	6	8	•	8	6	4	2
Thousands	Hundreds	Tens	Units		Tenths	Hundredths	Thousandths	Ten Thousandths

Decimal fractions are written in tenths, hundredths, thousandths, and ten-thousandths. Frequently, decimal fractions are used in drug dosing. The metric system is referred to as the *decimal system*. After decimal problems are solved, decimal

fractions are generally rounded off to tenths. ***If the hundredth column is 5 or greater, the tenth is increased by 1, e.g., 0.67 is rounded up to 0.7 (tenths).***
Decimal fractions are an integral part of the metric system. Tenths mean 0.1 or $\frac{1}{10}$, hundredths mean 0.01 or $\frac{1}{100}$, and thousandths mean 0.001 or $\frac{1}{1000}$. When a decimal is changed to a fraction, the denominator is based on the number of digits to the right of the decimal point (0.8 is $\frac{8}{10}$, 0.86 is $\frac{86}{100}$).

EXAMPLES

PROBLEM 1: 0.5 is $\frac{5}{10}$, or 5 tenths.
PROBLEM 2: 0.55 is $\frac{55}{100}$, or 55 hundredths.
PROBLEM 3: 0.555 is $\frac{555}{1000}$, or 555 thousandths.

Multiplying Decimals

To multiply decimal numbers, multiply the multiplicand by the multiplier. Count how many numbers (spaces) are to the right of the decimals in the problem. Mark off the number of decimal spaces in the answer (right to left) according to the number of decimal spaces in the problem. Answers are rounded off to the nearest **tenths.**

EXAMPLES

```
  1.34   multiplicand
  2.3    multiplier
  402
 2680
 3.082   or   3.1 (rounded off in tenths)
```

Answer: 3.1. Because 8 is greater than 5, the "tenth" number is increased by 1.

Dividing Decimals

To divide decimal numbers, move the decimal point in the divisor to the right to make a whole number. The decimal point in the dividend is also moved to the right according to the number of decimal spaces in the divisor. Answers are rounded off to the nearest **tenths.**

EXAMPLES

$$\text{Dividend} \div \text{Divisor}$$

$$2.46 \div 1.2 \quad \text{or} \quad \frac{2.46}{1.2} =$$

```
                     2.05 = 2.1
(divisor) 1.2 )2.4 60 (dividend)
                  2 4
                     60
                     60
                      0
```

PRACTICE PROBLEMS: III Decimals

Answers can be found on page 12.

Round off to the nearest tenths.

1. Multiply decimals.

   a. $6.8 \times 0.123 =$

   b. $52.4 \times 9.345 =$

_____

_____

2. Divide decimals.

   a. $69 \div 3.2 =$

   c. $100 \div 4.5 =$

_____

_____

   b. $6.63 \div 0.23 =$

   d. $125 \div 0.75 =$

_____

_____

3. Change decimals to fractions.

   a. $0.46 =$

   b. $0.05 =$

   c. $0.012 =$

_____

_____

_____

4. Which has the greatest value: 0.46, 0.05, or 0.012? Which has the smallest value? _____

RATIO AND PROPORTION

A *ratio* is the relation between two numbers and is separated by a colon, e.g., 1:2 (1 is to 2). It is another way of expressing a fraction, e.g., $1:2 = \frac{1}{2}$.

Proportion is the relation between two ratios separated by a double colon (::) or equals sign (=).

To solve a ratio and proportion problem, the middle numbers *(means)* are multiplied and the end numbers *(extremes)* are multiplied. To solve for the unknown, which is X, the X goes to the left side and is followed by an equals sign.

EXAMPLES

PROBLEM 1: 1:2::2:X (1 is to 2, as 2 is to X)

   means
   extremes

   X = 4 (1 X is the same as X)

Answer: 4 (1:2::2:4)

PROBLEM 2: 4:8 :: X:12

   8 X = 48
   X = $\frac{48}{8}$ = 6

Answer: 6 (4:8::6:12)

PROBLEM 3: A ratio and proportion problem may be set up as a fraction.

Ratio and Proportion   Fraction

2 : 3 :: 4 : X $\dfrac{2}{3} = \dfrac{4}{X}$ (cross multiply)

2 X = 12   2 X = 12

X = $^{12}/_2$ = 6   X = 6

Answer: 6. Remember to cross-multiply when the problem is set up as a fraction.

PRACTICE PROBLEMS: IV Ratio and Proportion

Answers can be found on page 16.

Solve for X.

1. 2 : 10 :: 5 : X

_____

2. 0.9 : 100 = X : 1000

_____

3. Change the ratio and proportion to a fraction and solve for X.
3 : 5 :: X : 10

_____

4. It is 500 miles from Washington, DC, to Boston, MA. Your car averages 22 miles per 1 gallon of gasoline. How many gallons of gasoline will be needed for the trip?

_____

PERCENTAGE

Percent (%) means 100. Two percent (2%) means 2 parts of 100, and 0.9% means 0.9 part (less than 1) of 100. A percent can be expressed as a fraction, a decimal, or a ratio.

EXAMPLES

Percent		Fraction	Decimal	Ratio
60%	=	$^{60}/_{100}$	0.6	60 : 100

Note: *To change a percent to a decimal, move the decimal point two places to the left. In the example, the decimal point comes before the whole number 60.*

PRACTICE PROBLEMS: V Percentage

Answers can be found on page 12.

Change percent to fraction, decimal, and ratio.

Percent	Fraction	Decimal	Ratio
1. 2%			
2. 0.33%			
3. 150%			
4. $\frac{1}{2}$% (0.5%)			
5. 0.9%			

ANSWERS

I Roman Numerals
1. $10 + 5 + 1 = 16$
2. $10 + 2 = 12$
3. $20 (10 + 10) + 4 (5 - 1) = 24$
4. $30 (10 + 10 + 10) + 9 (10 - 1) = 39$
5. $40 (50 - 10) + 5 = 45$
6. $100 - 10 = 90$

II Fractions (Round off to the nearest tenths unless otherwise indicated.)
1. **a.** $\frac{1}{50}$ has the greatest value.   **b.** $\frac{1}{150}$ has the lowest value.
2. **a.** 3   **c.** $7\frac{1}{3}$
   b. 4   **d.** $5\frac{2}{6}$ or $5\frac{1}{3}$

3. **a.** $\frac{2}{24} = \frac{1}{12}$

   c. $\dfrac{\overset{10}{\cancel{500}}}{\underset{7}{\cancel{350}}} \times 5 = \dfrac{50}{7} = 7.1$

   b. $12\frac{1}{5} \times 15\frac{1}{4} = \dfrac{180}{20} = 9$

   d. $\dfrac{\overset{2}{\cancel{400,000}}}{\underset{1}{\cancel{200,000}}} \times 3 = 6$

4. **a.** $\frac{2}{3} \div 6 = \frac{2}{3} \times \frac{1}{6}$
      $= \frac{2}{18} = \frac{1}{9}$

   d. $\frac{1}{150} \div \frac{1}{100} = \dfrac{1}{\underset{3}{\cancel{150}}} \times \dfrac{\overset{2}{\cancel{100}}}{1}$
      $= \frac{2}{3}$, or 0.666, or 0.67 or 0.7

   b. $\frac{1}{4} \div \frac{1}{5} =$
      $\frac{1}{4} \times \frac{5}{1} = \frac{5}{4} =$
      $1\frac{1}{4}$, or 1.25 or 1.3

   e. $\frac{1}{200} \div \frac{1}{300} = \frac{1}{200} \times \frac{300}{1} =$
      $\frac{300}{200} = 1\frac{1}{2}$, or 1.5

   c. $\dfrac{1}{6} \div \dfrac{1}{8} = \dfrac{1}{\underset{3}{\cancel{6}}} \times \dfrac{\overset{4}{\cancel{8}}}{1} = \dfrac{4}{3} = 1.33$ or 1.3

   f. $48\frac{1}{5} \div \frac{4}{1} = 48\frac{1}{5} \times \frac{1}{4}$
      $= \dfrac{48}{20} = 2.4$

5. a. $\frac{1}{4} = 4\overline{)1.00}$ $\dfrac{0.25}{}$ or 0.3   **b.** $\frac{1}{10} = 10\overline{)1.00}$ $\dfrac{0.10}{}$ or 0.1   **c.** $\frac{2}{5} = 5\overline{)2.00}$ $\dfrac{0.40}{}$ or 0.4

III Decimals

1. a. 0.8364, or 0.8

     0.123

     $\underline{6.8}$

     984

     $\underline{738}$

     0.8364, or 0.8 (round off in tenths: 3 hundredths is less than 5)

  b. 489.6780, or 489.7 (7 hundredths is greater than 5)

2. a. 21.56, or 21.6 (6 hundredths is greater than 5, so the tenth is increased by one)

  b. 28.826, or 28.8 (2 hundredths is *not* 5 or greater than 5, so the tenth is not changed)

  c. $100 \div 4.5 = 4.5\overline{)100.0} = 22.2$, or 22 (whole number)

  d. $125 \div 0.75 = 0.75\overline{)125.00} = 166.6$, or 167 (rounded off to whole number)

3. a. $\frac{46}{100}$ **b.** $\frac{5}{100}$ **c.** $\frac{12}{1000}$

4. 0.46 has the greatest value; 0.012 has the lowest value. Forty-six hundredths is greater than 12 thousandths.

IV Ratio and Proportion

1. $2X = 50$ **3.** $\frac{3}{5} = \frac{x}{10} = 5X = 30$

     $X = 25$ $X = 6$

2. $100X = 900$ **4.** 1 gal : 22 miles :: X gal : 500

       $X = 9$ $22X = 500$

                                             $X = 22.7$ gal

                     22.7 gallons of gasoline are needed.

V Percentage

	Percent	Fraction	Decimal	Ratio
1.	2	$\frac{2}{100}$	0.02	2:100
2.	0.33 or 0.3	$\frac{0.33}{100}$ or $\frac{33}{10,000}$	0.0033	0.33:100, or 33:10,000
3.	150	$\frac{150}{100}$	1.50	150:100
4.	0.5	$\frac{0.5}{100}$ or $\frac{5}{1000}$	0.005	0.5:100, or 5:1000
5.	0.9	$\frac{0.9}{100}$ or $\frac{9}{1000}$	0.009	0.9:100, or 9:1000

POST-MATH TEST

The math test is composed of five sections: Roman and Arabic numerals, fractions, decimals, ratios and proportions, and percentages. There are 60 questions. A passing score is 54 or more correct answers (90%). A nonpassing score is 7 or more incorrect answers. Answers to the Post-Math Test can be found on page 16.

Roman and Arabic Numerals

Convert Roman numerals to Arabic numerals.

1. vii

4. xiv

_____

_____

2. xi

5. xliii, or XLIII

_____

_____

3. xvi

_____

Convert Arabic numerals to Roman numerals.

6. 4

9. 37

_____

_____

7. 18

10. 62

_____

_____

8. 29

_____

Fractions

Which fraction has the larger value?

11. $\frac{1}{100}$ or $\frac{1}{150}$?

_____

12. $\frac{1}{3}$ or $\frac{1}{2}$?

_____

Reduce improper fractions to whole or mixed numbers.

13. $\frac{45}{9} =$

14. $\frac{74}{3} =$

_____

_____

Change a mixed number to an improper fraction.

15. $5\frac{2}{3} =$

_____

Change fractions to decimals.

16. $\frac{2}{3} =$ (reduce to tenths)

_____

17. $\frac{1}{12} =$ (reduce to tenths)

_____

Multiply fractions.

18. $\frac{7}{8} \times \frac{4}{6} =$ (reduce to lowest terms
or to tenths)

_____

19. $2\frac{3}{5} \times \frac{5}{8} =$

_____

Divide fractions.

20. $\frac{1}{2} \div \frac{1}{3} =$

_____

22. $\frac{1}{8} \div \frac{1}{12} =$

_____

21. $6\frac{3}{4} \div 3 =$

_____

23. $20\frac{3}{4} \div \frac{1}{6} =$

_____

Decimals

Round off decimal numbers to tenths.

24. $0.87 =$

_____

26. $0.42 =$

_____

25. $2.56 =$

_____

Change decimals to fractions.

27. $0.68 =$

_____

29. $0.012 =$

_____

28. $0.9 =$

_____

30. $0.33 =$

_____

Multiply decimals (round off to tenths or whole numbers).

31. $0.34 \times 0.6 =$

_____

32. $2.123 \times 0.45 =$

_____

Divide decimals.

33. $3.24 \div 0.3 =$

_____

34. $69.4 \div 0.23 =$

_____

Ratio and Proportion

Change ratios to fractions.

35. $3:4 =$ **37.** $65:90 =$

36. $1:175 =$ **38.** $0.9:100 =$

Solve ratio and proportion problems.

39. $2:3::8:X$

40. $0.5:20::X:100$

41. $3:100 = X:1000$

42. $5:25 = 10:X$

Change ratios and proportions to fractions and solve.

43. $1:2::4:X$

44. $5:50::X:300$

45. $0.9:10 = X:100$

Percentage

Change percents to fractions.

46. $3\% =$ **47.** $27\% =$ **48.** $1.2\% =$ **49.** $5.75\% =$

Change percents to decimals (round off to tenths, hundredths, or thousandths).

50. 8% =   **52.** 0.9% =   **54.** 0.25% =

51. 15% =   **53.** 3.5% =   **55.** 0.45% =

Change percents to ratios.

56. 35% =   **58.** 4% =   **60.** 0.45% =

57. 12.5% =   **59.** 0.9% =

ANSWERS   Post-Math Test

Roman and Arabic Numerals

1. 7   **3.** 16   **5.** 43   **7.** $\overline{\text{xviii}}$ **9.** xxxvii

2. 11   **4.** 14   **6.** $\overline{\text{iv}}$ **8.** $\overline{\text{xxix}}$ **10.** LXII

Fractions

11. $\frac{1}{100}$

12. $\frac{1}{2}$

13. 5

14. $24\frac{2}{3}$

15. $\frac{17}{3}$

16. 0.66, or 0.7

17. 0.08 or 0.1

18. $\frac{28}{48}$ or $\frac{7}{12}$ or 0.58 or 0.6

19. $\frac{13}{\cancel{5}_1} \times \frac{\cancel{5}^1}{8} =$
$\frac{13}{8} = 1\frac{5}{8}$

20. $\frac{1}{2} \times \frac{3}{1} =$
$\frac{3}{2} = 1\frac{1}{2}$

21. $\frac{\cancel{27}^9}{4} \times \frac{1}{\cancel{3}_1} =$
$\frac{9}{4} = 2\frac{1}{4}$

22. $\frac{1}{\cancel{8}_2} \times \frac{\cancel{12}^3}{1} =$
$\frac{3}{2} = 1\frac{1}{2}$

23. $\frac{83}{\cancel{4}_2} \times \frac{\cancel{6}^3}{1} =$
$\frac{249}{2} = 124.5$ or 125 whole number

Decimals

24. 0.9

25. 2.6

26. 0.4

27. $\frac{68}{100}$

28. $\frac{9}{10}$

29. $\frac{12}{1000}$

30. $\frac{33}{100}$

31. 0.204 or 0.2

32. 0.95535, or 0.96, or 1

33. 10.8

34. 301.739, or 301.7

Ratio and Proportion

35. $\frac{3}{4}$

36. $\frac{1}{175}$

37. $\frac{65}{90}$

38. $\frac{9}{1000}$

39. 12

40. 2.5

41. 30

42. 50

43. $\frac{1}{2} \times \frac{4}{x} =$ (cross multiply)
X = 8

44. $\frac{\frac{1}{\cancel{5}}}{\cancel{50}_{10}} = \frac{X}{300}$
10 X = 300
X = 30

45. $\frac{0.9}{10} = \frac{X}{100}$
10 X = 90
X = 9

Percentage

46. $\frac{3}{100}$

47. $\frac{27}{100}$

48. $\frac{12}{1000}$

49. $\frac{575}{10,000}$

50. 0.08 or 0.1

51. 0.15

52. 0.009

53. 0.035

54. 0.0025

55. 0.0045

56. 35:100

57. 12.5:100, or 125:1000

58. 4:100

59. 0.9:100, or 9:1000

60. 0.45:100, or 45:10,000

Additional practice problems are available on the enclosed CD-ROM in the "Mathematics Review" section.

PART II

SYSTEMS, CONVERSION, AND METHODS OF DRUG CALCULATION

Systems Used for Drug Administration

OBJECTIVES

- Identify the system of measurement accepted worldwide and the system of measurement used in home settings.
- List the basic units and subunits of weight, volume, and length of the metric system.
- Explain the rules for changing grams to milligrams and milliliters to liters.
- Give abbreviations for the frequently used metric units and subunits.
- List the basic units in the apothecary system for weight and volume.
- Give the abbreviations for the apothecary and household units of measurement.
- List the basic units of measurement for volume in the household system.
- Convert units of measurement within the metric system, within the apothecary system, and within the household system.

OUTLINE

The three systems used for measuring drugs and solutions are the metric, apothecary, and household systems. The metric system, developed in 1799 in France, is the chosen system for measurements in the majority of European countries. The metric system, also referred to as *the decimal system,* is based on units of 10. Since the enactment of the Metric Conversion Act of 1975, the United States has been moving toward the use of this system. The intention of the act is to adopt the International Metric System worldwide. The metric system is known as the *International System of Units,* abbreviated as SI units. Eventually, it will be the only system used in drug dosing.

The apothecary system dates back to the Middle Ages and has been the system of weights and measurements used in England since the seventeenth century. It was brought to the United States from England. The system is also referred to as *the fractional system* because anything less than one is expressed in fractions. In the United States, the apothecary system is rapidly being phased out and is being replaced by the metric system. You may omit the apothecary system if you desire.

Standard household measurements are used primarily in home settings. With the trend toward home care, conversions to household measurements may gain importance.

METRIC SYSTEM

The metric system is a decimal system based on multiples of 10 and fractions of 10. There are three basic units of measurements. These basic units are as follows:

Gram (g, gm, G, Gm): unit for weight
Liter (l, L): unit for volume or capacity
Meter (m, M): unit for linear measurement or length

Prefixes are used with the basic units to describe whether the units are larger or smaller than the basic unit. The prefixes indicate the size of the unit in multiples of 10. The prefixes for basic units are as follows:

Prefix for Larger Unit		**Prefix for Smaller Unit**	
Kilo	1000 (one thousand)	Deci	0.1 (one-tenth)
Hecto	100 (one hundred)	Centi	0.01 (one-hundredth)
Deka	10 (ten)	Milli	0.001 (one-thousandth)
		Micro	0.000001 (one-millionth)
		Nano	0.000000001 (one-billionth)

Abbreviations of metric units that are frequently written in drug orders are listed in Table 1-1. Lowercase letters are usually used for abbreviations rather than capital letters.

The metric units of weight, volume, and length are given in Table 1-2. Meanings of the prefixes are stated next to the units of weight. Note that the larger units are 1000, 100, and 10 times the basic units (in bold type) and the smaller units differ by factors of 0.1, 0.01, 0.001, 0.000001, and 0.000000001.

TABLE 1-1

Metric Units and Abbreviations

	Names	Abbreviations
Weight	Kilogram	kg, Kg
	Gram	g, gm, G, Gm
	Milligram	mg, mgm
	Microgram	mcg
	Nanogram	ng
Volume	Kiloliter	kl, kL
	Liter	l, L
	Deciliter	dl, dL
	Milliliter	ml, mL
Length	Kilometer	km, Km
	Meter	m, M
	Centimeter	cm
	Millimeter	mm

TABLE 1-2

Units of Measurement in the Metric System With Their Prefixes

Weight Per Gram	Meaning
*1 kilogram (kg) = 1000 grams	One thousand
1 hectogram (hg) = 100 grams	One hundred
1 dekagram (dag) = 10 grams	Ten
*1 gram (g) = 1 gram	One
1 decigram (dg) = 0.1 gram ($\frac{1}{10}$)	One tenth
1 centigram (cg) = 0.01 gram ($\frac{1}{100}$)	One hundredth
*1 milligram (mg) = 0.001 gram ($\frac{1}{1000}$)	One thousandth
*1 microgram (mcg) = 0.000001 gram ($\frac{1}{1,000,000}$)	One millionth
*1 nanogram (ng) = 0.000000001 gram ($\frac{1}{1,000,000,000}$)	One billionth

Volume Per Liter	Length Per Meter
*1 kiloliter (kl) = 1000 liters	1 kilometer (km) = 1000 meters
1 hectoliter (hl) = 100 liters	1 hectometer (hm) = 100 meters
1 dekaliter (dal) = 10 liters	1 dekameter (dam) = 10 meters
*1 liter (l, L) = 1 liter	1 metric (m) = 1 meter
*1 deciliter (dl) = 0.1 liter	1 decimeter (dm) = 0.1 meter
1 centiliter (cl) = 0.01 liter	1 centimeter (cm) = 0.01 meter
*1 milliliter (ml) = 0.001 liter	1 millimeter (mm) = 0.001 meter

*Commonly used units of measurements.

The size of a basic unit can be changed by multiplying or dividing by 10. Micrograms and nanograms are the exceptions: one (1) milligram = 1000 micrograms, and one (1) microgram = 1000 nanograms. Micrograms and nanograms are changed by 1000 instead of by 10.

Conversion Within the Metric System

Drug administration often requires conversion within the metric system to prepare the correct dosage. Two basic methods are given for changing larger to smaller units and smaller to larger units.

METHOD A

To change from a *larger* unit to a *smaller* unit, multiply by 10 for each unit decreased, or move the decimal point one space to the right for each unit changed.

When changing three units from larger to smaller, such as from gram to milligram (a change of three units), multiply by 10 three times (or by 1000), or move the decimal point three spaces to the right.

Change 1 gram (g) to milligrams (mg):

a. $1 \times 10 \times 10 \times 10 = 1000$ mg

b. $1 \text{ g} \times 1000 = 1000$ mg

or

c. $1 \text{ g} = 1.000$ mg (1000 mg)

When changing two units, such as kilogram to dekagram (a change of two units from larger to smaller), multiply by 10 twice (or by 100), or move the decimal point two spaces to the right.

Change 2 kilograms (kg) to dekagrams (dag):

a. $2 \times 10 \times 10 = 200$ dag

b. $2 \text{ kg} \times 100 = 200$ dag

or

c. $2 \text{ kg} = 2.00$ dag (200 dag)

When changing one unit, such as liter to deciliter (a change of one unit from larger to smaller), multiply by 10, or move the decimal point one space to the right.

Change 3 liters (L) to deciliters (dl):

a. $3 \times 10 = 30$ dl
b. $3 \text{ L} \times 10 = 30$ dl

or

c. $3 \text{ L} = 3.0$ dl (30 dl)

A micro unit is one thousandth of a milli unit, and a nano unit is one thousandth of a micro unit. To change from a milli unit to a micro unit, multiply by 1000, or move the decimal place three spaces to the right. Changing micro units to nano units involves the same procedure, mulitplying by 1000 or moving the decimal place three spaces to the right.

EXAMPLES

PROBLEM 1: Change 2 grams (g) to milligrams (mg).

$$2 \text{ g} \times 1000 = 2000 \text{ mg}$$
or
$$2 \text{ g} = 2.000 \text{ mg} \ (2000 \text{ mg})$$

PROBLEM 2: Change 10 milligrams (mg) to micrograms (mcg).

10 mg × 1000 = 10,000 mcg)

or

10 mg = 10.000 mcg (10,000 mcg)

PROBLEM 3: Change 4 liters (L) to milliliters (ml).

4 L × 1000 = 4000 ml

or

4 L = 4.000 ml (4000 ml)

PROBLEM 4: Change 2 kilometers (km) to hectometers (hm).

2 km × 10 = 20 hm

or

2 km = 2.0 hm (20 hm)

METHOD B

To change from a *smaller* unit to a *larger* unit, divide by 10 for each unit increased, or move the decimal point one space to the left for each unit changed.

When changing three units from smaller to larger, divide by 1000, or move the decimal point three spaces to the left.

Change 1500 milliliters (ml) to liters (L):

a. 1500 ml ÷ 1000 = 1.5 L

or

b. 1500 ml = 1 500. L (1.5 L)

When changing two units from smaller to larger, divide by 100, or move the decimal point two spaces to the left.

Change 400 centimeters (cm) to meters (m):

a. 400 cm ÷ 100 = 4 m

or

b. 400 cm = 4 00. m (4 m)

When changing one unit from smaller to larger, divide by 10, or move the decimal point one space to the left.

Change 150 decigrams (dg) to grams (g):

a. 150 dg ÷ 10 = 15 g

or

b. 150 dg = 15 0. g (15 g)

EXAMPLES

PROBLEM 1: Change 8 grams to kilograms (kg).

8 g ÷ 1000 = 0.008 kg

or

8 g = 008. kg (0.008 kg)

PROBLEM 2: Change 1500 milligrams (mg) to decigrams (dg).

1500 mg ÷ 100 = 15 dg

or

1500 mg = 15 00. dg (15 dg)

PROBLEM 3: Change 750 micrograms (mcg) to milligrams (mg).

750 mcg ÷ 1000 = 0.75 mg

or

750 mcg = 750. mg (0.75 mg)

PROBLEM 4: Change 2400 milliliters (ml) to liters (L).

2400 ml ÷ 1000 = 2.4 L

or

2400 ml = 2 400. L (2.4 L)

PRACTICE PROBLEMS: I Metric System

Answers can be found on page 30.

1. Conversion from larger units to smaller units: *Multiply* by 10 for each unit changed (multiply by 10, 100, 1000), or move the decimal point one space to the *right* for each unit changed (move one, two, or three spaces), Method A.

   a. 7.5 grams to milligrams

   _____

   b. 10 milligrams to micrograms

   _____

   c. 35 kilograms to grams

   _____

   d. 2.5 liters to milliliters

   _____

   e. 1.25 liters to milliliters

   _____

   f. 20 centiliters to milliliters

   _____

   g. 18 decigrams to milligrams

   _____

   h. 0.5 kilograms to grams

   _____

2. Conversion from smaller units to larger units: *Divide* by 10 for each unit changed (divide by 10, 100, 1000), or move the decimal point one space to the *left* for each unit changed (move one, two, or three spaces), Method B.

a. 500 milligrams to grams

_____

b. 7500 micrograms to milligrams

_____

c. 250 grams to kilograms

_____

d. 4000 milliliters to liters

_____

e. 325 milligrams to grams

_____

f. 100 milliliters to deciliters

_____

g. 2800 milliliters to liters

_____

h. 75 millimeters to centimeters

_____

APOTHECARY SYSTEM

The apothecary system is seldom used. The student may skip this part of Chapter 1, as advised by the faculty or school.

The apothecary system of measurement was the common system used by most practitioners prior to the universal acceptance of the International Metric System. Now, all pharmaceuticals are manufactured using the metric system, and the apothecary system is no longer included on any drug labels. All medication should be prescribed and calculated using metric measures, but occasionally the use of the fluid ounce or grains may be found. In those rare circumstances, nurses should have a general understanding of the apothecary system.

The basic unit of weight in the apothecary system is the grain (gr), and the basic unit of fluid volume is the minim (m); these are the smaller units in the apothecary system. As a safety issue, please note that the abbreviation for minim, m, must not be mistaken for milliliter, ml. Larger units of measurement for weight and fluid volume are the dram (dr) and the ounce (oz). In the apothecary system, Roman numerals are written in lowercase letters, e.g., gr x, to express numbers.

Table 1-3 gives the equivalents of units of dry weight (grain, dram, ounce) and units of liquid volume (minim, fluid dram, fluid ounce). The apothecary

TABLE 1-3

Abbreviations and Units of Measurement in the Apothecary System

Abbreviations			
Weight		**Liquid Volume**	
grain	gr	quart	qt
ounce	oz	pint	pt
dram*	dr	fluid ounce	fl oz
		fluid dram	fl dr
		minim†	ℳ

Basic Equivalent Units			
Weight		**Liquid Volume†**	
Larger units	*Smaller units*	*Larger units*	*Smaller units*
1 ounce	= 480 grains	1 quart	= 2 pints
1 ounce	= 8 drams	1 pint	= 16 fluid ounces
1 dram	= 60 grains	1 fluid ounce	= 8 fluid drams
		1 fluid dram	= 60 minims
		1 minim†	= 1 drop (gt)

*Drams and minims are rarely used for drug administration; however, know their symbols.
†Liquid volume of basic units is frequently used.
Note: Constant values are the numbers of the smaller equivalent units.

system uses fluid ounces and fluid drams to differentiate between liquid volume and dry weight. In clinical practice, units of liquid volume are commonly seen as dram and ounce. Often, the term *fluid,* which is the correct labeling of liquid volume, is dropped. However, the proper names for units of dry weight and units of liquid volume are used in this text.

The most common drugs prescribed in the past with use of the apothecary system designation are listed with their metric equivalent:

Aspirin gr x (650 mg)
Codeine gr ½ (30 mg)
Phenobarbital gr ¼ (15 mg)
Nitroglycerin gr ¹⁄₁₅₀ (0.4 mg)

Conversion Within the Apothecary System

It is often necessary to change units within the apothecary system. The method applied when changing larger units to smaller units is as follows:

METHOD C

To change a *larger* unit to a *smaller* unit, multiply the constant value found in Table 1-3 by the number of the larger unit.

NOTE

The constant values are the basic equivalent numbers of the smaller units given in Table 1-3. You might want to memorize these equivalents or refer to the table as needed.

EXAMPLES

PROBLEM 1: 2 drams (dr) = _____ grains (gr).
1 dr = 60 gr (60 is the constant value, dry weight)
$2 \times 60 = 120$ gr

PROBLEM 2: 3 pints (pt) = _____ fluid ounces (fl oz).
1 pt = 16 fl oz (16 is the constant value)
$3 \times 16 = 48$ fl oz

PROBLEM 3: 3 fluid ounces (fl oz) = _____ fluid drams (fl dr).
1 fl oz = 8 fl dr (8 is the constant value)
$3 \times 8 = 24$ fl dr

The method applied when smaller units are changed to larger units is as follows:

METHOD D

To change a *smaller* unit to a *larger* unit, divide the constant value found in Table 1-3 into the number of the smaller unit.

EXAMPLES

PROBLEM 1: 30 grains (gr) = _____ dram (dr).
1 dr = 60 gr (60 is the constant value)
$30 \div 60 = \frac{1}{2}$ dr

PROBLEM 2: 80 fluid ounces (fl oz) = _____ pints (pt).
1 pt = 16 fl oz (16 is the constant value)
$80 \div 16 = 5$ pt

PROBLEM 3: 2 fluid drams (fl dr) = _____ fluid ounces (fl oz).
1 fl oz = 8 fl dr (8 is the constant value)
$2 \div 8 = \frac{1}{4}$ fl oz

PRACTICE PROBLEMS: II Apothecary System

Answers can be found on page 31.

1. Give the abbreviations for the following:

   a. grain = _____

   b. dram = _____

   c. fluid dram = _____

   d. drop = _____

   e. fluid ounce = _____

   f. pint = _____

   g. quart = _____

2. Give the equivalent using Method C, changing larger units to smaller units.

   a. dr v = _____ gr

   b. fl oz v = _____ fl dr

   c. qt iii = _____ pt

   d. pt ii = _____ fl oz

3. Give the equivalent using Method D, changing smaller units to larger units.

   a. gr 240 = _____ dr

   b. dr xvi = _____ oz

   c. fl dr xxiv = _____ fl oz

   d. ℳ xv = _____ gtt

HOUSEHOLD SYSTEM

The use of household measurements is on the increase because more patients/clients are being cared for in the home. The household system of measurement is not as accurate as the metric system because of a lack of standardization of spoons, cups, and glasses. A teaspoon (t) is considered 5 ml, although it could represent anywhere from 4 to 6 ml. Three household teaspoons are equal to one tablespoon (T). A drop size can vary with the size of the lumen of the dropper. Basically, a drop and a minim are considered equal. Again, household measurements must be considered approximate measurements. Some of the household units are the same as the apothecary units, because there is a blend of these two systems.

The community health nurse may use and teach the household units of measurements to patients/clients.

Table 1-4 gives the commonly used units of measurement in the household system. You might want to memorize the equivalents in Table 1-4 or refer to the table as needed.

Conversion Within the Household System

For changing larger units to smaller units and smaller units to larger units within the household system, the same methods that applied to the apothecary system can be used. With household measurements, a fluid ounce is usually indicated as an ounce.

METHOD E

To change a *larger* unit to a *smaller* unit, multiply the constant value found in Table 1-4 by the number of the larger unit.

TABLE 1-4

Units of Measurement in the Household System

1 drop (gt) (gtt)	= 1 minim (m̥)
1 teaspoon (t)	= 60 drops (gtt) (gtts) 5 ml
1 tablespoon (T)	= 3 teaspoons (t)
1 ounce (oz)	= 2 tablespoons (T)
1 coffee cup (c)	= 6 ounces (oz)
1 medium size glass	= 8 ounces (oz)
1 measuring cup	= 8 ounces (oz)

Note: Constant values are the numbers of the smaller equivalent units.

NOTE

The constant values are the numbers of the smaller units in Table 1-4.

EXAMPLES

PROBLEM 1: 2 medium-size glasses = _____ ounces (oz).
  1 medium glass = 8 fl oz (8 is the constant value)
  $2 \times 8 = 16$ oz

PROBLEM 2: 3 tablespoons (T) = _____ teaspoons (t).
  1 T = 3 t (3 is the constant value)
  $3 \times 3 = 9$ t

PROBLEM 3: 5 ounces (oz) = _____ tablespoons (T).
  1 oz = 2 T (2 is the constant value)
  $5 \times 2 = 10$ T

PROBLEM 4: 2 teaspoons (t) = _____ drops (gtt).
  1 t = 60 gtt (60 is the constant value)
  $2 \times 60 = 120$ gtt

METHOD F

To change a *smaller* unit to a *larger* unit, divide the constant value found in Table 1-4 into the number of the smaller unit.

EXAMPLES

PROBLEM 1: 120 drops (gtt) = _____ teaspoons (t).
  1 t = 60 gtt (60 is the constant value)
  $120 \div 60 = 2$ t

PROBLEM 2: 6 teaspoons (t) = _____ tablespoons (T).
  1 T = 3 t (3 is the constant value)
  $6 \div 3 = 2$ T

PROBLEM 3: 18 ounces (oz) = _____ coffee cups (c).

1 c = 6 oz (6 is the constant value)

18 ÷ 6 = 3 c

PROBLEM 4: 4 tablespoons (T) = _____ ounces (oz).

1 oz = 2 T (2 is the constant value)

4 ÷ 2 = 2 oz

PRACTICE PROBLEMS: III Household System

Answers can be found on page 31.

1. Give the equivalents using Method E, changing larger units to smaller units.

   a. 2 glasses = _____ oz

   b. 3 ounces = _____ T

   c. 4 tablespoons = _____ t

   d. 1½ coffee c (cups) = _____ oz

   e. ½ teaspoon = _____ gtt

2. Give the equivalents using Method F, changing smaller units to larger units.

   a. 9 teaspoons = _____ T

   b. 6 tablespoons = _____ oz

   c. 90 drops = _____ t

   d. 12 ounces = _____ coffee c (cups)

   e. 24 ounces = _____ medium-size glasses

ANSWERS

I Metric System

1. a. 7.5 g to mg

      7.5 g × 1000 = 7500 mg

      or

      7.500 mg (7500 mg)

   b. 10,000 mcg

   c. 35,000 g

   d. 2500 ml

   e. 1250 ml

   f. 200 ml

   g. 1800 mg

   h. 500 g

2. a. 500 mg to g

      500 ÷ 1000 = 0.5 g

      or

      500 mg = 500. g (0.5 g)

   b. 7.5 mg

   c. 0.25 kg

   d. 4 L

   e. 0.325 g

   f. 1 dl

   g. 2.8 L

   h. 7.5 cm

II Apothecary System

Abbreviations	Equivalents	Equivalents
1. a. grain = gr	**2. a.** dr v = _____ gr	**3. a.** gr 240 = _____ dr
b. dram = dr	5 × 60 = 300 gr	240 ÷ 60 = 4 dr
c. fluid dram = fl dr	**b.** 40 fl dr	**b.** 2 oz
d. drop = gt (gtt)	**c.** 6 pt	**c.** 3 fl oz
e. fluid ounce = fl oz	**d.** 32 fl oz	**d.** 15 gtt (gtts)
f. pint = pt		
g. quart = qt		

III Household System

1. a. 2 glasses = _____ oz
  2 × 8 = 16 oz
b. 6 T
c. 12 t
d. 9 oz
e. 30 gtt (gtts)

2. a. 9 teaspoons = _____ T
  9 ÷ 3 = 3 T
b. 3 oz
c. 1½ t
d. 2 c
e. 3 glasses

SUMMARY PRACTICE PROBLEMS

Make conversions within the three systems. Answers are on page 32.

1. Metric system

   a. 30 mg = _____ mcg

   b. 3 g = _____ mg

   c. 6 L = _____ ml

   d. 1.5 kg = _____ g

   e. 10,000 mcg = _____ mg

   f. 500 mg = _____ g

   g. 2500 ml = _____ L

   h. 125 g = _____ kg

   i. 120 mm = _____ cm

   j. 5 m = _____ cm

2. Apothecary system

   a. 90 gr = _____ dr

   b. fl dr iv = _____ fl oz

   c. fl oz 2½ = _____ fl dr

   d. 8 pt = _____ qt

3. Household system

    a. 12 t = _____ T

    b. 5 glasses = _____ oz

    c. 3 T = _____ t

    d. 2 coffee c (cups) = _____ oz

    e. 30 oz = _____ coffee c (cups)

    f. 4 oz = _____ T

ANSWERS   Summary Practice Problems

1. a. 30,000 mcg
  b. 3000 mg
  c. 6000 ml
  d. 1500 g
  e. 10 mg
  f. 0.5 g
  g. 2.5 L
  h. 0.125 kg
  i. 12 cm
  j. 500 cm

2. a. 1.5 dr
  b. ½ or s̄s̄ fl oz
  c. 20 fl dr
  d. 4 qt

3. a. 4 T
  b. 40 oz
  c. 9 t
  d. 12 oz
  e. 5 coffee c (cups)
  f. 8 T

Additional information is available on the enclosed CD-ROM in the "Introducing Drug Measures" section.

Conversion Within the Metric, Apothecary, and Household Systems

OBJECTIVES

- State rules for converting drug dosage by weight between the apothecary and metric systems.
- Convert grams/milligrams to grains and grains to grams/milligrams.
- Convert drug dosage by weight from one system to another system by using the ratio method.
- State rules for converting drug dosage by volume among the metric, apothecary, and household systems.
- Convert liters/milliliters to ounces/pints and milliliters to drams, tablespoons, and teaspoons.

OUTLINE

Today, conversion within the metric system is more common than conversion within the metric-apothecary systems. If the faculty find that the apothecary system is not being used in their institutions, they may wish to omit apothecary equivalents and conversion in Table 2-1 and the part in Chapter 2 that relates to the apothecary system.

Drug doses are usually ordered in metric units (grams, milligrams, liters, and milliliters). Although the apothecary system is being phased out, some physicians still order drug doses by apothecary units. To calculate a drug dose, **the same unit of measurement must be used.** Therefore, the nurse must know the metric and apothecary equivalents by memorizing a conversion table or by using methods for converting from one system to the other, if necessary. After the conversion is made, the dosage problem can be solved. Some authorities state that it is easier to *convert to the unit used on the container (bottle)*. If the physician ordered phenobarbital gr ½ and the bottle is labeled 30 mg, then the conversion would be from grains to milligrams.

Metric and apothecary equivalents are approximations, e.g., 1 gram equals 15.432 grains. When values are unequal, they should be rounded off to the nearest whole number (1 gram = 15 grains).

Dosage conversion tables are available in many institutions; however, when you need a conversion table, one might not be available. Nurses should memorize metric and apothecary equivalents or should be able to convert from one system to the other by using calculation methods.

UNITS, MILLIEQUIVALENTS, AND PERCENTS

Units, milliequivalents, and percents are measurements and are used to indicate the strength or potency of certain drugs. When a drug is developed, its strength is based on chemical assay or biological assay. Chemical assay denotes strength by weight, e.g., milligrams or grains. Biological assays are used for drugs in which the chemical composition is difficult to determine. Biological assays assess potency by determining the effect that one unit of the drug can have on a laboratory animal. Units mainly measure the potency of hormones, vitamins, anticoagulants, and some antibiotics. Drugs that were once standardized by units and were later synthesized to their chemical composition may still retain units as an indication of potency, e.g., insulin.

Milliequivalents measure the strength of an ion concentration. Ions are given primarily for electrolyte replacement. They are measured in milliequivalents (mEq), one of which is $\frac{1}{1000}$ of the equivalent weight of an ion. Potassium chloride (KCl) is a common electrolyte replacement and is ordered in milliequivalents.

Percents, the concentrations of weight dissolved in a volume, are always expressed as units of mass per units of volume. Common concentrations are g/ml, g/L, and mg/ml. These concentrations, expressed as percentages, are based on the definition of a 1% solution as 1 g of a drug in 100 ml of solution. Dextrose 50% in a 50-ml pre-filled syringe is a concentration of 50 g of dextrose in 100 ml of water. Calcium gluconate 10% in a 30-ml bottle is a concentration of 10 g of calcium gluconate in 100 ml of solution. Proportions can also express concentrations. A solution that is 1:100 has the same concentration as a 1% solution. Epinephrine 1:1000 means that 1 g of epinephrine was dissolved in a 1000-ml solution.

Units, milliequivalents, and percents cannot be directly converted into the metric, apothecary, or household system.

METRIC, APOTHECARY, AND HOUSEHOLD EQUIVALENTS

Knowing how to convert drug doses among the systems of measurement is essential in the clinical setting. In discharge teaching for individuals receiving liquid medication, converting metric to household measurement may be important.

Table 2–1 gives the metric and apothecary equivalents by weight and the metric, apothecary, and household equivalents by volume.

Remember, conversion from one system to another is an approximation. Memorize Table 2–1, refer to Table 2–1, or use the methods that follow in the text for system conversion.

TABLE 2-1

Approximate Metric, Apothecary, and Household Equivalents

	Metric System	Apothecary System	Household System
Weight	1 kg; 1000 g	2.2 lb	2.2 lb
	30 g	1 oz	
	15 g	4 dr	
	1 g; 1000 mg*	15 (16) gr	
	0.5 g; 500 mg	7½ gr	
	0.3 g; 300 mg	5 gr	
	0.1 g; 100 mg	1½ gr	
	0.06 g; 60 (65) mg*	1 gr	
	0.03 g; 30 (32) mg	½ gr	
	0.01 g; 10 mg	⅙ gr	
	0.6 mg	1/100 gr	
	0.4 mg	1/150 gr	
	0.3 mg	1/200 gr	
Volume	1 L; 1000 ml	1 qt; 32 fl oz	1 qt
	0.5 L; 500 ml	1 pt; 16 fl oz	1 pt
	0.24 L; 240 ml	8 oz	1 glass
	0.18 L; 180 ml	6 oz	1 c
	30 ml	1 oz or 8 dr	2 T or 6 t
	15 ml	½ oz or 4 dr	1 T
	4-5 ml		1 t
	4 ml	1 dr or 60 minims (ℳ)	1 t
	1 ml	15 (16) ℳ	15-16 gtt
Height	2.54 cm	1 inch	1 inch
Length	0.0254 m	1 inch	—
Distance	25.4 mm	1 inch	1 inch

*Equivalents commonly used for computing conversion problems by ratio.
Note: ½ may be written as s͞s.

CONVERSION IN METRIC AND APOTHECARY SYSTEMS BY WEIGHT

Grams and Grains: 1 g = 15 gr

a. To convert grams to grains, *multiply* the number of grams by 15, the constant value.

b. To convert grains to grams, *divide* the number of grains by 15, the constant value.

EXAMPLES

PROBLEM 1: Change 2 grams to grains.

$$2 \times 15 = 30 \text{ gr (grains)}$$

PROBLEM 2: Change 60 grains to grams.

$$60 \div 15 = 4 \text{ g (grams)}$$

Grains and Milligrams: 1 gr = 60 mg

a. To convert grains to milligrams, *multiply* the number of grains by 60, the constant value.

b. To convert milligrams to grains, *divide* the number of milligrams by 60, the constant value.

EXAMPLES

PROBLEM 1: Change 3 grains to milligrams

$$3 \times 60 = 180 \text{ mg (milligrams)}$$

PROBLEM 2: Change 300 milligrams to grains.

Note: *325 milligrams may be ordered instead of 300. Round off to the whole number. One grain is equivalent to 60, 64, or 65 milligrams. In this situation, you may want to divide by 65 instead of rounding off to the whole number.*

$$300 \div 60 = 5 \text{ gr (grains)}$$
or
$$325 \div 65 = 5 \text{ gr}$$
or
$$325 \div 60 = 5.43 \text{ gr, or 5 gr (0.43 is less than 0.5)}$$

Ratio and Proportion

Multiply the means (numbers that are closest to each other) by the extremes (numbers that are farthest from each other). You are solving for X, so X goes first.

If it is difficult for you to recall these methods, then use the ratio and proportion method to convert from one system to another.

you must MEMORIZE

Metric Equivalence:
1 gram (g) = 1000 milligrams (mg)
1 milligram (mg) = 1000 micrograms (mcg)
Metric-Apothecary Equivalence:
1 gram (g) = 15 grains (gr)
1 grain (gr) = 60 milligrams (mg)

EXAMPLES

PROBLEM 1: Convert 2.5 grams to grains.

Known   Desired
g: gr :: g :gr
1 :15 :: 2.5 :X

means

extremes

X = 37.5 gr

PROBLEM 2: Convert 10 grains to milligrams.

Known   Desired
gr :mg   :: gr :mg
1 :60(65) :: 10 :X

X = 600 mg or 650 mg

Note: *Because conversion gives approximate values, the answer could be 600 mg or 650 mg. If the problem uses 1 gr = 60 mg, the answer is 600 mg. However, the bottle may be labeled 10 gr = 650 mg. Both 600 mg and 650 mg are correct.*

PRACTICE PROBLEMS: I Conversion by Weight

Answers can be found on page 41.

Grams and Grains

1. 10 g = _____ gr   **4.** 0.03 g = _____ gr

2. 0.5 g = _____ gr   **5.** 3 gr = _____ g

3. 0.1 g = _____ gr   **6.** 1½ gr = _____ g

Grains and Milligrams

1. 4 gr = _____ mg   **5.** 150 mg = _____ gr

2. 1½ gr = _____ mg   **6.** 30 mg = _____ gr

3. 7½ gr = _____ mg   **7.** 15 mg = _____ gr

4. ½ gr = _____ mg   **8.** 0.6 mg = _____ gr

Ratio and Proportion: Grams, Milligrams, and Grains

1. 2.5 g = _____ mg   **4.** 500 mg = _____ g

2. 0.5 g = _____ gr   **5.** 1 gr = _____ g

3. 100 mg = _____ g   **6.** ¼ gr = _____ mg

CONVERSION IN METRIC, APOTHECARY, AND HOUSEHOLD SYSTEMS BY LIQUID VOLUME

Liters and Ounces: 1 L = 32 oz

a. To convert liters and quarts to ounces, *multiply* the number of liters by 32, the constant value.

b. To convert ounces to liters or quarts, *divide* the number of ounces by 32, the constant value.

EXAMPLES

PROBLEM 1: Change 3 liters to ounces.
$$3 \text{ L} \times 32 = 96 \text{ oz}$$
PROBLEM 2: Change 64 ounces to liters.
$$64 \text{ oz} \div 32 = 2 \text{ L (liters)}$$

Ounces and Milliliters: 1 oz = 30 ml

a. To convert ounces to milliliters, *multiply* the number of ounces by 30, the constant value.

b. To convert milliliters to ounces, *divide* the number of milliliters by 30, the constant value.

EXAMPLES

PROBLEM 1: Change 5 ounces to milliliters.
$$5 \text{ oz} \times 30 = 150 \text{ ml (milliliters)}$$
PROBLEM 2: Change 120 milliliters to ounces.
$$120 \text{ ml} \div 30 = 4 \text{ oz}$$

Milliliters and Drops: 1 ml = 15 drops (gtt) (number of drops may vary according to the size of the dropper)

a. To convert milliliters to drops, *multiply* the number of milliliters by 15, the constant value.

b. To convert drops to milliliters, *divide* the number of minims or drops by 15, the constant value.

EXAMPLES

PROBLEM 1: Change 4 milliliters to drops.
$$4 \text{ ml} \times 15 = 60 \text{ minims or 60 drops}$$
PROBLEM 2: Change 10 drops (gtt) to milliliters.
$$10 \text{ gtt} \div 15 = \tfrac{2}{3} \text{ ml or 0.667 ml or 0.7 ml (in tenths)}$$

Ratio and Proportion

The ratio method is useful when smaller units are converted within the three systems.

If it is difficult for you to recall these methods, then use the ratio and proportion method to convert from one system to the other.

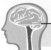 *you must* **MEMORIZE**

30 ml = 1 oz = 8 dr = 2 T = 6t

These are equivalent values.

EXAMPLES

PROBLEM 1: Change 20 ml to teaspoons.

Known Desired
ml : t :: ml : t
30 : 6 :: 20 : X

30 X = 120
X = 4 t (teaspoons)

PROBLEM 2: Change 15 ml to tablespoons.

Known Desired
ml : T :: ml : T
30 : 2 :: 15 : X
30 X = 30
X = 1 T (tablespoon)

PROBLEM 3: Change 5 oz to tablespoons.

Known Desired
oz : T :: oz : T
1 : 2 :: 5 : X
X = 10 T (tablespoons)

PRACTICE PROBLEMS: II Conversion by Liquid Volume

Answers can be found on pages 41 and 42.

Liters and Ounces (Round to the nearest tenths.)

1. 2.5 L = _____ oz (fl oz)

3. 40 oz (fl oz) = _____ L

2. 0.25 L = _____ oz

4. 24 oz = _____ L

Ounces and Milliliters

1. 4 oz (fl oz) = _____ ml

4. 45 ml = _____ oz

2. 6½ oz = _____ ml

5. 150 ml = _____ oz

3. ½ oz = _____ ml

6. 15 ml = _____ oz

Milliliters and Drops

1. 1.5 ml = _____ gtt

3. 20 gtt = _____ ml

2. 12 ♍ = _____ gtt

4. 8 gtt = _____ ml

CONVERSION IN METRIC, APOTHECARY, AND HOUSEHOLD SYSTEMS BY LENGTH

Inches and Meters: 1 inch = 0.0254 meter (constant value)

a. To convert inches to meters, **multiple** the number of inches by 0.0254, the constant value.

b. To convert meters to inches, **divide** the number of meters by 0.0254, the constant value.

EXAMPLES

PROBLEM 1: Change 12 inches to meters (m)

12 inches × 0.0254 = 0.3048 or 0.305 meter or 0.3 meter

PROBLEM 2: Change 0.6 meter to inches

0.6 meter ÷ 0.0254 = 23.6 inches

Inches and Centimeters: 1 inch = 2.54 centimeters (constant value)

a. To convert inches to centimeters, multiply the number of inches by 2.54, the constant value.

b. To convert centimeters to inches, divide the numbers of centimeters by 2.54, the constant value.

EXAMPLES

PROBLEM 1: 12 inches to centimeters (cm)

12 inches × 2.54 = 30.48 cm (centimeters) or 30.5 cm

PROBLEM 2: Change 60 cm to inches

60 cm ÷ 2.54 = 23.6 inches

Note: When multiplying or dividing, move the decimal point 3 places and round off the third number when the next number is 5 or greater, e.g. 0.3048 to 0.305

PRACTICE PROBLEMS: III Conversion by Length

Answers can be found on page 42.

Inches to Meters (Change feet to inches, e.g., 6 ft 2 inches = 74 inches.)

1. 6 ft 2 inches = _____m

2. 5 ft 2 inches = _____m

3. 6 ft 5 inches = _____m

4. 2 ft 10 inches = _____m

5. 4 ft 7 inches = _____m

Inches to Centimeters

1. 2 inches = _____cm

2. 3 inches = _____cm

3. ½ inch =_____cm

4. 6 inches = _____cm

5. 8 inches = _____cm

ANSWERS

I Conversion by Weight

Grams and Grains

1. $10 \times 15 = 150$ gr

2. $0.5 \times 15 = 7.5$ or $7\frac{1}{2}$ gr

3. $0.1 \times 15 = 1.5$ or $1\frac{1}{2}$ gr

4. $0.03 \times 15 = 0.45$ or 0.5 gr

5. $3 \div 15 = 0.2$ g

6. $1.5 \div 15 = 0.1$ g

Grains and Milligrams

1. $4 \times 60 = 240$ mg

2. $1.5 \times 60 = 90$ (100) mg

3. $7.5 \times 60 = 450$ mg

4. $0.5 \times 60 = 30$ mg

5. $150 \div 60 = 2.5$ or $2\frac{1}{2}$ gr

6. $30 \div 60 = 0.5$ or $\frac{1}{2}$ gr

7. $15 \div 60 = \frac{1}{4}$ gr

8. $0.6 \div 60 =$

$$60\overline{)0.60}^{.01} = 0.01 \text{ or } \frac{1}{100} \text{ gr}$$

Ratio and Proportion: Grams, Milligrams, and Grains

1. g: mg :: g :mg

   1:1000::2.5: X

   X = 2500 mg

   or

   Move decimal point three spaces to the right (conversion within the metric system).

   2.5 g = 2.500 mg

2. g:gr :: g:gr

   1:15::0.5:X

   X = 7.5 or $7\frac{1}{2}$ gr

3. mg :g::mg:g

   1000:1::100:X

   1000 X = 100

   X = 0.1 g

4. mg :g:: mg:g

   1000:1::500:X

   1000 X = 500

   X = 0.5 g

5. g: gr::g:gr

   1:15::X:1

   15 X = 1

   X = 0.06 g

6. gr:mg:: gr :mg

   1 :60 ::0.25:X

   X = 60 × 0.25

   X = 15 mg

II Conversion by Liquid Volume

Liters and Ounces

1. 2.5 L × 32 = 80 oz

2. 0.25 L × 32 = 8 oz

3. 40 oz ÷ 32 = 1.25 L or 1.3 L

4. 24 oz ÷ 32 = 0.75 L or 0.8 L

Ounces and Milliliters
1. 4 oz × 30 = 120 ml
2. 6.5 oz × 30 = 195 ml
3. 0.5 oz × 30 = 15 ml

4. 45 ml ÷ 30 = 1½ oz or 1.5 oz
5. 150 ml ÷ 30 = 5 oz
6. 15 ml ÷ 30 = ½ oz or 0.5 oz

Milliliters and Drops
1. 1.5 ml × 15 = 22.5 or 23 gtt
2. 12 ml × 1 = 12 gtt (1 ml = 1 gtt)

3. 20 gtt ÷ 15 = 1.3 ml
4. 8 gtt ÷ 15 = 0.5 ml

III Conversion by Length
Inches to Meters
1. 74 inches × 0.0254 = 1.879 m
2. 62 inches × 0.0254 = 1.575 m
3. 77 inches × 0.0254 = 1.956 m

4. 34 inches × 0.0254 = 0.864 m
5. 55 inches × 0.0254 = 1.397 m

Inches to Centimeters
1. 2 inches × 2.54 = 5.08 cm
2. 3 inches × 2.54 = 7.62 cm
3. ½ inch × 2.54 = 1.27 cm

4. 6 inches × 2.54 = 15.24 cm
5. 8 inches × 2.54 = 20.32 cm

SUMMARY PRACTICE PROBLEMS:

Before dosage problems can be completed, one system of measurement must be selected. If a medication is ordered in one system and the drug label is in another system, then conversion to one of the systems is necessary. As previously stated, it may be easier to convert to the system used on the drug label.

There are three methods of conversion for the three systems: (1) memorization of a conversion table, (2) conversion methods, and (3) ratio method. You need to convert not only within three systems but also within the same system if units are not the same, e.g., grams and milligrams. Again, units of measurement *must* be the same to solve problems.

REMEMBER

Multiply when converting from larger to smaller units, and *divide* when converting from smaller to larger units.

Weight: Metric and Apothecary Conversion

Fill in the blanks with the correct terms, and make the conversions.

1. To convert grams to grains, (multiply/divide)_____ the number of grams by _____; to convert grains to grams, (multiply/divide) _____ the number of grains by _____.

a. 2 g = _____ gr

b. 7½ gr (gr v̄īīss̄) = _____ g

c. 3 gr = _____ g

d. 0.02 g = _____ gr

e. 150 gr = _____ g

f. 0.06 g = _____ gr

2. To convert grains to milligrams, (multiply/divide) _____ the

   number of grains by_____; to convert milligrams to grains,

   (multiply/divide) _____ the number of milligrams

   by _____.

   a. 3 gr (gr ⅲ) = _____ mg   **d.** 5 gr = _____ mg

   b. 10 mg = _____ gr   **e.** 7½ gr = _____ mg

   c. ¼ gr = _____ mg   **f.** 0.4 mg = _____ gr

3. Ratio and proportion.
   Remember: 1 g or 1000 mg = 15 gr; 60 (65) mg = 1 gr

   a. Change 5 g to gr

   _____

   b. Change 120 mg to gr

   _____

Volume: Metric, Apothecary, and Household Conversion

4. To convert liters and quarts to ounces, (multiply/divide) the number of liters

   by _____; to convert ounces to liters and quarts, (multiply/

   divide) the number of ounces by _____.

   a. 3 L = _____ fl oz   **d.** ½ L = _____ oz

   b. 1½ qt − _____ oz   **e.** 8 oz = _____ L or qt

   c. 64 fl oz = _____ qt   **f.** 24 oz = _____ qt

5. To convert ounces to milliliters, (multiply/divide) _____ the

   number of ounces by _____; to convert milliliters to ounces,

   (multiply/divide) the number of milliliters by _____.

   a. 1½ oz = _____ ml   **d.** 75 ml = _____ oz

   b. 15 ml = _____ fl oz   **e.** 3 fl oz = _____ ml

   c. 60 ml = _____ oz   **f.** 8 oz = _____ ml

6. To convert milliliters to drops, (multiply/divide) _____ the

   number of milliliters by _____; to convert drops to milliliters

   (multiply/divide) the number of drops by _____.

   a. 15 ml = _____ gtt   **d.** 4 ml = _____ gtt

   b. 10 gtt = _____ ml   **e.** 30 gtt = _____ ml

   c. 18 gtt = _____ ml   **f.** ½ ml = _____ gtt

7. Ratio and proportion.

REMEMBER

30 ml = 1 oz = 8 dr = 2 T = 6 t (fl oz and oz have been used interchangeably with liquids)

    a. Change 16 oz to L or qt

    _____

    b. Change 1½ oz to T

    _____

    c. Change 1 T to t

    _____

    d. Change 20 ml to t

    _____

    e. Change 2½ oz to ml

    _____

    f. Change 4 oz to ml

    _____

8. Patient intake for lunch included a carton of milk (8 oz), cup of coffee (6 oz), small glass of apple juice (4 oz), and jello (4 oz). How many milliliters (ml) did the client consume?

9. Add 8-hour intake: IV: 30 ml/hr; 230 ml in IV medications. PO intake: juice 4 oz; tea 6 oz; water 3 oz; jello 4 oz; gingerale 5 oz, and milk 8 oz.

10. Add 8-hour intake: IV: 60 ml/hr; 250 ml in IV medications. PO intake: juice 4 oz; water 3 oz; jello 2 oz; and broth 4 oz.

ANSWERS   Summary Practice Problems

1. multiply, 15; divide, 15
    a. 2 g × 15 = 30 gr
    b. 7.5 gr ÷ 15 = ½ or 0.5 g
    c. 3 gr ÷ 15 = 0.2 g

    d. 0.02 g × 15 = 0.3 or ⅓ gr
    e. 150 gr ÷ 15 = 10 g
    f. 0.06 g × 15 = 0.9 or 1 gr (round off to 1)

2. multiply, 60; divide, 60
    a. 3 gr × 60 = 180 mg
    b. 10 mg ÷ 60 = $\frac{10}{60}$ = ⅙ gr
    c. 0.25 gr × 60 = 15 mg

    d. 5 gr × 60 = 300 mg
    e. 7.5 gr × 60 = 450 mg
    f. 0.4 mg ÷ 60 = $\frac{4}{600}$ = $\frac{1}{150}$ gr or 0.4 gr

3. Ratio and proportion
    Known   Desired
    a. g : gr :: g : gr
       1 : 15 :: 5 : X
          X = 75 gr

b. gr:mg:: gr :mg

    1 : 60 :: X :120

     60 X = 120

       X = 2 gr

       or

  mg: gr ::mg:gr

   60: 1 ::120:X

    60 X = 120

      X = 2 gr

4. multiply, 32; divide, 32

  a. 3 L × 32 = 96 oz

  b. 1.5 qt × 32 = 48 oz

  c. 64 oz ÷ 32 = 2 qt

  d. 0.5 L × 32 = 16 oz

  e. 8 oz ÷ 32 = $\frac{8}{32}$ = $\frac{1}{4}$ L or $\frac{1}{4}$ qt or 0.25 or 0.3 qt

  f. 24 oz ÷ 32 = $\frac{24}{32}$ = $\frac{3}{4}$ qt or 0.75 or 0.8 qt

5. multiply, 30; divide, 30

  a. 1$\frac{1}{2}$ oz × 30 = 45 ml

  b. 15 ml ÷ 30 = $\frac{15}{30}$ = $\frac{1}{2}$ oz or 0.5 oz

  c. 60 ml ÷ 30 = 2 oz

  d. 75 ml ÷ 30 = 2$\frac{1}{2}$ oz or 2.5 oz

  e. 3 oz × 30 = 90 ml

  f. 8 oz × 30 = 240 ml

6. multiply, 15; divide, 15

  a. 15 ml × 15 = 225 gtt

  b. 10 gtt ÷ 15 = $\frac{10}{15}$ = $\frac{2}{3}$ ml or 0.67 or 0.7 ml

  c. 18 gtt ÷ 15 = 1$\frac{1}{5}$ ml or 1.2 ml

  d. 4 ml × 15 = 60 gtt

  e. 30 gtt ÷ 15 = 2 ml

  f. $\frac{1}{2}$ ml × 15 = 7.5 gtt or 8 gtt

7. Ratio and proportion

Known   Desired

  a. L:oz::L:oz

     1:32::X:16

    32 X = 16

      X = $\frac{1}{2}$ L

  b. oz:T::oz:T

     1:2::1$\frac{1}{2}$:X

      X = 3 T

  c. T:t::T:t

     2:6::1:X

    2 X = 6

      X = 3 t

  d. ml:t::ml:t

    30:6::20:X

   30 X = 120

     X = 4 t

  e. oz:ml::oz:ml

    1:30::2$\frac{1}{2}$:X

     X = 75 ml

  f. oz:ml::oz:ml

    1:30::4:X

     X = 120 ml

8. (1 ounce = 30 ml)

$$
\begin{aligned}
\text{Milk} &= 240 \text{ ml} \\
\text{Coffee} &= 180 \text{ ml} \\
\text{Apple juice} &= 120 \text{ ml} \\
\text{Jello} &= \underline{120 \text{ ml}} \\
&\ 660 \text{ ml}
\end{aligned}
$$

The patient's intake for lunch is 660 ml.

9.

$$
\begin{aligned}
\text{IV: } 30 \text{ ml} \times 8 \text{ hr} &= 240 \text{ ml} \\
\text{IV medications} &= 230 \text{ ml} \\
\text{Juice (4 oz} \times 30 \text{ ml)} &= 120 \text{ ml} \\
\text{Tea} &= 180 \text{ ml} \\
\text{Water} &= 90 \text{ ml} \\
\text{Jello} &= 120 \text{ ml} \\
\text{Ginger ale} &= 150 \text{ ml} \\
\text{Milk} &= \underline{240 \text{ ml}} \\
&1370 \text{ ml}
\end{aligned}
$$

10.

$$
\begin{aligned}
\text{IV: } 60 \text{ ml/hr} \times 8 \text{ hr} &= 480 \text{ ml} \\
\text{IV medications} &= 250 \text{ ml} \\
\text{Juice} &= 120 \text{ ml} \\
\text{Water} &= 90 \text{ ml} \\
\text{Jello} &= 60 \text{ ml} \\
\text{Broth} &= \underline{120 \text{ ml}} \\
&1120 \text{ ml}
\end{aligned}
$$

 Additional information is available on the enclosed CD-ROM in the "Introducing Drug Measures" section.

Interpretation of Drug Labels, Drug Orders, Bar Codes, MAR and eMAR, Automation of Medication Dispensing Administration, "6 Rights," and Abbreviations

OBJECTIVES

- Identify brand names, generic names, drug forms, dosages, expiration dates, and lot numbers on drug labels.
- Give examples of drugs with "look-alike" drug names.
- Name the components of a drug order.
- Explain the computer-based medication administration system.
- Explain the use of the bar code for unit dose drug.
- Identify drug information for charting.
- Name the "6 rights" in drug administration, and give examples of each.
- Use the chart related to the "6 rights."
- Provide meanings of abbreviations: drug form, drug measurement, and routes and times of drug administration.

OUTLINE

INTERPRETATION OF DRUG LABELS

Pharmaceutical companies label drugs with their brand name of the drug in large letters and the generic name in smaller letters. The form of the drug (tablet, capsule, liquid, or powder) and dosage are printed on the drug label.

Many of the calculation problems in this book use drug labels. By using drug labels, the student can practice solving drug problems that are applicable to clinical practice. The student should know what information is on a drug label and how this information is used in drug calculations. All drug labels provide seven basic items of data: (1) brand (trade) name, (2) generic name, (3) dosage, (4) form of the drug, (5) expiration date, (6) lot number, and (7) name of the manufacturer.

EXAMPLES

DRUG LABEL

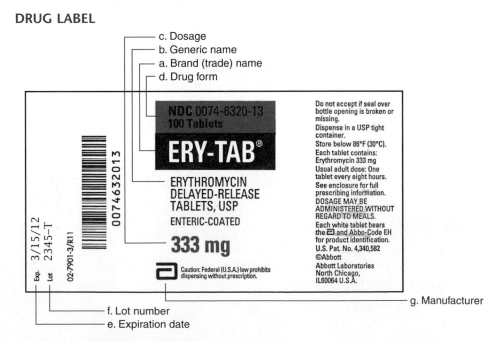

c. Dosage
b. Generic name
a. Brand (trade) name
d. Drug form

NDC 0074-6320-13
100 Tablets

ERY-TAB®

ERYTHROMYCIN
DELAYED-RELEASE
TABLETS, USP

ENTERIC-COATED

333 mg

Caution: Federal (U.S.A.) law prohibits dispensing without prescription.

Do not accept if seal over bottle opening is broken or missing.
Dispense in a USP tight container.
Store below 86°F (30°C).
Each tablet contains: Erythromycin 333 mg
Usual adult dose: One tablet every eight hours.
See enclosure for full prescribing information.
DOSAGE MAY BE ADMINISTERED WITHOUT REGARD TO MEALS.
Each white tablet bears the ⊐ and Abbo-Code EH for product identification.
U.S. Pat. No. 4,340,582
©Abbott
Abbott Laboratories
North Chicago,
IL60064 U.S.A.

g. Manufacturer

f. Lot number
e. Expiration date

Exp. 3/15/12
Lot 2345-T
02-7901-3/R11

a. The brand (trade) name is the commercial name given by the pharmaceutical company (manufacturer of the drug). It is printed in large, bold letters.

b. The generic name is the chemical name given to the drug, regardless of the drug manufacturer. It is printed in smaller letters, usually under the brand name.

c. The dosage strength is the drug dose per drug form (tablet, capsule, liquid) as stated on the label.

d. The form of the drug (tablet, capsule, liquid) relates to the dosage strength.

e. The expiration date refers to the length of time the drug can be used before it loses its potency. Drugs should not be administered after the expiration date. The nurse must check the expiration date of all drugs that he or she administers.

f. The lot number identifies the drug batch in which the medication was produced. Occasionally, a drug is recalled according to the lot number.

g. The manufacturer is the pharmaceutical company that produces the brand name drug.

Examples of drug labels are given, and practice problems for reading drug labels follow the examples.

EXAMPLES

ORAL DRUG (SOLID FORM)

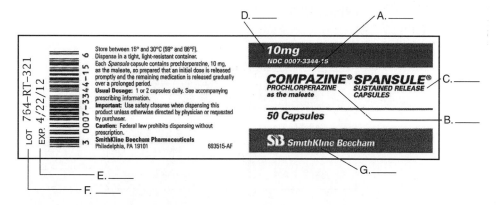

a. Brand (trade) name is Compazine.
b. Generic name is prochlorperazine.
c. Drug form is a sustained release capsule (SR capsule).
d. Dosage is 10 mg per capsule.
e. Expiration date is 4/22/12 (after this date, the drug should be discarded).
f. Lot number is 764-RT-321.
g. Manufacturer is SmithKline Beecham Pharmaceuticals.

EXAMPLES

ORAL DRUG (LIQUID FORM)

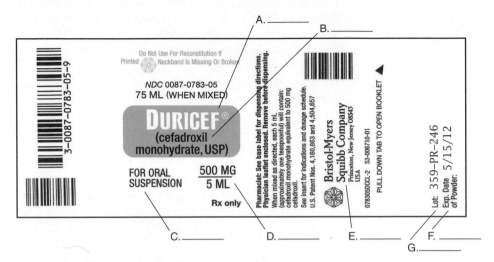

a. Brand (trade) name is Duricef.
b. Generic name is cefadroxil monohydrate.
c. Drug form is oral suspension.
d. Dosage is 500 mg per 5 ml.
e. Manufacturer is Bristol-Myers Squibb Company.
f. Expiration date is 5/15/12.
g. Lot number is 359-PR-246.

EXAMPLES

INJECTABLE DRUG

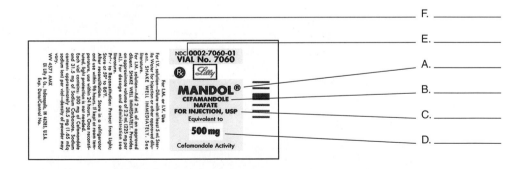

a. Brand name is Mandol.
b. Generic name is cefamandole nafate.
c. Drug form is drug powder that must be reconstituted in a liquid form for use (circular paper).

d. Dosage is 500 mg drug powder.

e. Drug container is vial.

f. IV: Reconstitute by using at least 5 ml of sterile water for injection, which then must be diluted in 50 to 100 ml of IV fluids.

IM: 2 ml of a diluent should be added. The total amount of the drug would then equal 2.2 ml. The powder increases the liquid form by 0.2 ml.

PRACTICE PROBLEMS: I Interpretation of Drug Labels

Answers can be found on page 71.

1.

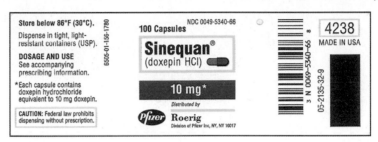

a. Brand (trade) name _____   d. Dosage _____

b. Generic name _____   e. Manufacturer _____

c. Drug form _____

2.

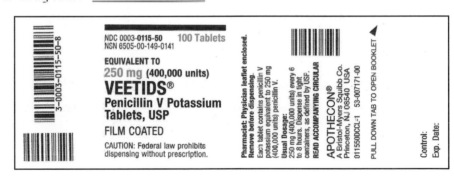

a. Brand (trade) name_____

b. Generic name_____

c. Drug form_____

d. Dosage _____ mg _____ units

e. Manufacturer _____

3.

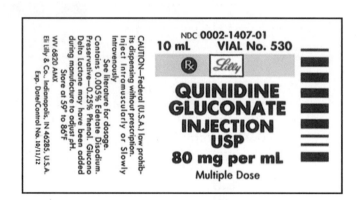

a. Brand (trade) name _____

b. Generic name _____

c. Drug form _____

d. Dosage _____

e. Lot number _____

f. Expiration date _____

g. Manufacturer _____

4.

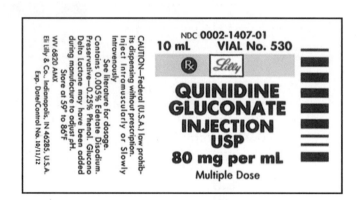

a. Brand (trade) name _____

b. Generic name _____

c. Drug form _____

d. Drug container _____

e. Dosage _____

5.

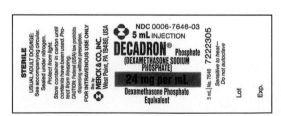

a. Brand (trade) name _____

b. Generic name _____

c. Drug form _____

d. Dosage _____

6.

NDC 0015-7225-20
EQUIVALENT TO
1 gram NAFCILLIN
**NAFCILLIN SODIUM
FOR INJECTION, USP**
Buffered-For IM or IV Use
CAUTION: Federal law prohibits
dispensing without prescription.
APOTHECON®
A BRISTOL-MYERS SQUIBB COMPANY

When reconstituted with 3.4 mL
diluent, (SEE INSERT-INTRAMUS-
CULAR ROUTE), each vial contains
4 mL solution. Each mL of solution
contains nafcillin sodium, as the
monohydrate, equivalent to 250 mg
nafcillin, buffered with 10 mg sodium
citrate. Read accompanying circular
for complete stability data.
Usual Dosage: Adults—500 mg every
4 to 6 hours. Read accompanying
circular for directions for IM or IV
use.
APOTHECON®
A Bristol-Myers Squibb Company
Princeton, NJ 08540 USA
722520DRL-2

Cont:
Exp. Date: 11/30/12

a. Brand name _____

b. Generic name_____

c. Drug form_____

d. Drug label suggests adding _____ diluent

e. Method of administration _____

f. Dosage 1 gram = _____ ml

g. Expiration date _____

h. Manufacturer_____

Military Time versus Traditional (Universal) Time

Many nursing settings currently are using military time, a 24-hour clock, when administering medications and treatments. For example, in military time, 3 AM is 0300 and 3 PM is 1500; 7:15 AM is 0715 and 7:30 PM is 1930. The AM hours are the same as on the traditional clock, and for hours after 12 noon, 12 is added to the PM hours; see Figure 3-1. The use of the 24-hour clock reduces drug administration errors.

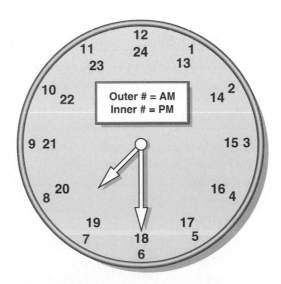

FIGURE 3-1 Military clock.

DRUG DIFFERENTIATION

Some drugs with similar names, such as quinine and quinidine, have different chemical drug structures. Extreme care must be exercised when administering drugs that "look alike" or that have similar spellings.

EXAMPLES

PERCOCET

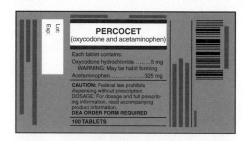

PERCODAN

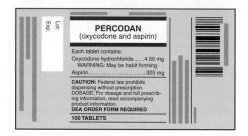

Percocet contains oxycodone and acetaminophen, whereas Percodan contains oxycodone and aspirin. A patient may be allergic to aspirin or should not take aspirin; therefore it is important that the patient be given Percocet. *Read the drug labels carefully.*

EXAMPLES

HYDROXYZINE AND HYDRALAZINE
Hydroxyzine is an antianxiety drug, and hydralazine is an antihypertensive drug.

EXAMPLES

QUINIDINE AND QUININE
Quinidine sulfate is an antidysrhythmic drug, and quinine sulfate is an antimalarial drug.

Drug Orders

Medication orders may be prescribed and written by a physician (MD), an osteopathic physician (DO), a dentist (DDS), a podiatrist (DPM), or a licensed health care provider (HCP), e.g., a nurse practitioner, who has been given authority by the state to write prescriptions. Drug prescriptions in private practice or in clinics are written on a small prescription pad and are filled by a pharmacist at a drug store or hospital (Figure 3-2). For hospitalized patients, the drug orders may be written on a doctor's order sheet and signed by the physician or licensed health care provider (Figure 3-3), or a computerized drug order system may be used. If the order is given by telephone (TO), the order must be cosigned by the physician within 24 hours. Most health care institutions have policies concerning verbal or telephone drug orders. The nurse must know and follow the institution's policy.

Roger J. Smith, Jr., M.D.
678 Apple Street
Wilmington, Delaware 19810

(123) 456-7891

Name _____ Age _____
Address _____ Date _____

R~x~

Generic permitted
Label _____   _____ M.D.
Safety cap _____
Refill _____ times

FIGURE 3-2 Prescription pad medication order.

CITY HOSPITAL Dover, Delaware		PATIENT'S NAME Room #
Date	Time	Patient's Orders
12/2/09	0900	Zoloft 75mg, po, daily

FIGURE 3-3 Patient's orders.

The basic components of a drug order are (1) date and time the order was written, (2) drug name, (3) drug dosage, (4) route of administration, (5) frequency of administration, and (6) physician's or health care provider's signature. It is the nurse's responsibility to follow the physician's or health care provider's order, but if any one of these components is missing, the drug order is incomplete and cannot be carried out. If the order is illegible, is missing a component, or calls for an inappropriate drug or dosage, clarification must be obtained before the order is carried out.

Examples of drug orders and their interpretation are as follows:

6/3/09   9:10A   Digoxin 0.25 mg, po, daily
(give 0.25 mg of digoxin by mouth daily)

Ibuprofen 400 mg, po, q4h, PRN
(give 400 mg of ibuprofen by mouth every 4 hours as needed)

Cefadyl 500 mg, IM, q6h
(give 500 mg of Cefadyl intramuscularly every 6 hours)

Prednisone 5 mg, po, q8h × 5 days
(give 5 mg of prednisone by mouth every 8 hours for 5 days)

PRACTICE PROBLEMS: II Interpretation of Drug Orders

Answers can be found on page 72.

Interpret these drug orders. For abbreviations that you do not know, see the section on abbreviations later in this chapter.

1. Tetracycline 250 mg, po, q6h

_____

2. HydroDIURIL 50 mg, po, daily

_____

3. Meperidine 50 mg, IM, q3–4h, PRN

_____

4. Ancef 1 g, IV, q8h

_____

5. Prednisone 10 mg, tid × 5 days

_____

List what is missing in the following drug orders.

6. Codeine 30 mg, po, PRN for pain _____

TABLE 3-1

Types of Drug Orders

Types/Description	Examples
Standing orders: A standing order may be typed or written on the doctor's order sheet. It may be an order that is given for a number of days, or it may be a routine order for all patients who had the same type of procedure. Standing orders may include PRN orders.	Erythromycin 250 mg, po, q6h, 5 days Demerol 50 mg, IM, q3-4h, PRN, pain Colace 100 mg, po, hs, PRN
One-time (single) orders: One-time orders are given once, usually at a specified time.	Preoperative orders: Meperidine 75 mg, IM, 7:30 AM Atropine SO$_4$ 0.4 mg, IM, 7:30 AM
PRN orders: PRN orders are given at the patient's request and at the nurse's discretion concerning safety and need.	Pentobarbital 100 mg, hs (bedtime) PRN Darvocet-N, tab 1, q4h, PRN
STAT orders: A STAT order is for a one-time dose of drug to be given immediately.	Regular insulin 10 units, subQ, STAT

7. Digoxin 0.25 mg, daily _____

8. Ceclor 125 mg, po_____

9. TheoDur 200 mg _____

10. Penicillin V K 200,000 units, for days _____

_____

There are four types of drug orders: (1) standing order, (2) one-time (single) order, (3) PRN (whenever necessary) order, and (4) STAT (immediate) order (Table 3-1). Many of the drugs ordered for nonhospitalized patients are normally standing orders that can be renewed (refilled) for 6 to 12 months. Narcotic orders are *not* automatically refilled; if the narcotic use is extended, the physician writes another prescription or calls the pharmacy.

UNIT-DOSE DISPENSING SYSTEM (UDDS)

The unit-dose drug dispensing system (UDDS) was developed to reduce medication errors, reduce the waste of medication, and improve the efficiency of the nurse when administering medication. The UDDS has almost replaced the ward stock system (Table 3-2). In the ward stock system, bulk drug supplies were delivered to the medication room in each patient area. In the medication room, the nurse would prepare the patient's dose from the large multidose containers or multiple-dose vials; the correct dosage of medication must be taken from the container each time and labeled. In unit-dose dispensing,

TABLE 3-2		

Methods of Drug Distribution

	Stock Drug Method	Unit-Dose Method
Description	Drug is stored in a large container on the floor and is dispensed from the container for all patients.	Drug is packaged in single doses by the pharmacy for 24-hour dosing.
Advantages	Drug is always available, which eliminates time spent waiting for drug to arrive from the pharmacy. Cost efficiency is enhanced by having large quantities of the drug.	Fewer drug errors are made. Packaging saves the nurse time otherwise spent in preparing the drug dose. Correct dose is provided with *no* calculation needed. Drug is billed for specific number of doses.
Disadvantages	Drug error is more prevalent because the drug is "poured" by many persons. More drugs are available to choose from; this may cause error. Drug expiration date on the container may be missed.	Time delay is seen in receipt of drug from the pharmacy. If doses are contaminated or damaged, they are not immediately replaceable.

the pharmacy can provide individual doses in packets or containers for each patient. The pharmacy buys the drugs in bulk and repackages the medication in individual dose packets labeled with the drug name, dosage, and usually a bar code. Many variations are seen in ways that drugs are stored and delivered to patient care areas. Unit-dose cart cabinets (Figure 3-4) with individualized drawers labeled with the patient's name, room number, and bed number are most common. Each drawer is filled with 24 hours of medication as prescribed by the physician and filled and verified by the pharmacist. The drawers may be refilled or exchanged every 24 hours. When the nurse administers medication, the patient's drawer is accessed, and the appropriate drug is withdrawn.

Unit-dose dispensing has eliminated the need for many drug calculations that were essential with the ward stock system. Drug manufacturers are working to develop single doses for all medications but extra packaging is costly. In addition, not all medications that are prescribed for a patient are dosed in the exact amount manufactured. Therefore, the nurse must master manual calculations and must have working knowledge of the process and formulas needed for medications to be given safely.

COMPUTER-BASED DRUG ADMINISTRATION (CBDA)

Computer-based drug administration (CBDA) is a technological software system that is designed to prevent medication errors. The concept began when the Centers for Disease Control and Prevention (CDC) reported a rise in the

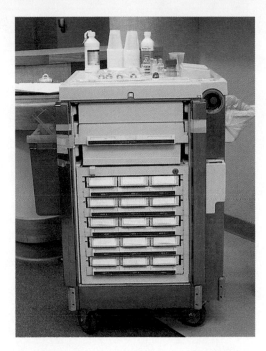

FIGURE 3-4 Unit dose cabinet. (From Clayton, B. D., Stock, Y. N., & Harroun, R. D. [2007]. *Basic pharmacology for nurses*. 14th ed. St. Louis: Mosby).

number of medication-related deaths between 1983 and 1993. Since that time, the National Coordinating Council for Medication Error Reporting and Prevention has made several recommendations regarding the causes of medication errors; one example of its proposed changes is the bar coding of medications. The federal government through the Department of Veterans Affairs Hospitals has developed a software program that automates the medication administration process to improve accuracy and efficiency in documentation. Currently, this system is composed of the Computerized Prescriber Order System (CPOS), the Bar Code Administration System (BCMA), the electronic Medication Administration Record (eMAR), and the Pharmacy Information System (PIS), will be expanded to track medications in all forms and to include the whole process of prescribing, administering, monitoring, and documenting.

COMPUTERIZED PRESCRIBER ORDER SYSTEM (CPOS)

The process begins with the Computerized Prescriber Order (entry) System (CPOS), by which the physician or health care provider selects medication from a scrolling list; see Figure 3-5. Once the medication is chosen, the next screen displays all the possible doses, routes, and schedules; see Figure 3-6. Once the physician selects those components of the order, he or she can view the screen and make changes. If the screen information is correct, the physician signs the order with his or her personal electronic code, and the order is sent through the PIS, where the order is processed.

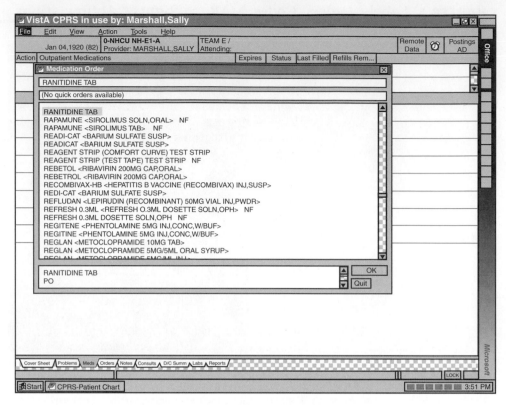

FIGURE 3-5 Medication screen for scrolling.

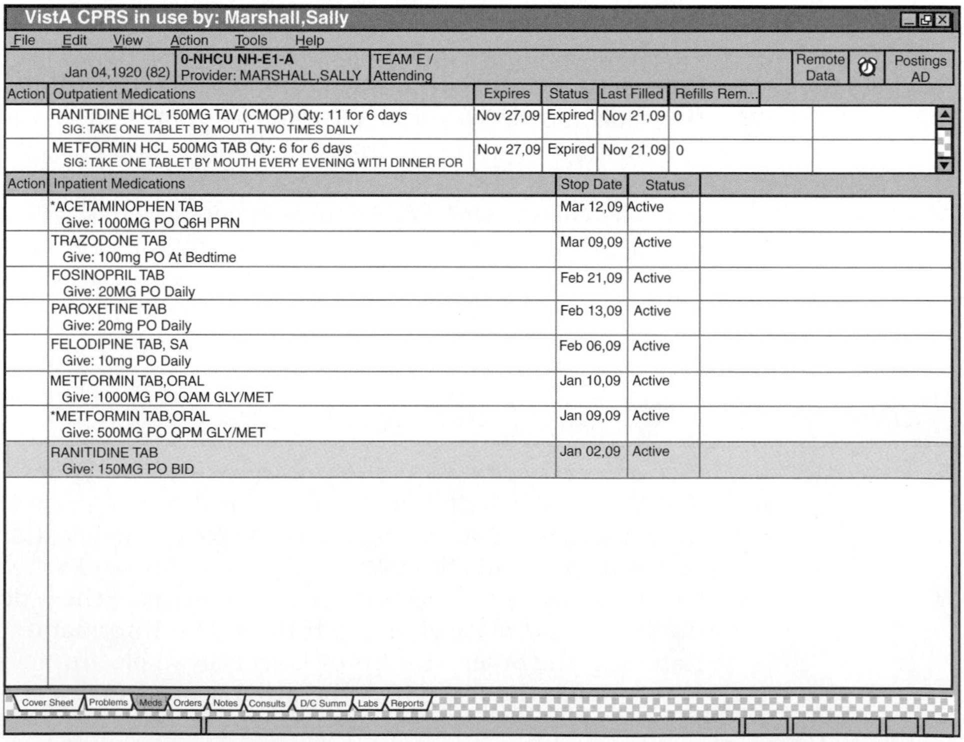

FIGURE 3-6 Medications chosen, doses, routes, and time.

Bar Code Medication Administration

Bar codes are mandatory on medication packaging produced by drug suppliers. Pharmacies can buy drugs in bulk and repackage the medication individually in cellophane envelopes or packets for the unit dose, with each drug and dose having a specific bar code number. The pharmacy delivers bar-coded drugs to hospital units at specified times, and drugs are kept in special carts within designated areas in patient care locations.

When the nurse is ready to administer the medications, she/he accesses the bar code medication administration system (BCMA), which displays the medication record screen, and uses the bar code reader to scan the patient's wrist band and the bar code on the drug; see Figures 3-7 and 3-8.

The software validates the correct patient, drug, and dosage, along with the right route and time. The software is intended to enhance patient safety by clarifying orders, improving communication, and augmenting clinical judgment.

Medication Administration Record (MAR and eMAR)

Documentation for the Medication Administration Record (MAR) should be completed immediately after medications are given. Failing to do so may result in (1) forgetting to chart/document, or (2) administration of drugs by another

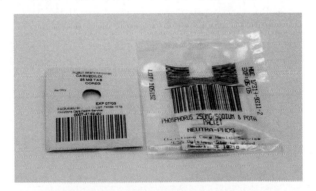

FIGURE 3-7 Bar code for unit drug dose.

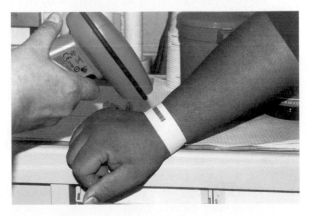

FIGURE 3-8 Bar code reader. It is used to scan the patient's wristband.

nurse who thought that the drugs were not given. Although the MAR may vary among health care facilities, all include basic information, such as the patient's name, identification number, date of birth, location, allergies, sex, and date of admission. Drug information on the MAR that is common to all records includes the following: (1) date the drug was ordered, (2) drug name, (3) dosage, (4) route of administration, (5) frequency of administration, (6) date and time the drug was given, and (7) the nurse's signature and initials. Handwritten MARs (Figure 3-9) should be avoided because of the high risk of transcription error.

The electronic medication administration record (eMAR) (Figure 3-10) is the counterpart to BCMA. It is a paperless system that displays on the computer screen the medications to be administered and the appropriate times for each. The nurse uses his or her own specific code to log on to the system, and when the drug is scanned, it is documented as given.

Automation of Medication Dispensing Administration

Automated dispensing cabinets (ADCs) are medication cabinets that store, dispense, and track drugs in patient areas. They were developed to reduce medication errors, increase pharmacy and nursing efficiency, increase security, support efforts to maintain The Joint Commission and regulatory compliance and control costs. ADCs permit nurses to access the system with a user ID, personal password, or biometric fingerprint scan to obtain medication in the patient area without having to wait for medication to come from a centralized pharmacy. The three most common dispensing systems are the Pyxis® MedStation™ system (Figure 3-11), Omnicell OmniRx®, and the AcuDose-Rx®. These systems support storage of vials, ampules, unit-dose packages, prefilled syringes, liquid cups, pre-mixed IVs, large volume IVs, and other forms of packing. Now almost 90% of all ADCs are linked to the pharmacy information system's patient medication profile; this ensures that the nurse accesses only medication for a specific patient.

THE "6 RIGHTS" IN DRUG ADMINISTRATION

To provide safe drug administration, the nurse should practice the "6 rights": the right patient, the right drug, the right dose, the right time, the right route, right documentation (see "Checklist"). Four additional rights could be added: the right assessment, the right of the patient to know the reason for administration of the drug, the right of the patient to refuse to take a medication, and right evaluation.

Right Patient

The patient's identification band should always be checked before a medication is given. The nurse should do the following:

- Verify patient by checking his or her identification bracelet/armband.
- Ask the patient his or her name. Do not call the patient by name. Some individuals answer to any name. Ask for his or her date of birth (this may or may not be required).
- Check the name on the patient's medication label.

HOPE HOSPITAL				Patient's Name *John Smith* 123-24-8449						

HOPE HOSPITAL

Medication Administration Record (MAR)

Patient's Name *John Smith*
123-24-8449

Age: *78*

Room# *6033*

Nurse's signature/Title	Initial
Joyce L. Kee, RN	JK
Sally Marshall, RN	SM
Jane Jones, LPN	JJ

Allergies:

Penicillin

DATE ORDER	STOP DATE	Medication Dose – Route – Frequency	HOUR	Date, Initial, HT Rate, BP												
				5/16		5/17		5/18		5/19						
5/16		Digoxin 0.25 mg, po, daily	8	JK	92	JK	86	JK	88	SM	84					
5/16	5/20 @ 24h	Prednisone 5 mg, po q8h X 5 days	8	JK		JK		JK		SM						
			16	SM		JJ		SM		JK						
			24	JJ		SM		JJ		JJ						
5/16		Atenolol 50 mg, po, daily	8	JK	152/110	JK	146/90	JK	148/72	SM	145/75					

One-Time/PRN/STAT Medications				
Date	Medication/Dose Route/Frequency	Time/ Initial	Reason	Result
5/18	Ibuprofen 400 mg, po q4h, PRN	9:30 A SM	Leg pain	10:30A Relief from pain

FIGURE 3-9 Medication Administration Record (MAR).

THURSDAY 10/12/09 - 0700 thru FRIDAY 10/13/09 - 0659	ST ANNE HOSPITAL

Meyer, Lois M.   Unit#:
 WESOF W303-2
 Age: 72   Sex: F   Admitted: 10/12/09
              Ht: 152.40 cm   Wt: kg
 Primary Dx: CP
	MEDICATION ADMINISTRATION RECORD
	 Acct#: Page: 1
	 Attending Dr: Thomas Smith, MD
	 Run Date/Time: 10/12/09 - 2237
	                    DOB: 06/23/1934

ALLERGIES: Drug: PCN. ERYTHROMYCIN. IV DYE
                 Other: NO ALLERGIES RECORED
               Pharmacy: IODINE (INCLUDES RADIOPAQUE AGENTS W/IODINE). MACROLIDE ANTIBIOTICS, PENICILLINS

Init	IV Flushes: Routine		0700-1459	1500-2259	2300-0659
	Sodium Chloride 0.9% **IV** Flush peripheral IV lines with 5 mls 0.9 NS q 8 hours and central lines per protocol.		Time _____ Init _____ # Flushed_____	Time _____ Init _____ # Flushed_____	Time _____ Init _____ # Flushed_____

Init	SCHED MEDS	DOSE		0700-1459	1500-2259	2300-0659
	DOCUSATE SODIUM (DOCUSATE SODIUM) START: 10/12 D/C: 11/11/09 AT 2244	**100 MG**	PO Q12 RX 002306792			
	PRAVACHOL (PRAVASTATIN SODIUM) Give at: BEDTIME START: 10/12 D/C: 11/11/09 AT 2244	**80 MG**	PO RX 002306793			
	METOPROLOL TARTRATE (METOPROLOL TARTRATE) HOLD FOR SBP<110 OR HR<55 Check apical rate and BP before drug admin. START: 10/12 D/C: 11/11/09 AT 2244	**50 MG**	PO Q12 RX 002306794			
	ACCUPRIL (QUINAPRIL HCL) HOLD FOR SBP<120 START: 10/12 D/C: 11/11/09 AT 2244	**40 MG**	PO Q12 RX 002306795			
	NITROGLYCERIN 2% (NITROGLYCERIN 2%) HOLD FOR SBP<100 START: 10/12 D/C: 11/11/09 AT 2244	**1 INCH**	TP Q6 RX 002306796			0000 0600
	ALPRAZOLAM (ALPRAZOLAM) START: 10/12 D/C: 10/14/09 AT 1601	**0.25 MG**	PO Q8 RX 002306791			0000

Init	PRN MEDS	DOSE		0700-1459	1500-2259	2300-0659
	NITROSTAT 25 TABS/BOTTLE (NITROGLYCERIN) Chest discomfort. May repeat q 5 min x 3. If no relief after 3 doses. Stat ECG & call Physician. START: 10/12 D/C: 11/11/09 at 1833	**0.4 MG**	SL STAT RX 002306718 PRN			

FIGURE 3-10 Electronic Medication Administration Record (eMAR).

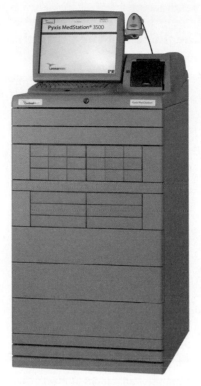

FIGURE 3-11 Pyxis® MedStation™ system. (From Cardinal Health, San Diego, CA.)

Right Drug

To avoid error, the nurse should do the following:

- Check the drug label three times: (1) at first contact with the drug bottle, (2) before pouring the drug, and (3) after pouring the drug.
- Check that the drug order is complete and legible. If it is not, contact the physician or charge nurse.
- Know the drug action.
- Check the expiration date. Discard an outdated drug, or return the drug to the pharmacy.
- If the patient questions the drug, recheck drug and drug dose. If in doubt, seek another health care provider's advice, e.g., pharmacist, physician, licensed health care provider. Some generic drugs differ in shape or color.

Right Dose

Stock drugs and unit doses are the two methods frequently used for drug distribution. Not all health care institutions use the unit-dose method (drugs prepared by dose in the pharmacy or by the pharmaceutical company). If the institution uses the unit-dose method, drugs in bottles should *not* be administered without the consent of the physician or pharmacist. The nurse should

- Be able to calculate drug dose using the ratio and proportion, basic formula, fractional equation, or dimensional analysis method.

Checklist for the "6 Rights" in Drug Administration

Right Patient
- Check patient's identification bracelet. ❏
- Ask the patient his or her name. ❏
- Check the name on the patient's medication label. ❏

Right Drug
- Check that the drug order is complete and legible. ❏
- Check the drug label three times. ❏
- Check the expiration date. ❏
- Know the drug action. ❏

Right Dose
- Calculate the drug dose. ❏
- Know the recommended dosage range for the drug. ❏
- Recalculate the drug dose with another nurse if in doubt. ❏

Right Time
- Administer drug at the specified time(s). ❏
- Document any delay or omitted drug dose. ❏
- Administer with food drugs that irritate gastric mucosa. ❏
- Administer antibiotics at even intervals (q6h, q8h). ❏

Right Route
- Know the route for administration of the drug. ❏
- Use aseptic techniques when administering a drug. ❏
- Document the injection site on the patient's chart. ❏

Right Documentation
- Place nurse's initials on MAR sheet or eMAR.
- Document that the patient refused or the drug was omitted by circling the nurse's initials. ❏
- Indicate on the MAR whether the drug dose was delayed and the time it was given. ❏

- Know how to calculate drug dose by body weight (kg) or by body surface area (BSA; m^2). Doses of potent drugs (e.g., anticancer agents) and doses for children are frequently determined by body weight or BSA.
- Know the recommended dosage range for the drug. Check the *Physicians' Desk Reference,* the *American Hospital Formulary, Nursing Drug* references, computerized drug reference programs, or other drug references. If the nurse believes that the dose is incorrect or is not within the therapeutic range, he or she should notify the charge nurse, physician, or pharmacist and should document all communications.
- Recalculate drug dose if in doubt, or have a colleague recheck the dose.

- Question drug doses that appear to be incorrect.
- Have a colleague check the drug dose of potent or specified drugs such as insulin, digoxin, narcotics, and anticancer agents. This procedure is required by some facilities.

Right Time

The drug dose should be given at a specified time to maintain a therapeutic drug serum level. Too-frequent dosing can cause drug toxicity, and missed doses can nullify the drug action and its effect. The nurse should

- Administer the drug at the specified time(s). Drugs can be given ½ hour before or after the time prescribed.
- Omit or delay a drug dose according to specific circumstance, e.g., laboratory and diagnostic tests. Notify the appropriate personnel of the reason.
- Administer drugs that are affected by foods, e.g., tetracycline, 1 hour before or 2 hours after meals.
- Administer drugs that can irritate the gastric mucosa, e.g., potassium or aspirin, with food.
- Know that drugs with a long half-life (t½), e.g., 20 to 36 hours, are usually given once per day. Drugs with a short half-life, e.g., 1 to 6 hours, are given several times a day.
- Administer antibiotics at even intervals (e.g., q8h [8-4-12] rather than tid [8-12-4]; q6h [6-12-6-12] rather than qid [8-12-4-8]) to maintain a therapeutic drug serum level.

Right Route

The right route is necessary for appropriate absorption of the medication. The more common routes of absorption are (1) oral (by mouth, po) tablet, capsule, pill, liquid, or suspension; (2) sublingual (under the tongue for venous absorption, *not* to be swallowed); (3) buccal (between gum and cheek); (4) topical (applied to the skin); (5) inhalation (aerosol sprays); (6) instillation (in nose, eye, ear, rectum, or vagina); (7) and four parenteral routes: intradermal, subcutaneous, intramuscular, and intravenous. The nurse should

- Know the drug route. If in doubt, check with the pharmacy. Ointment for the eye should have "ophthalmic" written on the tube. Drugs given sublingually (e.g., nitroglycerin tablet) should *not* be swallowed, because the effect of the drug would be lost.
- Administer injectables (subcutaneous and intramuscular) at appropriate sites (see Chapter 8).
- Use aseptic technique when administering drugs. Sterile technique is required with parenteral routes.
- Document on the patient's chart or on another designated sheet the injection site used.

Right Documentation

Document on the MAR the time the drug was administered and the nurse's initials. To avoid overdosing or underdosing of drug, administration of medication should be recorded immediately.

- Put your initials on the MAR sheet at the proper space immediately after administering the drug.
- Refused drug: Circle your initials and document on the nurse's notes or on the MAR if space is provided.
- Omitted drug: Circle your initials and document on the nurse's notes or on the MAR if space is provided. Document why the drug was omitted, such as the client was on nothing by mouth because of a laboratory or diagnostic test.
- Delay in administering drug should be documented on the nurse's notes or the MAR sheet. If the drug is to be administered once a day and is delayed, document the time the drug is given. If the drug is to be given every 4 hours, call the health care provider for direction on when the drug should be administered.

Other *rights* may include right assessment, right to educate the patient, right evaluation, and right to refuse drug.

ABBREVIATIONS

The Joint Commission (TJC)

In 2005, The Joint Commission (TJC) (formerly known as the Joint Commission on Accreditation of Healthcare Organization [JCAHO]) issued a new list of abbreviations that should not be used but written out to avoid misinterpretation. Below is the "Do Not Use" abbreviation list, followed by a list of abbreviations that could possibly be included in future "Do Not Use" lists.

Lists of acceptable abbreviations follow TJC lists in three categories: drug measurements and drug forms, routes of drug administration, and times of administration.

Abbreviation	**Use Instead**
q.d., Q.D.	Write "daily" or "every day."
q.o.d., Q.O.D.	Write "every other day."
U	Write "unit."
IU	Write "international unit."
MS, MSO$_4$	Write "morphine sulfate."
MgSO$_4$	Write "magnesium sulfate."
.5 mg	Write "0.5 mg," use zero before a decimal point when the dose is less than a whole.
1.0 mg	Write "1 mg," do not use a decimal point or zero after a whole number.

The following abbreviations could possibly be included in future Joint Commission "Do Not Use" lists. These abbreviations are as follows:

Abbreviation	Use Instead
c.c.	Use "ml" (milliliter).
μg	Use "mcg" (microgram).
>	Write "greater than."
<	Write "less than."
Drug name abbreviations	Write out the full name of the drug.
Apothecary units	Use metric units.
@	Write "at."

Selected abbreviations are listed below. These are frequently used in drug therapy and must be known by the nurse.

Drug Measurements and Drug Forms

Abbreviation	Meaning
cap	capsule
dr	dram
elix	elixir
g, gm, G, GM	gram
gr	grain
gtt	drops
kg	kilogram
l, L	liter
m^2	square meter
mcg	microgram
mEq	milliequivalent
mg	milligram
mL, ml	milliliter
m, min	minim
oz	ounce
pt	pint
qt	quart
SR	sustained release
s̄s̄	one half
supp	suppository
susp	suspension
T.O.	telephone order
T, tbsp	tablespoon
t, tsp	teaspoon
V.O.	verbal order

Routes of Drug Administration

Abbreviation	Meaning
A.D., ad	right ear
A.S., as	left ear
A.U., au	both ears
ID	intradermal
IM	intramuscular
IV	intravenous
IVPB	intravenous piggyback
KVO	keep vein open
L	left
NGT	nasogastric tube
O.D., od	right eye
O.S., os	left eye
O.U., ou	both eyes
PO, po, os	by mouth
®	right
SC, subc, sc, SQ, subQ	subcutaneous
SL, sl, subl	sublingual
TKO	to keep open
Vag	vaginal

Times of Administration

Abbreviation	Meaning
AC, ac	before meals
ad lib	as desired
B.i.d., b.i.d.	twice a day
$\bar{c}$	with
hs	hour of sleep
NPO	nothing by mouth
PC, pc	after meals
PRN, p.r.n.	whenever necessary, as needed
q	every
qAM	every morning
qh	every hour
q2h	every 2 hours
q4h	every 4 hours
q6h	every 6 hours
q8h	every 8 hours
$\bar{s}$	without
SOS	once if necessary: if there is a need
Stat	immediately
T.i.d., t.i.d.	three times a day

Please refer to The Joint Commission website at *www.jointcommission.org* and Institute for Safe Medication practices at *www.ismp.org* for more detailed safety information.

PRACTICE PROBLEMS: III Abbreviations

Answers can be found on page 72.

If you have more than two incorrect answers, review the abbreviations and meanings. Then quiz yourself again.

1. cap _____

2. SR _____

3. fl oz _____

4. g, G _____

5. gr _____

6. L _____

7. ml _____

8. mcg _____

9. mg _____

10. oz _____

11. T _____

12. t _____

13. IM _____

14. IV _____

15. KVO _____

16. subQ _____

17. c̄ _____

18. A.C., ac _____

19. NPO _____

20. P.C., pc _____

21. q4h _____

22. Qid, qid, q.i.d. _____

23. Tid, tid, t.i.d. _____

24. Bid, bid, b.i.d. _____

25. STAT _____

ANSWERS

I Interpretation of Drug Labels

1. **a.** Sinequan
   b. doxepin
   c. capsule
   d. 10 mg per capsule
   e. Pfizer/Roerig
2. **a.** Veetids
   b. penicillin V potassium
   c. tablet
   d. 250 mg per tablet; 400,000 units per tablet
   e. Apothecon

3. **a.** Amoxil
   b. amoxicillin
   c. liquid for oral suspension when reconstituted
   d. 200 mg/5 ml
   e. Lot #T54325
   f. Expiration date: 11/15/12
   g. SmithKline Beecham
4. **a.** quinidine gluconate
   b. quinidine gluconate (same as brand name)
   c. liquid for injection
   d. vial (multiple-dose vial), total amount is 10 ml per vial
   e. 80 mg per ml

5. **a.** Decadron phosphate
   b. dexamethasone sodium phosphate
   c. liquid for injection
   d. 24 mg per ml
6. **a.** nafcillin sodium
   b. nafcillin sodium (same as brand name)
   c. drug powder to be reconstituted
   d. 3.4 ml diluent
   e. IM or IV
   f. 1 gram = 4 ml
   g. 11/30/12
   h. Apothecon

II Interpretation of Drug Orders

1. Give 250 mg of tetracycline by mouth every 6 hours
2. Give 50 mg of HydroDIURIL by mouth every day
3. Give 50 mg of meperidine intramuscularly every 3 to 4 hours whenever necessary
4. Give 1 g of Ancef intravenously every 8 hours
5. Give 10 mg of prednisone three times a day for 5 days
6. frequency of administration
7. route of administration
8. frequency of administration
9. route and frequency of administration
10. route and frequency of administration and stop date

III Abbreviations

1. capsule
2. sustained release
3. fluid ounce
4. gram
5. grain
6. liter
7. milliliter
8. microgram
9. milligram
10. ounce
11. tablespoon
12. teaspoon
13. intramuscular
14. intravenous
15. keep vein open
16. subcutaneous
17. with
18. before meals
19. nothing by mouth
20. after meals
21. every 4 hours
22. four times a day
23. three times a day
24. two times a day
25. immediately

 Additional information is available on the enclosed CD-ROM in the "Safety in Medication Administration" section.

Alternative Methods for Drug Administration

OBJECTIVES

■ Recognize the various methods for drug administration.

■ Explain the steps (methods) in drug administration when the various methods are used.

OUTLINE

Numerous methods are used to administer medications, in addition to the oral (tablets, capsules, liquid) and parenteral (subcutaneous, intramuscular, intravenous) routes. Alternative methods for drug administration include transdermal patches; inhalation sprays; nasal sprays and drops; eye drops and ointments; ear drops; pharyngeal (throat) sprays, mouthwashes, and lozenges; topical lotions, creams, and ointments; rectal suppositories; and vaginal suppositories, creams, and ointments.

TRANSDERMAL PATCH

Purpose

The transdermal patch contains medication (Figure 4-1); the patch is applied to the skin for slow, systemic absorption, usually over 24 hours. Use of the transdermal route avoids the gastrointestinal problems associated with some oral medications and provides a more consistent drug level in the patient's blood.

METHOD

Transdermal Patch

1. Cleanse the skin area where the patch will be applied. The area can be the chest, abdomen, arms, or thighs. Avoid areas that have hair. Wear gloves.
2. Remove the transparent cover (inside) of the patch. Do not touch the inside of the patch.
3. Apply the patch to the chosen area with the dull, plastic side up.

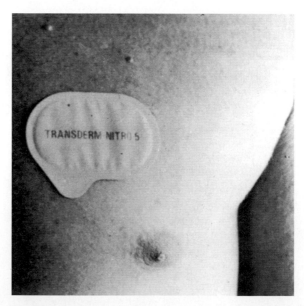

FIGURE 4-1 Transdermal nitrogycerin patch. (From Summit Pharmaceutical)

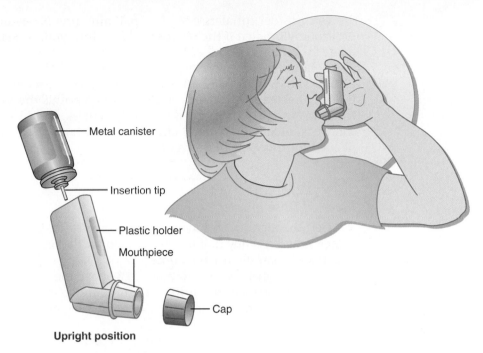

Metal canister

Insertion tip

Plastic holder

Mouthpiece

Cap

Upright position

FIGURE 4-2 Technique for using the aerosol inhaler. (From Kee, J. L., Hayes, E. R., & McCuistion, L. E. [2006]. *Pharmacology: a nursing process approach.* 5th ed. Philadelphia: W. B. Saunders.)

TYPES OF INHALATION

Purpose

The drug inhaler delivers the prescribed dose to be absorbed by the mucosal lining of the respiratory tract (Figure 4-2). The drug categories for respiratory inhalation are bronchodilators, which dilate bronchial tubes; glucocorticoids, which are anti-inflammatory agents; and mucolytics, which liquefy bronchial secretions.

Types

Inhalers can be divided into four groups; metered-dose inhalers (MDIs), MDI inhalers with spacers, dry powder inhalers, and nebulizers. Standard MDIs use a pressurized gas that expels the medication. Press the canister and inhale fully at the same time. Breath-activated MDIs are another type, in which the dose is triggered by inhaling through the mouthpiece; they require less coordination.

Spacer devices are used with MDIs and act as a reservoir to hold the medication until it is inhaled. These devices have a one-way valve that prevents the aerosol from escaping. Good coordination is not needed to use a spacer device.

Dry powder inhalers contain small amounts of medications that have to be strongly inhaled if the powder is to get into your lungs. This method is difficult for children younger than 6.

Nebulizers are devices that convert medication into a fine mist. The medication is usually prescribed in a prefilled dosette, which is placed in a nebulizer connected to a small compressor that aerosols the medication. The medication is inhaled via mouthpiece or face mask. Nebulizers are the choice for the weak, elderly, and small children and infants because no coordination is needed for this type of delivery.

METHOD

Metered-Dose Inhaler

1. Insert the medication canister into the plastic holder. If the inhaler has not been used recently or if it is being used for the first time, test spray before administering the metered dose.
2. Shake the inhaler well before using. Remove the cap from the mouthpiece.
3. Instruct the patient to breathe out through the mouth, expelling air. Place the mouthpiece into the patient's mouth, holding the inhaler upright (see Figure 4-2).
4. Instruct the patient to keep his or her lips securely around the mouthpiece and inhale. While the patient is inhaling, push the top of the medication canister once.
5. Instruct the patient to hold his or her breath for a few seconds. Remove the mouthpiece and take your finger off the canister. Tell the patient to exhale slowly.
6. If a second dose is required, wait 1 to 2 minutes, and repeat steps 3 to 5.
7. Cleanse the mouthpiece.

METHOD

Metered-Dose Inhaler With Spacer

This method is similar to MDI with the following additions; see Figure 4-3.
1. Start to inhale as soon as the canister is depressed.
2. Check that the valve opens and closes with each breath.
3. Wash spacer as directed by manufacturer.
NOTE: For steroid inhalers, rinsing and gargling is necessary to remove residual steroid medication, thus preventing a sore throat or fungal overgrowth and infection.

NASAL SPRAY AND DROPS

Purpose

Most drugs in nasal spray and drop containers are intended to relieve nasal congestion caused by upper respiratory tract infection and polyps by shrinking swollen nasal membranes. Types of drugs given by this method are vasoconstrictors and glucocorticoids.

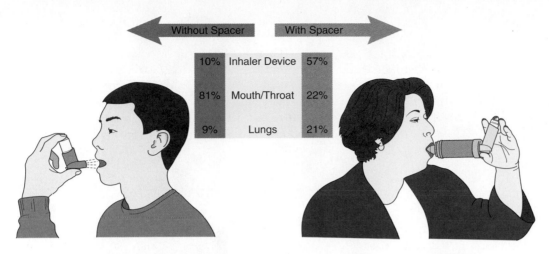

FIGURE 4-3 Distribution of medication with and without a spacer.

METHOD

Nasal Spray

1. Instruct the patient to sit with his or her head tilted slightly back or slightly forward, according to the directions on the spray container (Figure 4-4).
2. Insert the tip of the container into one nostril and occlude the other nostril.
3. Instruct the patient to inhale as you squeeze the drug spray container. Repeat with the same nostril if ordered.
4. Repeat the procedure with the other nostril if ordered.
5. Encourage the patient to keep his or her head tilted for several minutes until the drug action is effective. The nose should not be blown until the head is upright.
6. Drink fluid after spray if steroid is used to avoid overgrowth.

METHOD

Nose Drops

1. Place the patient in an upright position with his or her head tilted back.
2. Insert the dropper into the nostril without touching the nasal membranes.
3. Instill 2 drops of medications or the amount prescribed.
4. Instruct the patient to keep his or her head back for 5 minutes and to breathe through the mouth.
5. Cleanse the dropper.
6. For the medication to reach the sinuses, the patient should be in the supine position with head turned to one side and then the other, so the medication can reach the frontal and maxillary sinuses. For the medication to reach the ethmoidal and sphenoidal sinuses, the patient's head is lowered below his or her shoulders (Figure 4-5).

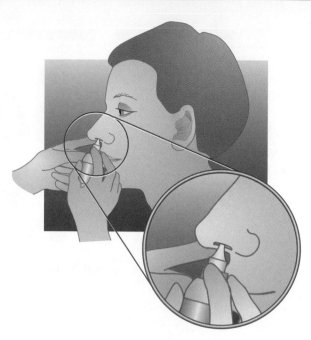

FIGURE 4-4 Administering nasal spray. (From Kee, J. L., Hayes, E. R., & McCuistion, L. E. [2006]. *Pharmacology: a nursing process approach.* 5th ed. Philadelphia: W. B. Saunders.)

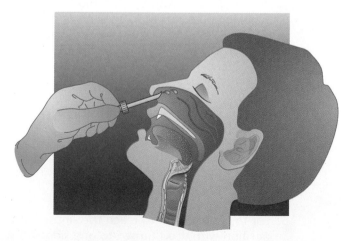

FIGURE 4-5 Administering nose drops. (From Kee, J. L., Hayes, E. R., & McCuistion, L. E. [2006]. *Pharmacology: a nursing process approach.* 5th ed. Philadelphia: W. B. Saunders.)

EYE DROPS AND OINTMENT

Purpose

Eye medications are prescribed for various eye disorders, such as glaucoma, infection, and allergies, and for eye examination and eye surgery.

METHOD

Eye Drops

1. Instruct the patient to lie or sit with his or her head tilted back.
2. Instruct the patient to look up toward the ceiling and away from the dropper. Pull down the lower lid of the affected eye (Figure 4-6). Place one drop of medication into the lower conjunctival sac. This prevents the drug from dropping onto the cornea.
3. Press gently on the medial nasolacrimal canthus (side closer to the nose) with a tissue to prevent systemic drug absorption.
4. If the other eye is affected, repeat the procedure in the other eye.
5. Inform the patient to blink one or two times and then to keep the eyes closed for several minutes. Use a tissue to blot away excess drug fluid.

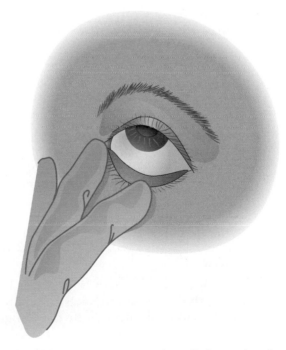

FIGURE 4-6 To administer eye drops, gently pull down the skin below the eye to expose the conjunctival sac. (From Kee, J. L., Hayes, E. R., & McCuistion, L. E. [2006]. *Pharmacology: a nursing process approach.* 5th ed. Philadelphia: W. B. Saunders.)

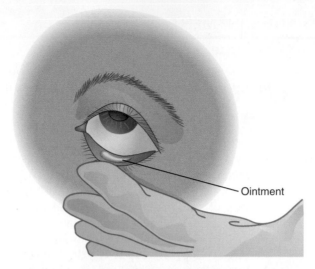

FIGURE 4-7 To administer eye ointment, squeeze a ¼-inch–wide strip of ointment onto the conjunctival sac. (From Kee, J. L., Hayes, E. R., & McCuistion, L. E. [2006]. *Pharmacology: a nursing process approach.* 5th ed. Philadelphia: W. B. Saunders.)

METHOD

Eye Ointment

1. Instruct the patient to lie or sit with his or her head tilted back.
2. Pull down the lower lid to expose the conjunctival sac of the affected eye (Figure 4-7).
3. Squeeze a strip of ointment about ¼-inch long (unless otherwise indicated) onto the conjunctival sac. Medication placed directly onto the cornea can cause discomfort or damage.
4. If the other eye is affected, repeat the procedure.
5. Instruct the patient to close his or her eyes for 2 to 3 minutes. The patient's vision may be blurred for a short time.

EAR DROPS

Purpose

Ear medication is frequently prescribed to soften and loosen the cerumen (wax) in the ear canal, for anesthetic effect, to immobilize insects in the ear canal, and to treat infection such as fungal infection.

METHOD

Ear Drops

1. Instruct the client to lie on the unaffected side or to sit upright with his or her head tilted toward the unaffected side.

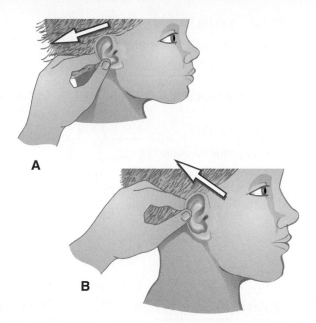

FIGURE 4-8 To administer ear drops, straighten the external ear canal by (A) pulling down and back on the auricle in children and (B) pulling up and back on the auricle in adults. (From Kee, J. L., Hayes, E. R., & McCuistion, L. E. [2006]. *Pharmacology: a nursing process approach.* 5th ed. Philadelphia: W. B. Saunders.)

2. Straighten the external ear canal (Figure 4-8), as follows:
   Adult: Pull the auricle of the ear up and back.
   Child: Pull the auricle of the ear down and back.
3. Instill the prescribed number of drops. Avoid contaminating the dropper.
4. Instruct the client to remain in this position for 2 to 5 minutes to prevent the medication from leaking out of the ear.

PHARYNGEAL SPRAY, MOUTHWASH, AND LOZENGE

Purpose

Sprays, mouthwashes, and lozenges can be prescribed to reduce throat irritation and for antiseptic and anesthetic effects. These methods are prescribed for a local effect on the throat and *not* for systemic use.

METHOD

Pharyngeal Spray

1. Instruct the patient to sit upright.
2. Place a tongue blade over the patient's tongue to prevent the tongue from becoming numb if an anesthetic is being administered.
3. Hold the spray pump nozzle outside the patient's mouth, and direct the spray to the back of the throat.

METHOD

Pharyngeal Mouthwash

1. Instruct the client to sit upright.
2. Instruct the client to swish the solution around the mouth, but *not* to swallow the solution, and then to spit it into an emesis basin or sink.

METHOD

Pharyngeal Lozenge

1. Instruct the patient to sit upright.
2. Instruct the patient to place the lozenge into his or her mouth and suck until it is fully dissolved. The lozenge should *not* be chewed or swallowed whole.

TOPICAL PREPARATIONS: LOTION, CREAM, AND OINTMENT

Purpose

Topical lotions, creams, and ointments are used to protect skin areas, prevent skin dryness, treat itching of skin areas, and relieve pain.

METHOD

Topical Lotion

1. Cleanse skin area with soap and water or other designated solution.
2. Shake the lotion container. Use clean gloves to apply the medicated lotion. Rub the lotion thoroughly into the skin unless otherwise indicated.

METHOD A

Topical Cream or Ointment

1. Cleanse the skin area.
2. Use clean or sterile glove(s) and a sterile tongue blade or gauze to apply the cream or ointment to the affected skin area. Use long, smooth strokes. A piece of sterile gauze can be placed over the medicated area after application to prevent soiling of clothing.

METHOD B

Topical Cream or Ointment

1. Cleanse the skin area. Apply gloves.
2. Squeeze a line of ointment from the tube onto your finger from the tip to the first skin crease; this is known as a fingertip unit (FTU) (Figure 4-9). One FTU weighs about 0.5 g.
3. Use the guidelines shown in Figure 4-10 to determine the number of FTUs to apply to various body areas.
4. Apply the medication to the affected area.

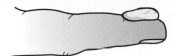

FIGURE 4-9 Fingertip unit: ointment squeezed from the tip of the finger to the first skin crease.

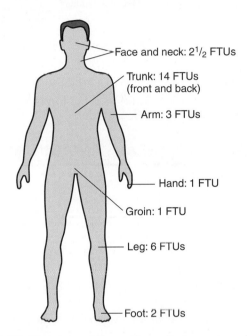

Face and neck: 2$\frac{1}{2}$ FTUs

Trunk: 14 FTUs
(front and back)

Arm: 3 FTUs

Hand: 1 FTU

Groin: 1 FTU

Leg: 6 FTUs

Foot: 2 FTUs

FIGURE 4-10 Number of fingertip units to various body areas.

RECTAL SUPPOSITORY

Purpose

Rectal medications are used to relieve vomiting when the client is unable to take oral medication, to relieve pain or anxiety, to promote defecation, and to administer drugs that could be destroyed by digestive enzymes.

METHOD

Rectal Suppository

1. Place the patient on his or her left side in the Sims' position (Figure 4-11).
2. Use gloves or a finger cot on the index finger.
3. Expose the anus by lifting the upper portion of the buttock.
4. Lightly lubricate the suppository with water-soluble lubricant, and insert the narrow (pointed) end of the suppository through the anal sphincter muscle.
5. Instruct the client to remain in a supine (side lying) position for 5 to 10 minutes.

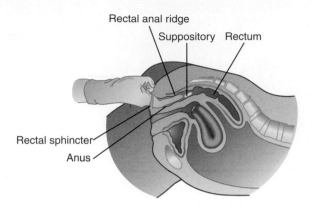

FIGURE 4-11 Inserting a rectal suppository. (From Kee, J. L., Hayes, E. R., & McCuistion, L. E. [2006]. *Pharmacology: a nursing process approach.* 5th ed. Philadelphia: W. B. Saunders.)

VAGINAL SUPPOSITORY, CREAM, AND OINTMENT

Purpose

Vaginal medications are used to treat vaginal infection or inflammation.

METHOD

Vaginal Suppository, Cream, and Ointment

1. Wear clean gloves.
2. Place the patient in the lithotomy position (knees bent with feet on the table or bed).
3. Place the vaginal suppository at the tip of the applicator.

or

   Connect the top of the vaginal cream or ointment tube with the tip of the applicator. Squeeze the tube to fill the applicator.
4. Lubricate the applicator with water-soluble lubricant if necessary.
5. Insert applicator downward first and then upward and backward (Figure 4-12).
6. The patient may use a light pad in the underwear to prevent soiling of clothing. Bedtime is the suggested time for vaginal drug administration.
7. Instruct the patient to avoid using tampons after insertion of the vaginal medication.

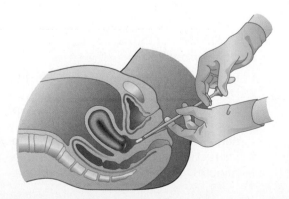

FIGURE 4-12 Inserting a vaginal suppository. (From Kee, J. L., Hayes, E. R., & McCuistion, L. E. [2006]. *Pharmacology: a nursing process approach.* 5th ed. Philadelphia: W. B. Saunders.)

Methods of Calculation

OBJECTIVES

- Determine the amount of drug needed for a specified time.
- Select a dosage formula, such as basic formula, ratio and proportion, fraction equation, or dimensional analysis, for solving drug dosage problems.
- Convert units of measurement to the same system and unit of measurement before calculating drug dosage.
- Calculate the dosage amount of tablets, capsules, and liquid volume (oral or parenteral) needed to administer the prescribed drug.

OUTLINE

Before drug dosage can be calculated, units of measurement must be converted to one system. If the drug is ordered in milligrams and comes in grains, then grains are converted to milligrams or milligrams are converted to grains.

Four methods for calculating drug dosages include basic formula, ratio and proportion, fractional equation, and dimensional analysis. The ratio and proportion and fractional equation methods are similar. For drugs that require individualized dosing, body weight and body surface area are used. When body weight and body surface area calculations are used, one of the first four methods for calculation is necessary to determine the amount of drug needed from the container.

At some institutions, the nurse orders enough medication doses for a designated period. If the order requires 2 tablets, qid (4 times a day) for 5 days, then the number of tablets needed would be 2 tablets × 4 times a day × 5 days = 40 tablets.

DRUG CALCULATION

The four methods as mentioned for drug calculations are (1) basic formula, (2) ratio and proportion, (3) fractional equation, and (4) dimensional analysis (factor labeling).

METHOD 1: BASIC FORMULA

The following formula is often used to calculate drug dosages. The basic formula (BF) is the most commonly used method, and it is easy to remember.

$$\frac{D}{H} \times V = \text{Amount to give}$$

D or desired dose: drug dose ordered by physician or health care providers (HCP).
H or on-hand dose: drug dose on label of container (bottle, vial, ampule)
V or vehicle: form and amount in which the drug comes (tablet, capsule, liquid)

EXAMPLES

PROBLEM 1: Order: erythromycin (ERY-TAB) 0.5 g, po, q8h.
Drug available:

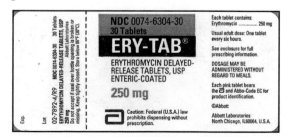

a. Both the dosage of the drug ordered and the dosage on the bottle are in the metric system; however, the units of measurement are different. Conversion is needed. To convert grams to milligrams, move the decimal point three spaces to the right (see Chapter 1, Metric System):

$$0.5 \text{ g} = 0.500 \text{ mg} = 500 \text{ mg}$$

b. BF: $\dfrac{D}{H} \times V = \dfrac{\overset{2}{\cancel{500}}}{\underset{1}{\cancel{250}}} \times 1 \text{ tab} = 2 \text{ tablets}$

Answer: erythromycin 0.5 g = 2 tablets

PROBLEM 2: Order: 0.5 g of ampicillin (Principen), po, bid.
Drug available:

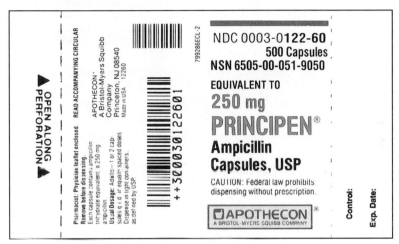

a. The unit of measurement that is ordered and the unit on the bottle are in the same system but in different units; therefore, conversion of units within the same system must be done first. To convert grams to milligrams, move the decimal point three spaces to the right (see Chapter 1, Metric System):

$$0.5 \text{ g} = 0.500 \text{ mg} = 500 \text{ mg}$$

b. BF: $\dfrac{D}{H} \times V = \dfrac{500}{250} \times 1 \text{ capsule} = \dfrac{\overset{2}{\cancel{500}}}{\underset{1}{\cancel{250}}} = 2 \text{ capsules}$

Answer: ampicillin (Principen) 0.5 g = 2 capsules

PROBLEM 3: Order: phenobarbital gr ii (2), STAT.
Drug available: phenobarbital 30 mg per tablet.
a. Before calculating drug dosage, convert to one unit of measurement. To convert grains to milligrams, *multiply* the number of grains by 60 (see Chapter 2, Grains and Milligrams):

$$2 \text{ gr} \times 60 = 120 \text{ mg}$$

b. BF: $\dfrac{D}{H} \times V = \dfrac{120}{30} \times 1 = \dfrac{120}{30} = 4 \text{ tablets}$

Answer: phenobarbital gr ii = 4 tablets

PROBLEM 4: Order: meperidine (Demerol) 35 mg, IM, STAT.
Drug available:

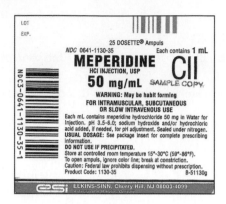

a. Conversion is not needed, because both are of the same unit of measurement.

b. BF: $\dfrac{D}{H} \times V = \dfrac{35}{50} \times 1 \text{ ml} = \dfrac{35}{50} = 0.7 \text{ ml}$

Answer: meperidine (Demerol) 35 mg = 0.7 ml

METHOD 2: RATIO AND PROPORTION

Ratio and proportion (RP) is the oldest method used for calculating dosage problems:

$$
\begin{array}{ccc}
\textit{Known} & & \textit{Desired} \\
H \quad : \quad V & :: & D \quad : \quad X \\
\text{on hand vehicle} & & \text{desired dose amount to give}
\end{array}
$$
means
extremes

H and **V**: On the left side of the equation are the known quantities, which are dose on hand and vehicle.
D and **X**: On the right side of the equation are the desired dose and the unknown amount to give.
Multiply the means and the extremes. Solve for **X**.

EXAMPLES

PROBLEM 1: Order: erythromycin (ERY-TAB) 0.5 g, po, q8h.
Drug available:

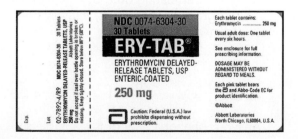

a. To convert grams to milligrams, move the decimal point three spaces to the right (see Chapter 1, Metric System):

$$0.5 \text{ g} = 0.\underset{\smile}{500} \text{ mg} = 500 \text{ mg}$$

b. RP: H : V :: D : X
250 mg:1 tab::500 mg:X tab

250 X = 500
X = 2 tablets

Answer: erythromycin 0.5 g = 2 tablets

Note: With ratio and proportion, the ratio on the left (milligrams to tablets) has the same relation as the ratio on the right (milligrams to tablets); the only difference is values.

PROBLEM 2: Order: aspirin (ASA) gr X, PRN.
 Drug available: aspirin 325 mg per tablet.

a. To convert to one system and unit of measurement. Convert grains to milligrams, *multiply* the number of grains by 60 (65) (see Chapter 2, Grains and Milligrams).

$$10 \text{ gr} \times 60 \text{ (65)} = 600 \text{ or } 650 \text{ mg}$$

or

gr: mg   :: gr:mg
1 :60 (65):: 10: X
X = 600 or 650 mg

b. RP: H : V ::   D   :   X
325 mg:1 tablet:: 600 (650) mg:X tablet
325 X = 600 (650)
X = 1.8 tablets or 2 tablets
(round off or use 650 instead of 600)

Answer: aspirin gr x = 2 tablets

PROBLEM 3: Order: amoxicillin 75 mg, po, qid.
 Drug available:

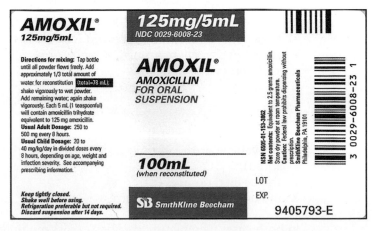

a. Conversion is not needed because both use the same unit of measurement.

b. RP: H   : V ::   D   : X

     125 mg : 5 ml :: 75 mg : X ml

          125 X = 375

              X = 3 ml

Answer: amoxicillin 75 mg = 3 ml

PROBLEM 4: Order: meperidine (Demerol) 60 mg, IM, STAT.
                Drug available:

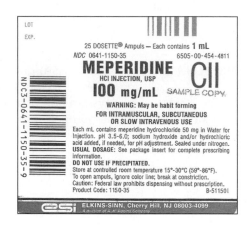

a. Conversion is not needed: the same unit of measurement is used.

b. RP: H   : V ::   D   : X

     100 mg : 1 ml :: 60 mg : X ml

         100 X = 60

           X = 0.6 ml

Answer: meperidine (Demerol) 60 mg = 0.6 ml

METHOD 3: FRACTIONAL EQUATION

The fractional equation (FE) method *is similar* to ratio and proportion, except it is written as a fraction. Instead of the = sign, an X may be used to remind students to cross multiply.

$$\frac{H}{V} = \frac{D}{X} \text{ or } \frac{H}{V} \times \frac{D}{X} =$$

H: the dosage on hand or in the container
V: the vehicle or the form in which the drug comes (tablet, capsule, liquid)
D: the desired dosage
X: the unknown amount to give

In both cases whether using = or X, cross multiply and solve for X.

EXAMPLES

PROBLEM 1: Order: kanamycin sulfate (Kantrex) 1 g, po, q6h × 3days.
Drug available:

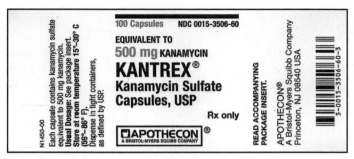

a. Convert grams to milligrams. Move the decimal point three spaces to the right.

$$1.0 \text{ g} = 1.\underset{\curvearrowright}{000} \text{ mg} = 1000 \text{ mg}$$

b. FE: $\dfrac{H}{V} = \dfrac{D}{X}$ $\qquad \dfrac{500 \text{ mg}}{1 \text{ capsule}} = \dfrac{1000}{X}$

(Cross multiply) $\qquad 500 \text{ X} = 1000$

$$X = 2$$

Answer: kanamycin 1 g = 2 capsules

PROBLEM 2: Order: valproic acid (Depakene) 100 mg, po, tid.
Drug available: valproic acid (Depakene) 250 mg/5 ml suspension.

a. No unit conversion is needed.

b. FE: $\dfrac{H}{V} = \dfrac{D}{X}$ $\qquad \dfrac{250}{5} = \dfrac{100}{X}$

(Cross multiply) $\qquad 250 \text{ X} = 500$

$$X = 2 \text{ ml}$$

Answer: valproic acid (Depakene) 100 mg = 2 ml

PROBLEM 3: Order: atropine gr ¹⁄₁₀₀, IM, STAT.
Drug available:

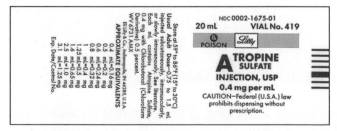

a. Two systems are involved: apothecary (grains) and metric (milligrams). Because the drug preparation is in milligrams, convert grains to milligrams (see Table 2-1 or Table 5-1; 0.6 mg = gr ¹⁄₁₀₀).

| TABLE 5-1 | | |

Metric and Apothecary Conversions*

	Metric	Apothecary
Grams (g)	Milligrams (mg)	Grains (gr)
1	1000	15
0.5	500	$7\frac{1}{2}$
0.3	300 (325)	5
0.1	100	$1\frac{1}{2}$
0.06	60 (64 or 65)	1
0.03	30 (32)	$\frac{1}{2}$
0.015	15 (16)	$\frac{1}{4}$
0.010	10	$\frac{1}{6}$
0.0006	0.6	$\frac{1}{100}$
0.0004	0.4	$\frac{1}{150}$
0.0003	0.3	$\frac{1}{200}$

Liquid (Approximate)

30 ml = 1 oz = 2 tbsp (T) = 6 tsp (t)
15 ml = $\frac{1}{2}$ oz = 1 T = 3 t
1000 ml = 1 quart (qt) = 1 liter (L)
500 ml = 1 pint (pt)
5 ml = 1 tsp (t)
4 ml = 1 fl dr
1 ml = 15 minims = 15 drops (gtt) (gtts)

*Metric and apothecary equivalents frequently used in drug dosage conversions.

Also, you could use the RP method:

$$gr:mg :: gr : mg$$
$$1:60 :: \frac{1}{100} : X$$
$$X = \frac{60}{100}$$
$$X = 0.6 \text{ mg}$$

b. FE: $\dfrac{H}{V} = \dfrac{D}{X}$ $\dfrac{0.4}{1} = \dfrac{0.6}{X}$

(Cross multiply) 0.4 X = 0.6
                            X = 1.5 ml

Answer: atropine gr $\frac{1}{100}$ = 1.5 ml

METHOD 4: DIMENSIONAL ANALYSIS

Dimensional Analysis (DA) is a calculation method known as units and conversions. The advantage of DA is that it decreases the number of steps required to calculate a drug dosage. It is set up as one equation.

1. Identify the unit/form (tablet, capsule, ml) of the drug to be calculated. If the drug comes in tablet, then tablet = (equal sign)

2. The known dose and unit/form from the **drug label** follow the equal sign, Example Order: Amoxicillin 500 mg. On the drug label: 250 mg per 1 capsule.

$$\text{capsule} = \frac{1 \text{ cap}}{250 \text{ mg}}$$
$$\text{(drug label)}$$

3. The milligram value (250 mg) is the **denominator** and it must match the NEXT **numerator,** which is 500 mg (desired dose or order). The NEXT denominator would be 1 (one) or blank.

$$\text{capsule} = \frac{1 \text{ cap} \times \cancel{500} \cancel{\text{mg}}^{\,2}}{\cancel{250} \cancel{\text{mg}}_{\,1} \times 1} =$$

4. Cancel out the mg, 250 and 500. What remains is the capsule and 2. Answer: 2 capsules.

When conversion is needed between milligrams (drug label) and grams (order), then a conversion factor is needed, which appears **between** the drug dose on hand (drug label) and the desired dose (order). You should REMEMBER the following:

Metric Equivalent   **Metric-Apothecary Equivalent**
1 g = 1000 mg   1 g = 15 gr
1 mg = 1000 mcg   1000 mg = 15 gr
                                        1 gr = 60 mg

EXAMPLE

Order: Amoxicillin 0.5 g.

Available: 250 mg − 1 capsule (drug label). A conversion is needed between grams and milligrams. Remember, 250 mg is the denominator; therefore, 1000 mg (conversion factor, which is 1000 mg = 1 g) is the NEXT numerator and 1 g becomes the NEXT denominator. The third numerator is 0.5 g (desired dose), and the denominator is 1 (one) or blank.

$$\text{capsule} = \frac{1 \text{ cap} \times \cancel{1000} \cancel{\text{mg}}^{\,4} \times 0.5 \cancel{\text{g}}}{\cancel{250} \cancel{\text{mg}}_{\,1} \times 1 \cancel{\text{g}} \times 1 \text{ (or blank)}} = 2 \text{ capsules}$$
$$\text{(drug label)} \quad \text{(conversion)} \quad \text{(drug order)}$$

If conversion from grams to milligrams is not needed, then the middle step can be omitted. The following are formulas for dimensional analysis (DA):

$$\text{V (form of drug)} = \frac{\text{V (drug form)} \times \text{D (desired dose)}}{\text{H (on hand) (drug label)} \times 1 \text{ or blank (drug order)}} =$$

For conversion: V (form of drug) =

$$\frac{\text{V (drug form)} \times \text{C (H)} \times \text{D (desired dose)}}{\text{H (on hand)} \times \text{C (D)} \times 1 \text{ (or blank)}}$$
$$\text{(drug label)} \quad \text{(conversion} \quad \text{(drug order)}$$
$$\text{factor)}$$

As with other methods for calculation, the three components are **D, H,** and **V.** With dimensional analysis, the conversion factor is built into the equation and is included when the units of measurements of the drug order and the drug container differ. If the two are of the same units of measurement, the conversion factor is eliminated from the equation.

EXAMPLES

PROBLEM 1: Order: kanamycin (Kantrex) 1 g, po, q6h × 3 days.
                     Drug available:

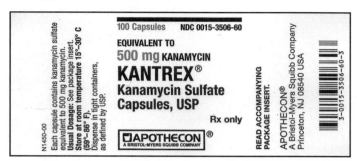

Drug label: 500 mg = 1 capsule
1 g (from drug order)
Conversion factor: 1 g = 1000 mg

$$\text{DA: cap} = \frac{1 \text{ cap}}{500 \text{ mg}} \times \frac{\overset{2}{1000 \text{ mg}}}{1 \text{ g}} \times \frac{1 \text{ g}}{1}$$

               (drug label)   × (conversion factor) × (drug order)
               (cancel units and numbers from numerator and denominator)

$$1 \text{ cap} \times 2 = 2 \text{ caps}$$

Answer: kanamycin 1 g = 2 capsules

PROBLEM 2: Order: acetaminophen (Tylenol) gr XV, po, PRN.
                     Drug available:

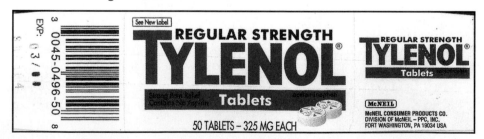

Drug label: 325 mg = 1 tablet
15 gr (from drug order)
Conversion factor: 1000 mg = 15 gr
How many tablet(s) would you give?

$$\text{DA: tab} = \frac{1 \text{ tab} \times 1000 \cancel{mg} \times \cancel{15} \cancel{gr}}{325 \cancel{mg} \times \cancel{15} \cancel{gr} \times 1} = \frac{1000}{325} = 3.07 \text{ tab or 3 tab (cannot round off in tenths for tablets)}$$

Answer: acetaminophen gr XV = 3 tablets

Tylenol is also available in 500-mg tablets (extra strength tablets).

PROBLEM 3: Order: ciprofloxacin (Cipro) 500 mg, po, q12h.
Drug available:

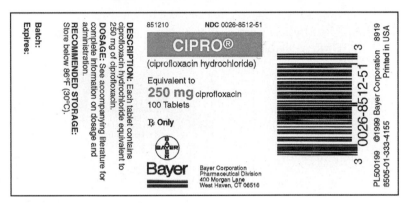

No conversion factor is needed because both are stated in milligrams (mg).

$$\text{DA: tab} = \frac{1 \text{ tab} \times \overset{2}{\cancel{500}} \cancel{mg}}{\underset{1}{\cancel{250}} \cancel{mg} \times 1} = 2 \text{ tablets}$$

Answer: Cipro 500 mg = 2 tablets

SUMMARY PRACTICE PROBLEMS

Solve the following calculation problems using Method 1, 2, 3, or 4. To convert units within the metric system (grams to milligrams), refer to Chapter 1. To convert apothecary to metric units and vice versa, refer to Chapter 2 or Table 5-1. For reading drug labels, refer to Chapter 3. Several of the calculation problems have drug labels. Drug dosage and drug form are printed on the drug label.

Extra practice problems are available in the chapters on oral drugs, injectable drugs, and pediatric drug administration.

1. Order: doxycycline hyclate (Vibra-Tab), po, initially 200 mg; then 50 mg, po, bid.
   Drug available: **Use one of the four methods to calculate dosage.**

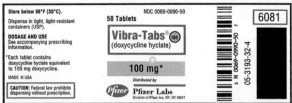

   a. How many tablet(s) would you give as the initial dose? _____

   b. How many tablets would you give for *each* dose after the initial

      dose? _____

2. Order: sulfisoxazole (Gantrisin) 1 g.
   Drug available: sulfisoxazole (Gantrisin) 250 mg per tablet.
   a. How many tablet(s) would you give? _____

3. The physician ordered erythromycin 500 mg, po, q8h, for 7 days.
   Drug available:

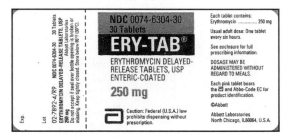

   a. How many tablets would you order for 7 days? _____

   b. How many tablets would you give every 8 hours? _____

4. Order: clarithromycin (Biaxin) 100 mg, po, q6h.
   Drug available:

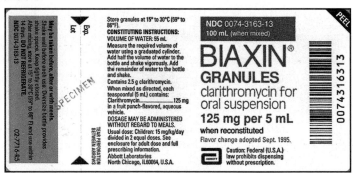

a. How many milliliters should the patient receive per dose? _____

5. Order: phenytoin (Dilantin) 50 mg, po, bid.
Drug available:

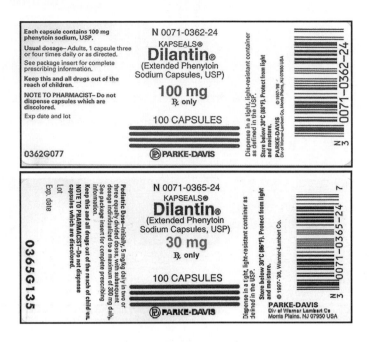

a. Which Dilantin container would you select? _____

b. How many Dilantin capsules would you give per dose? _____

6. Order: methyldopa (Aldomet) 150 mg, po, tid.
Drug available:

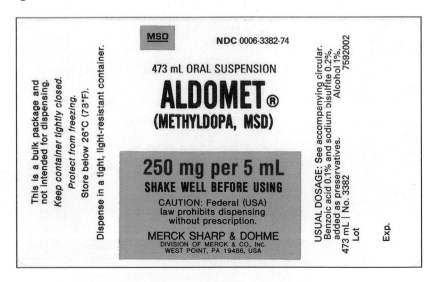

How many milliliters would you give per dose? _____

7. Order: dexamethasone (Decadron) 0.5 mg, po, qid.
Drug available:

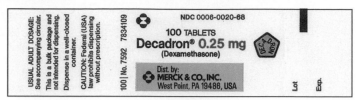

a. How many tablets would you give per dose? _____

b. How many milligrams would the patient receive per day? _____

8. Order: diltiazem (Cardizem) SR 120 mg, po, bid for hypertension.
Drugs available:

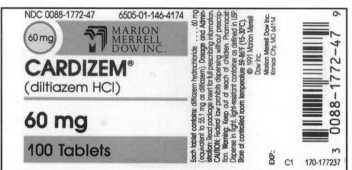

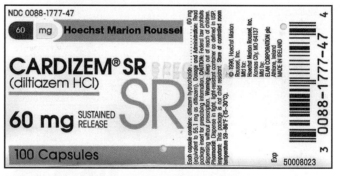

a. Which drug bottle should be selected?

b. How many tablet(s) should the patient receive per dose? _____

9. Order: cimetidine (Tagamet) 0.2 g, po, qid.
   Drug available:

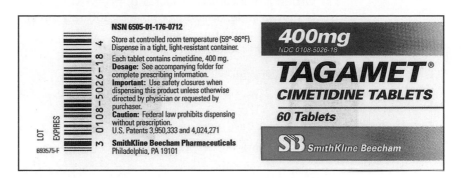

How many tablet(s) would you give per dose? _____

10. Order: codeine gr 1, po, STAT.
    Drug available:

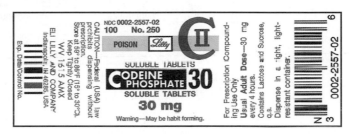

How many tablet(s) should the patient receive? _____

11. Order: methylprednisolone (Medrol) 75 mg, IM.
    Drug available: Medrol 125 mg per 2 ml per ampule.

How many milliliters would you give? _____

12. Order: atropine sulfate 0.3 mg, IM, STAT.
    Available:

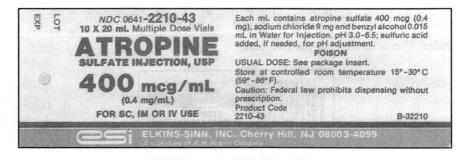

   a. How many milliliters should the patient receive?
   b. What type of syringe would you use to administer the atropine sulfate?

Additional Dimensional Analysis (Factor Labeling)

13. Order: aminocaproic acid 1.5 g, po, STAT.
    Drug available: aminocaproic acid 500 mg tablet.
    Drug label: 500 mg = tablet
    Conversion factor: 1 g = 1000 mg

    How many tablet(s) would you give? _____

14. Order: ampicillin (Principen) 50 mg/kg/day, po, in 4 divided doses (q6h).
    Patient weighs 88 pounds, or 40 kg (88 ÷ 2.2 = 40 kg).
    Drug available:

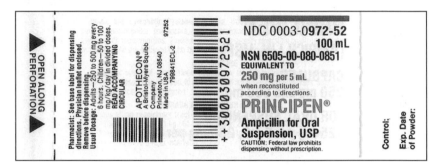

    Drug label: 250 mg = 5 ml
    Conversion factor: none (both are in milligrams)

    a. How many milligrams per day should the patient receive? _____

    b. How many milligrams per dose should the patient receive? _____

    c. How many milliliters should the patient receive per dose (q6h)?

    _____

15. Order: cimetidine (Tagamet) 0.8 g, po, bedtime.
    Drug available:

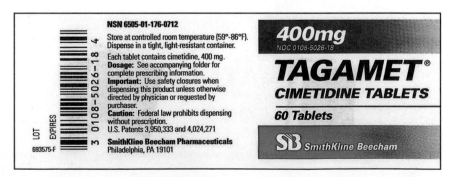

    Drug label: 400 mg = 1 tablet
           0.8 g (drug order)
    Conversion factor: 1 g = 1000 mg (units of measurements are not the same; conversion factor is needed)

    How many tablet(s) would you give? _____

16. Order: codeine gr i (1), po, STAT.
Drug available:

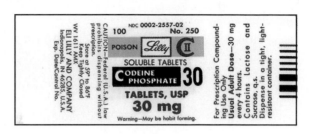

Drug label: 30 mg = 1 tablet
gr 1/1 (drug order)
Conversion factor: 1 gr = 60 mg

How many tablet(s) would you give? _____

17. Order: amikacin (Amikin) 250 mg, IM, q6h.
Drug available:

Drug label: 1 g = 4 ml
250 mg/1 (drug order)
Conversion factor: 1 g = 1000 mg

How many milliliters would you give? _____

ANSWERS Summary Practice Problems

1. **a.** *Initially:*

BF: $\dfrac{D}{H} \times V = \dfrac{200}{100} \times 1 =$

2 tablets

or
FE: $\dfrac{100}{1} \times \dfrac{200}{X} =$

$100X = 200$

$X = 2$ tablets

or
RP: H :V ::   D   :X
     100 mg:1 :: 200 mg:X

$100 X = 200$

$X = 2$ tablets

or
DA: No conversion factor

$$\text{Tablet(s)} = \frac{1 \text{ tab} \times \overset{2}{\cancel{200 \text{ mg}}}}{\underset{1}{\cancel{100 \text{ mg}}} \times 1} = 2 \text{ tablets}$$

b. *Daily:*

BF: $\dfrac{D}{H} \times V = \dfrac{50}{100} \times 1 =$

$\frac{1}{2}$ tablet

or
FE: $\dfrac{100}{1} \times \dfrac{50}{X} =$

(Cross multiply) $100X = 50$

$X = \frac{1}{2}$ tablet

or RP: H :V :: D :X
100 mg:1 :: 50 mg:X

$100\,X = 50$

$X = \frac{1}{2}$ tablet

or DA: No conversion factor

Tablet(s) $= \dfrac{1 \text{ tab} \times \overset{1}{\cancel{50} \text{ mg}}}{\underset{2}{\cancel{100} \text{ mg}} \times \quad 1} = \frac{1}{2}$ tablets

2. 4 tablets
3. **a.** 2 tablets $\times$ 3 doses per day $\times$ 7 days = 42 tablets
   b. 2 tablets every 8 hours

4. BF: $\dfrac{D}{H} \times V = \dfrac{100}{\underset{25}{\cancel{125}}} \times \overset{1}{\cancel{5}} = \dfrac{100}{25} = 4$ ml

   or RP: H : V :: D : X
   125 : 5 :: 100 : X
   125 X = 500
   $X = \dfrac{500}{125} = 4$ ml

   or
   DA: ml $= \dfrac{5 \text{ ml} \times \overset{4}{\cancel{100} \text{ mg}}}{\underset{5}{\cancel{125} \text{ mg}} \times \quad 1} = \dfrac{20}{5} = 4$ ml

   or
   FE: $\dfrac{125}{\cancel{5}} \times \dfrac{100}{X} =$
   (Cross multiply) $125X = 500$
   $X = 4$ ml

5. **a.** The nurse could *not* use either of the Dilantins.
   b. A capsule *cannot* be cut in half. The physician should be notified. Dilantin dose should be changed.

6. BF: $\dfrac{D}{H} \times V = \dfrac{150}{\underset{50}{\cancel{250}}} \times \overset{1}{\cancel{5}}$

   $\dfrac{150}{50} = 3$ ml

   or RP: H :V :: D :X
   250 : 5 :: 150 : X
   250 X = 750
   X = 3 ml

7. **a.** BF: $\dfrac{D}{H} \times V = \dfrac{0.5}{0.25} \times 1$

   $0.25 \overline{)0.50}^{\,2.} = 2$ tablets

   b. 2 mg

   or RP: H : V :: D : X
   0.25 : 1 tablet :: 0.5 : X tablets
   0.25 X = 0.5
   X = 2 tablets

8. **a.** Cardizem SR 60 mg
   b. 2 SR capsules per dose

9. Change grams to milligrams by moving the decimal three spaces to the right (see Chapter 1, Metric System).

0.2 g = 0.200 mg (200 mg)

BF: $\dfrac{D}{H} \times V = \dfrac{200}{400} \times 1$ tablet

$= \dfrac{200}{400} = \frac{1}{2}$ tablet

or RP: H : V :: D : X

400 mg : 1 tablet :: 200 mg : X tablet

400 X = 200

X $= \dfrac{200}{400} = 0.5$ or $\frac{1}{2}$ tablet

or DA: With conversion factor

Tablets $= \dfrac{1 \text{ tab } \times \overset{10}{\cancel{1000}} \text{ mg} \times 0.2 \cancel{g}}{\underset{4}{\cancel{400}} \text{ mg} \times \quad 1 \cancel{g} \quad \times \quad 1} = \dfrac{2.0}{4} = \frac{1}{2}$ tablet

10. Change grains to milligrams (see Chapter 2 or Table 5-1): 1 gr = 60 mg.

BF: $\dfrac{D}{H} \times V = \dfrac{60}{30} \times 1$

$= \dfrac{60}{30} = 2$ tablets

or RP: H : V :: D : X

30 mg : 1 tablet :: 60 mg : X tablet

30 X = 60

X = 2 tablets

11. BF: $\dfrac{D}{H} \times V = \dfrac{75}{125} \times 2$

$= \dfrac{150}{125} = 1.2$ ml

or RP: H : V :: D : X

125 : 2 :: 75 : X

125 X = 150

X = 1.2 ml

or FE: $\dfrac{125}{2} = \dfrac{75}{X}$ or $\dfrac{125}{2} \times \dfrac{75}{X}$

125 X = 150

X = 1.2 ml

or DA: No conversion factor needed

ml $= \dfrac{2 \text{ ml } \times \overset{3}{\cancel{75}} \text{ mg}}{\underset{5}{\cancel{125}} \text{ mg} \times \quad 1} = \dfrac{6}{5} = 1.2$ ml

12. a. BF: $\dfrac{D}{H} \times V = \dfrac{0.3 \text{ mg}}{0.4 \text{ mg}} \times 1$ ml =

0.75 ml

or FE: $\dfrac{0.4 \text{ mg}}{1} = \dfrac{0.3 \text{ mg}}{X} =$

0.4 mg X = 0.3 mg

X = 0.75 ml

or RP: H : V :: D : X

0.4 mg : 1 ml :: 0.3 mg : X

0.4 mg X = 0.3 mg

X = 0.75 ml

or DA: ml $= \dfrac{1 \text{ ml } \times 0.3 \cancel{\text{ mg}}}{0.4 \cancel{\text{ mg}} \times \quad 1} = \dfrac{0.3}{0.4} = 0.75$ ml

b. Tuberculin syringe or 3-ml syringe: between 0.7 ml and 0.8 ml (in tenths)

Additional Dimensional Analysis (Factor Labeling)

13. Tablets $= \dfrac{1 \text{ tablet} \times \overset{2}{\cancel{1000}} \cancel{mg} \times 1.5 \cancel{g}}{\underset{1}{\cancel{500}} \cancel{mg} \times 1 \cancel{g} \times 1} = \dfrac{3.0}{1} = 3 \text{ tablets}$

14. a. 50 mg/kg/day

$50 \times 40 = 2000 \text{ mg}$

b. 2000 mg ÷ 4 = 500 mg per dose.

c. ml $= \dfrac{5 \text{ ml} \times \overset{2}{\cancel{500}} \cancel{mg}}{\underset{1}{\cancel{250}} \cancel{mg} \times 1} = \dfrac{10}{1} = 10 \text{ ml}$

15. Tablets $= \dfrac{1 \text{ tablet} \times \overset{10}{\cancel{1000}} \cancel{mg} \times 0.8 \cancel{g}}{\underset{4}{\cancel{400}} \cancel{mg} \times 1 \cancel{g} \times 1} = \dfrac{10 \times 0.8}{4} = \dfrac{8}{4} = 2 \text{ tablets}$

16. Tablets $= \dfrac{1 \text{ tablet} \times \overset{2}{\cancel{60}} \cancel{mg} \times 1 \cancel{gr}}{\underset{1}{\cancel{30}} \cancel{mg} \times 1 \cancel{gr} \times 1} = 2 \text{ tablets}$

17. milliliters $= \dfrac{4 \text{ ml} \times 1 \cancel{g} \times \overset{1}{\cancel{250}} \cancel{mg}}{1 \cancel{g} \times \underset{4}{\cancel{1000}} \cancel{mg} \times 1} = \dfrac{4}{4} = 1 \text{ ml}$

 Additional practice problems are available on the enclosed CD-ROM in the "Methods of Calculating Dosages" section.

Methods of Calculation for Individualized Drug Dosing

OBJECTIVES

- State the differences between the weight formulas used for drug calculations.
- Calculate drug dosages according to body surface area.
- Calculate drug dosages according to body weight.
- List indications for use of ideal body weight, adjusted body weight, and lean body weight formulas.

OUTLINE

CALCULATION FOR INDIVIDUALIZED DRUG DOSING
Body Weight (BW)
Body Surface Area (BSA or m²)
Ideal Body Weight (IBW)
Adjusted Body Weight (ABW)
Lean Body Weight (LBW)

CALCULATION FOR INDIVIDUALIZED DRUG DOSING

The two methods for individualizing drug dosing are body weight (BW) and body surface area (BSA). Other formulas that are associated with drug dosing, especially in bariatrics, are ideal body weight (IBW) and lean body weight (LBW).

Body Weight (BW)

Drug dosing by actual body weight is the primary way medication is individualized for adults and children. Manufacturers supply dosing information in the package insert. The insert data provide the dosage based on the patient's weight in kilograms (kg). The first step is to convert pounds to kilograms (if necessary). The second step is to determine the drug dose per body weight by multiplying drug dose × body weight (BW) × frequency (day or per day in divided doses). The third step is to choose one of the four methods of drug calculation for the amount of drug to be given.

EXAMPLES

PROBLEM 1: Order: fluorouracil (5-FU), 12 mg/kg/day IV, not to exceed 800 mg/day. The adult weighs 140 pounds.

a. Convert pounds to kilograms. Divide number of pounds by 2.2.
   Remember: 1 kg = 2.2 lb

$$140 \div 2.2 = 64 \text{ kg}$$

b. Dosage/BW: mg × kg × 1 day =
   12 × 64 × 1   = 768 mg IV per day

Answer: fluorouracil (5-FU), 12 mg/kg/day = 768 mg or 750 to 800 mg

PROBLEM 2: Give cefaclor (Ceclor), 20 mg/kg/day in three divided doses. The child weighs 20 pounds.
Drug available:

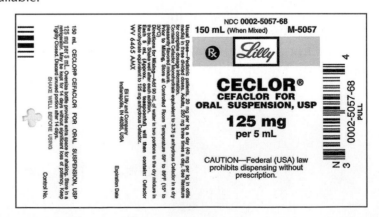

a. Convert pounds to kilograms

$$20 \div 2.2 = 9 \text{ kg}$$

b. Dosage/BW: 20 mg × 9 kg × 1 day = 180 mg per day.

180 mg ÷ 3 divided doses = 60 mg

BF: $\dfrac{D}{H} \times V = \dfrac{60}{125} \times 5 =$

$\dfrac{300}{125} = 2.4$ ml

or

RP: H : V :: D : X
125 : 5 :: 60 : X
125 X = 300
X = 2.4 ml

or
FE: $\dfrac{125}{5} = \dfrac{60}{X}$
125 X = 300
X = 2.4 ml

or
DA: ml = $\dfrac{\overset{1}{\cancel{5}} \text{ ml} \times \overset{12}{\cancel{60}} \text{ mg}}{\underset{\underset{5}{25}}{\cancel{125}} \text{ mg} \times 1} = \dfrac{12}{5} = 2.4$ ml

Answer: cefacelor (Ceclor) 20 mg/kg/day = 2.4 ml per dose three times per day

Body Surface Area (BSA or m²)

Body surface area is an estimated mathematical function of height and weight. BSA is considered to be the most accurate way to calculate drug dosages in that the correct dosage is more proportional to the surface area. BSA is commonly used in chemotherapy and some drug dosages are used for infants and children.

REMEMBER

Rounding Off Rule: Since calculators are used for working problems, round off at the final answer and not the steps in between. For BSA problems, round off answers to the nearest hundredth.

BSA With the Square Root

BSA can be calculated by using the square root and a fractional formula of height and weight divided by a constant, one for the metric system and another for inches and pounds. Now that calculators are readily available, research has shown that this method results in fewer errors than drawing intersecting lines on a nomogram. Conversion of weight and height to the same system of measure is necessary first.

BSA: Inch and Pound (lb) Formula

$$BSA = \sqrt{\dfrac{ht(in) \times wt(lb)}{3131}}$$

BSA: Metric Formula by Centimeters (cm) and Kilograms (kg)

$$BSA = \sqrt{\dfrac{ht(cm) \times wt(kg)}{3600}}$$

Do Not Have to Memorize this Formula

EXAMPLES

PROBLEM 1: Order: melphalon (Alkeran) 16 mg/m² q 2 weeks. Patient is 68 inches tall and weighs 172 pounds. Use the BSA inches and pounds formula.

a. BSA = $\sqrt{\dfrac{68 \text{ in} \times 172 \text{ lb}}{3131}}$

$$BSA = \sqrt{\frac{11696}{3131}}$$

BSA $= \sqrt{3.73}$
BSA $= 1.9$ m²

b. 16 mg $\times$ 1.9 m² = 30.4 mg/m² or 30 mg/m²

PROBLEM 2: Order: cisplatin (Platinol) 50 mg/m²/cycle IV. Patient weighs 84.5 kg and is 168 cm tall. Use the BSA metric formula.

a. $BSA = \sqrt{\dfrac{168 \text{ cm} \times 84.5 \text{ kg}}{3600}}$

$BSA = \sqrt{\dfrac{14196}{3600}}$

BSA $= \sqrt{3.94}$
BSA $= 1.99$ m²

b. 50 mg $\times$ 1.99 m² = 99 mg/m², or 100 mg/m²

BSA With a Nomogram

The BSA in square meters (m²) is determined by the person's height and weight and where these points intersect on the nomogram scale (Figures 6-1 and 6-2). The nomogram charts were developed from the square root formulas and were correlated with heights and weights to simplify drug dosing before calculators were readily available. When a nomogram is used, points on the scale must be carefully plotted. An error in plotting points or drawing intersecting lines can lead to reading of the incorrect BSA, resulting in dosing errors.

To calculate the dosage by BSA obtained with homogram, multiply the drug dose $\times$ m², e.g., 100 mg $\times$ 1.6 m² = 160 mg/m². The advantage of using the nomogram is that no conversions from pounds to kilograms or inches to centimeters are needed.

EXAMPLES

PROBLEM 1: Order: cyclophosphamide (Cytoxan) 100 mg/m²/day, po. Patient weighs 150 pounds and is 5'8" (68 inches) tall.
a. 68 inches and 150 pounds intersect the nomogram scale at 1.88 m² (BSA).
b. BSA: 100 mg $\times$ 1.9 m² = 190 mg/m²/day of Cytoxan.

$$1.88 \text{ m}^2 = 188 \text{ mg/m}^2/\text{day or } 190 \text{ mg/m}^2/\text{day}$$

PROBLEM 2: Order: cytarabine (cytosine arabinoside) 200 mg/m²/day IV $\times$ 5 days for a patient with myelocytic leukemia. The patient is 64 inches tall and weighs 130 pounds.
a. 64 inches and 130 pounds intersect the nomogram scale at 1.69 m² (BSA), or 1.7 m² (BSA) rounded off to the nearest tenth.
b. BSA: 200 mg $\times$ 1.69 m² = 340 mg/m² IV daily for 5 days.

$$1.69 \text{ m}^2 = 338 \text{ mg/m}^2 \text{ or } 340 \text{ mg/m}^2$$

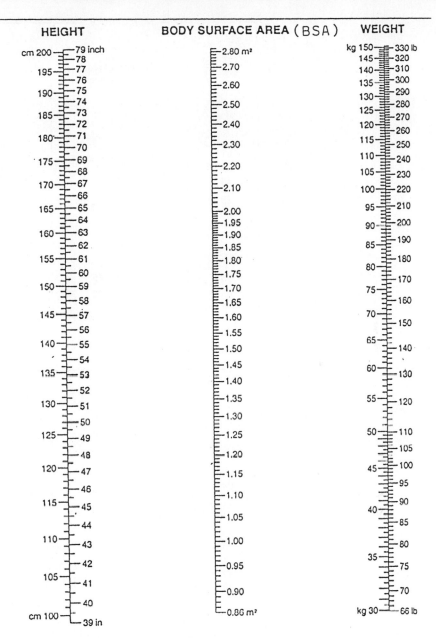

FIGURE 6-1 Body surface area (BSA) nomogram for adults. Directions: (1) find height, (2) find weight, (3) draw a straight line connecting the height and weight. Where the line intersects on the BSA column is the body surface area (m²). (From Deglin, H., Vallerand, A. H., & Russin, M. M. [1991]. *Davis' drug guide for nurses,* 2nd ed. Philadelphia: F. A. Davis, p. 1218. Used with permission from Lentner, C. [1991]. *Geigy scientific tables,* 8th ed., vol. 1, Basel, Switzerland: Ciba-Geigy, pp. 226-227.)

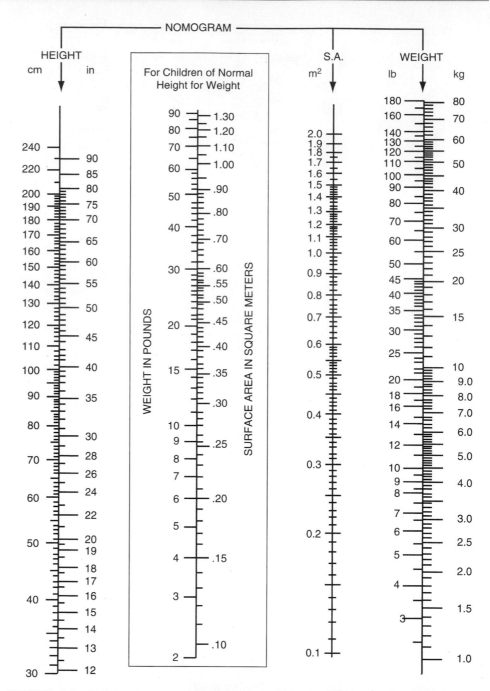

FIGURE 6-2 West nomogram for infants and children. Directions: (1) find height, (2) find weight, (3) draw a straight line connecting the height and weight. Where the line intersects on the SA column is the body surface area (m²). (From Behrman, R. E., Kliegman, R. M., & Jenson, H. B., editors. [2004]. *Nelson textbook of pediatrics,* 17th ed. Philadelphia: W. B. Saunders.)

Ideal Body Weight (IBW)

Drug dosing by ideal body weight (IBW) or lean body weight/mass (LBW)/(LBM) formulas is used for medications that are poorly absorbed and distributed throughout the body fat. The ideal body weight formula is based on height and can be adjusted for weight. The lean body weight/mass formula is based upon height and weight but is less frequently used because it may predict insufficient doses in obese patients.

IBW Formula
Male: 50 kg + 2.5 kg for **EACH** inch over 5 feet
Female: 45.5 kg + 2.3 kg for **EACH** inch over 5 feet

EXAMPLE

Female is 5 feet 2 inches (2 inches × 2.3 kg)
IBW: 45.5 kg + 2 (2.3 kg) = 45.5 kg + 4.6 kg = 50.1 kg

Adjusted Body Weight (ABW)

Adjusted body weight (ABW) is used for dosing some medication for obese individuals or pregnant women. The adjusted body weight formula uses both the ideal body weight and the actual body weight with adjustments for male and female.)

ABW Formula
Male: IBW + 0.3 (Actual Body Weight (kg) − IBW (kg)) = Adjusted Body Weight
Female: IBW + 0.2 (Actual Body Weight (kg) − IBW (kg)) = Adjusted Body Weight

EXAMPLE

Female is 5 feet 2 inches, weighs 100.5 kg, and is 55 years old.
(0.29569 × (100.5 kg) + (0.41813 × (62″ × 2.54 cm))) − 43.2933 =
29.71 + (0.41813 × 157.48) − 43.2933 =
29.71 + 65.84 − 43.2933 =
        95.55 − 43.2933 = 52.26 kg

Lean Body Weight (LBW)

Lean body weight (LBW) is the weight of bone, muscle, and organs without any fat. LBW is used for the dosing of some medications and can be used as an indicator of overall health for patients with chronic diseases.

LBW Formula

Lean body weight in kilograms (males over 16 years of age) = (0.32810 × [body weight in kg] + 0.33929 × [height in centimeters]) − 29.5336

Lean body weight in kilograms (women over 30) = (0.29569 × [body weight in kg] + 0.41813 × [height in centimeters]) − 43.2933

EXAMPLE

Female is 5 feet 2 inches and weighs 100.5 kg
    50.1 kg + 0.2 (100.5 − 50.1 kg) =
    50.1 kg + 0.2 (50.4 kg) =
    50.1 kg + 10.08 kg = 60.18 kg or 60.2 kg

SUMMARY PRACTICE PROBLEMS

Body Weight

1. Order: sulfisoxazole (Gantrisin) 50 mg/kg daily in 4 divided doses (q6h). Patient weighs 44 pounds.

   How many milligrams should the patient receive per dose? _____

2. Order: azithromycin (Zithromax), po. First day: 10 mg/kg/day; next 4 days: 5 mg/kg/day. Patient weighs 44 pounds.
   Drug available:

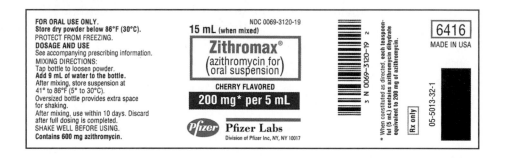

   a. How much does the child weigh in kilograms? _____

   b. How many milliliters should the child receive for the first day? _____

   c. How many milliliters should the child receive each day for the next

       4 days (second to fifth days)? _____

3. Order: ticarcillin disodium (Ticar), 200 mg/kg/day in 4 divided doses, IV. Patient weighs 176 pounds.
   Max dose: 24 g every day
   Drug available:

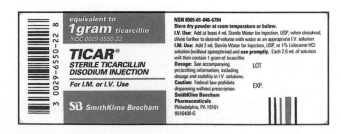

a. How many kilograms does the patient weigh? _____

b. How many milligrams per day _____ mg/day; and how many milligrams per dose? _____ mg, q6h; or how many grams per dose? _____ g, q6h.

4. Order: kanamycin (Kantrex) 15 mg/kg/day in 3 divided doses (q8h), IV. Drug is to be diluted in 100 ml of D₅W. Patient weighs 180 pounds. Drug available:

a. How many milligrams should the patient receive per day? _____

b. How many milligrams should the patient receive per dose? _____

c. How many milliliters of kanamycin should the patient receive per dose? _____

5. Order: sulfisoxazole (Gantrisin) 2 g/m² daily in 4 divided doses (q6h). The patient weighs 110 pounds and is 60 inches tall. Use nomogram.

How many milligrams should the patient receive per dose? _____

6. Order: doxorubicin (Adriamycin) 60 mg/m² IV per month. Patient weighs 120 pounds and is 5'2" (62 inches) tall. Use nomogram.

How many milligrams should the patient receive? _____

7. Order: etoposide (VePesid) 100 mg/m²/day × 5 days. Patient weighs 180 pounds and is 70 inches tall. Use nomogram. Drug available:

a. What is the BSA? _____

b. How many milligrams should the patient receive? _____

c. How many milliliters are needed? _____

PART III

CALCULATIONS FOR ORAL, INJECTABLE, AND INTRAVENOUS DRUGS

CHAPTER 7

Oral and Enteral Preparations With Clinical Applications

OBJECTIVES

- State the advantages and disadvantages of administering oral medications.
- Calculate oral dosages from tablets, capsules, and liquids using given formulas.
- Give the rationale for diluting and not diluting oral liquid medications.
- Explain the method for administering sublingual medication.
- Calculate the amount of drug to be given per day in divided doses.
- Determine the amount of tube feeding solution needed for dilution according to the percent ordered.
- Determine the amount of water needed to dilute liquid medication.

OUTLINE

Oral administration of drugs is considered a convenient and economical method of giving medications. Oral drugs are available as tablets, capsules, powders, and liquids. Oral medications are referred to as po (per os, or by mouth) drugs and are absorbed by the gastrointestinal tract, mainly from the small intestine.

There are some disadvantages in administering oral medications, such as (1) variation in absorption rate caused by gastric and intestinal pH and food consumption within the gastrointestinal tract; (2) irritation of the gastric mucosa causing nausea, vomiting, or ulceration (e.g., with oral potassium chloride); (3) retention or inactivation of the drug in the body because of reduced liver function; (4) destruction of drugs by digestive enzymes; (5) aspiration of drugs into the lungs by seriously ill or confused patients; and (6) discoloration of tooth enamel (e.g., with a saturated solution of potassium iodide [SSKI]). Oral administration is an effective way to give medications in many instances, and at times it is the route of choice.

Body weight and body surface area are discussed in Chapter 6. When solving drug problems that require body weight or body surface area, refer to Chapter 6.

Enteral nutrition and enteral medication are discussed toward the end of the chapter. Calculations of percent for enteral feeding solutions and enteral medication are also discussed.

TABLETS AND CAPSULES

Most tablets are scored and can be broken in halves and sometimes in quarters (Figure 7-1). Half of a tablet may be indicated when the drug does not come in a lesser strength. Half-tablets may not be broken equally; therefore, the patient may receive less than or more than the required dose. Also, crushing a drug tablet does not ensure that the patient will receive the entire drug dose. Some of the crushed tablet could be lost. Instead of halving or crushing a drug tablet, use the liquid form of the drug, if available, to ensure proper drug dosage.

Capsules are gelatin shells containing powder or time pellets. Caplets (solid-looking capsules) are hard-shell capsules. Time-release capsules should re-

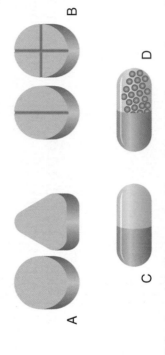

FIGURE 7-1 A and **B,** Shapes of tablets. **C** and **D,** Shapes of capsules. (From Kee, J. L., Hayes, E. R., & McCuistion, L. E. [2006]. *Pharmacology: A nursing process approach,* 5th ed. Philadelphia: W. B. Saunders.)

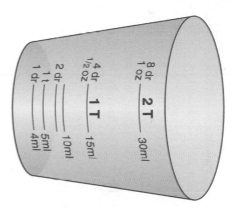

FIGURE 7-2 Medicine cup for liquid measurement. (From Kee, J. L., Hayes, E. R., & McCuistion, L. E. [2006]. *Pharmacology: A nursing process approach*, 5th ed. Philadelphia: W. B. Saunders.)

main intact and not be divided in any way. Many drugs that come in capsules also come in liquid form. When a smaller dose is indicated and is not available in tablet or capsule form, the liquid form of the drug is used (Figure 7-2).

Pill/Tablet Cutter

A pill or tablet cutter can be used to evenly split or divide a scored or unscored tablet. The pill cutter *cannot* be used to cut/divide enteric-coated tablets or capsules, time-released, sustained-released, or controlled-released capsules. Pill/tablet cutters can be purchased at a drug store (Figure 7-3).

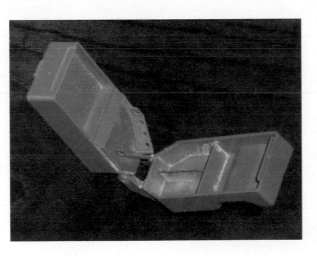

FIGURE 7-3 Pill/tablet cutter.

CAUTION

- Instead of breaking or crushing a tablet, use the liquid form if available.
- Time-release, sustained-release, or controlled-release capsules should not be crushed and diluted because the entire medication could be absorbed rapidly.
- Enteric-coated tablets must NOT be crushed because the medication could irritate the stomach. Enteric-coated tablets are absorbed by the small intestine.
- Tablets or capsules that are irritating to the gastric mucosa should be taken with 6 to 8 ounces of fluid, with meals, or immediately after meals.

Calculation of Tablets and Capsules

The following steps should be taken to determine the drug dose:

1. Check the drug order.
2. Determine the drug available (generic name, brand name, and dosage per drug form).
3. Set up the method for drug calculation (basic formula, ratio and proportion, fraction equation, or dimensional analysis).
4. Convert to like units of measurement within the same system before solving the problem. Use the unit of measure on the drug container to calculate the drug dose.
5. Solve for the unknown **(X)**.

Decide which of the methods of calculation you wish to use, and then use that same method for calculating all dosages. In the following examples, the basic formula, the ratio and proportion, fraction equation, and dimensional analysis methods are used (see Chapter 5).

Basic Formula (BF)

$$\frac{D \text{ (desired dose)}}{H \text{ (on-hand dose)}} \times V = \text{(vehicle)}$$

Ratio and Proportion (RP)

$$H : V :: D : X$$
on hand vehicle desired dose X

(Cross multiply)

Fraction Equation (FE)

$$\frac{H \text{ (on hand)}}{V \text{ (Vehicle)}} = \frac{D \text{ (desired dose)}}{X \text{ (unknown)}} \text{ or } \frac{H}{V} \times \frac{D}{X}$$

(Cross multiply)

Dimensional Analysis (DA)

$$V = \frac{V \times C \text{ (H)} \times D}{H \times C \text{ (D)} \times 1}$$

Note: C = conversion factor if needed.

EXAMPLES

PROBLEM 1: Order: pravastatin sodium (Pravachol) 20 mg, daily

Drug available:

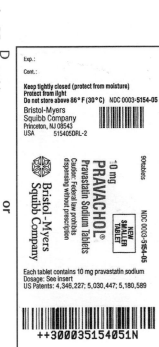

Methods: BF: $\dfrac{D}{H} \times V$

$\dfrac{20}{10} \times 1 = 2$ tablets

or

FE: $\dfrac{H}{V} \times \dfrac{D}{X} =$

$\dfrac{10}{1} \times \dfrac{20}{X} = 10X = 20$

$X = 2$ tablets

or

RP: $\quad$ H : V :: D : X

10 mg : 1 tab :: 20 mg : X tab

10 X = 20

X = 2 tablets

or

DA: no conversion factor

$$tab = \dfrac{1\ tab}{\cancel{10}\ mg} \times \dfrac{\overset{2}{\cancel{20}}\ mg}{1} = 2\ tablets$$

Answer: Pravachol 20 mg = 2 tablets, daily.

PROBLEM 2: Order: erythromycin (ERY-TAB) 0.5 g, qid (four times a day).

Drug available:

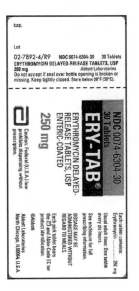

Note: Grams (g) and milligrams (mg) are units in the metric system. *Remember:* When changing grams (larger un t) to milligrams (smaller unit), move the decimal point three spaces to the right. Refer to Chapter 1, Table 2-1, or Table 5-1. Because the drug dose on the drug label is in milligrams, conversion should be from grams to milligrams.

Methods: 0.5 g = 0.500 mg or 500 mg

BF: $\dfrac{D}{H} \times V = \dfrac{500}{250} \times 1$

$= \dfrac{500}{250} = 2$ tablets

or
FE: $\dfrac{250}{1} \times \dfrac{500}{X}$

(Cross multiply) 250 X = 500

X = 2 tablets

or
RP: $\quad$ H $\quad$: $\quad$ V $\quad$ :: $\quad$ D $\quad$: $\quad$ X

250 mg:1 tab :: 500 mg:X tab

250 X = 500

X = 2 tablets

or
DA: tablet $= \dfrac{1 \text{ tab}}{\cancel{250} \text{ mg}} \times \dfrac{\cancel{1000} \text{ mg}}{1 \text{ g}} \times \dfrac{0.5 \text{ g}}{1}$

$4 \times 0.5 = 2$ tablets

Answer: ERY-TAB 0.5 g = 2 tablets

PROBLEM 3: Order: aspirin gr x, po, STAT.
Drug available: aspirin 325 mg per tablet.

Note: The dose is ordered in the apothecary system, gr x, and the label on the drug bottle is in the metric system (325 mg). Use Table 2-1 or Table 5-1 to convert units.

Methods: 325 mg = gr v (5) and 650 mg = gr x (10)

BF: $\dfrac{D}{H} \times V = \dfrac{10 \text{ gr}}{5 \text{ gr}} \times 1 = \dfrac{10}{5} = 2$ tablets

or
RP: $\quad$ H $\quad$: $\quad$ V $\quad$ :: $\quad$ D $\quad$: $\quad$ X

5 gr:1 tab :: 10 gr : X tab

5 X = 10

X = 2 tablets

or
FE: $\dfrac{H}{V} \times \dfrac{D}{X} =$

(Cross multiply) $\dfrac{325}{1} \times \dfrac{650}{X} =$

325X = 650

X = 2 tablets

or
BF: $\dfrac{D}{H} \times V = \dfrac{650 \text{ mg}}{325 \text{ mg}} \times 1 = \dfrac{650}{325} = 2$ tablets

or
DA: tablet $= \dfrac{1 \text{ tab}}{\underset{1}{\cancel{325}} \text{ mg}} \times \dfrac{\overset{3}{\cancel{1000}} \text{ mg}}{\underset{3}{\cancel{15}} \text{ gr}} \times \dfrac{\overset{2}{\cancel{10}} \text{ gr}}{1} = \dfrac{6}{3} = 2$ tablets

Answer: Aspirin gr x = 2 tablets.

LIQUIDS

Liquid medications come as tinctures, elixirs, suspensions, and syrups. Some liquid medications are irritating to the gastric mucosa and must be well diluted before being given (e.g., potassium chloride [KCl]). Usually, liquid cough medicines are not diluted. Medications in tincture form are always diluted or should be diluted.

Liquids are designed to be taken orally or through an enteral tube and are made palatable by the addition of sweetners such as suctrose, aspartame, saccharin, fructose, and sorbital. Unpalatable liquid drugs can be mixed with 30 to 60 ml of fruit juice.

CAUTION

- Concentrated liquid medication that can irritate the gastric mucosa should be diluted in *at least* 6 ounces of fluid, preferably 8 ounces of fluid.
- Liquid medication that can discolor the teeth *should be well diluted* and taken through a drinking straw.

Calculation of Liquid Medications

EXAMPLES

PROBLEM 1: Order: potassium chloride (KCl) 20 mEq, po, bid.
Drug available: liquid potassium chloride 10 mEq per 5 ml.

Methods: BF: $\dfrac{D}{H} \times V = \dfrac{20}{10} \times 5 = \dfrac{100}{10} = 10$ ml

or

RP: H : V :: D : X
10 mEq : 5 ml :: 20 mEq : X ml
10 X = 100
X = 10 ml

or

DA: no conversion factor

$$ml = \dfrac{5\ ml}{\cancel{10}\ mEq \times} \times \dfrac{\overset{2}{\cancel{20}}\ mEq}{1} = 10\ ml$$

Answer: Potassium chloride 20 mEq = 10 ml

PROBLEM 2: Order: amoxicillin (Amoxil) 0.25 g, po, tid.
Drug available:

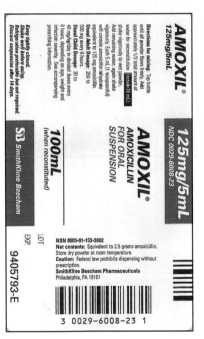

Change grams to milligrams: 0.25 g = 0.250 mg or 250 mg

Methods: BF: $\dfrac{D}{H} \times V = \dfrac{250}{125} \times 5 = \dfrac{1250}{125} = 10$ ml

or

RP: H : V :: D : X
125 mg:5 ml :: 250 mg:X ml
125 X = 1250
X = 10 ml

or

FE: $\dfrac{H}{V} \times \dfrac{D}{X} = \dfrac{125}{5} \times \dfrac{250}{X} =$

(Cross multiply) 125X = 1250
X = 10 ml

or

DA: ml = $\dfrac{5 \text{ ml}}{\cancel{125}\, \underset{1}{\cancel{mg}}} \times \dfrac{\overset{8}{\cancel{1000}}\, \cancel{mg}}{\underset{4}{\cancel{1}}\, \cancel{g}} \times \dfrac{\overset{1}{\cancel{0.25}}\, \cancel{g}}{1} = \dfrac{40}{4} = 10$ ml

Answer: Amoxil 0.25 g = 10 ml

PROBLEM 3: Give SSKI 300 mg, q6h, diluted in water.
Drug available: saturated solution of potassium iodide, 50 mg per drop (gt), drops (gtt).

Methods: BF: $\dfrac{D}{H} \times V = \dfrac{300}{50} \times 1 = \dfrac{300}{50} = 6$ gtt

or

RP: H : V :: D : X
50 mg:1 gt :: 300 mg:X gtt
50 X = 300
X = 6 gtt

or

DA: gtt = $\dfrac{1 \text{ gt}}{\underset{1}{\cancel{50}}\, \cancel{mg}} \times \dfrac{\overset{6}{\cancel{300}}\, \cancel{mg}}{1} = 6$ gtt

Answer: SSKI 300 mg = 6 gtt (drops)

SUBLINGUAL TABLETS

Few drugs are administered sublingually (tablet placed under the tongue). Sublingual tablets are small and soluble and are quickly absorbed by the numerous capillaries on the underside of the tongue.

 CAUTION

- A sublingual tablet (e.g., nitroglycerin [NTG]), should not be swallowed. If the drug is swallowed, the desired immediate action of the drug is decreased or lost.
- Fluids *should not* be taken until the drug has dissolved.

Calculation of Sublingual Medications

EXAMPLES

PROBLEM 1: Order: nitroglycerin (Nitrostat) 0.6 mg, sublingually (SL).

Drug available:

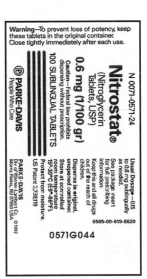

Note: The systems and weights must be the same. See Table 2-1 or Table 5-1. The label has both systems of measurement.

$$0.6 \text{ mg} = \text{gr } \tfrac{1}{100}$$

Methods: BF: $\dfrac{D}{H} \times V = \dfrac{0.6}{0.6} \times 1 = \dfrac{0.6}{0.6} = 1$ SL tablet

or

RP: H : V :: D : X

$\dfrac{1}{100}$ gr:1 tab :: $\dfrac{1}{100}$ gr:X tab

$\dfrac{1}{100}$ X = $\dfrac{1}{100}$

$X = \dfrac{1}{100} \times \dfrac{100}{1} = 1$ SL tablet

or

DA: no conversion factor

SL tab = $\dfrac{1 \text{ tab}}{0.6 \text{ mg}} \times \dfrac{\overset{1}{0.6 \text{ mg}}}{1} = 1$ SL tablet

Answer: nitroglycerin (Nitrostat) 0.6 mg = 1 SL tablet

PROBLEM 2: Order: isosorbide dinitrate (Isordil) 5 mg sublingually.

Drug available: Isordil 2.5 mg per tablet.

Methods: BF: $\dfrac{D}{H} \times V = \dfrac{5}{2.5} \times 1 = 2$ SL tablets

or

RP: H : V :: D : X   FE: $\dfrac{H}{V} \times \dfrac{D}{X} = \dfrac{2.5}{1} \times \dfrac{5}{X}$

2.5 mg:1 tab :: 5 mg:X tab

2.5 X = 5   (Cross multiply) 2.5X = 5

X = 2 SL tablets   X = 2 tablets

or

DA: no conversion factor

$$\text{SL tablet} = \frac{1\ \text{SL tab}}{2.5\ \overset{1}{\cancel{mg}}} \times \frac{\overset{2}{\cancel{5}}\ \cancel{mg}}{1} = 2\ \text{SL tablets}$$

Answer: Isordil 5 mg = 2 SL tablets

PRACTICE PROBLEMS: I Oral Medications

Answers can be found on pages 153-157.

For each question, calculate the correct dosage that should be administered.

1. Order: doxycycline hyclate (Vibra-Tabs) 50 mg, po, q12h
Drug available:

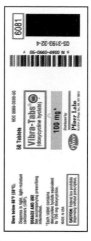

How many tablet(s) would you give for each dose? _____

2. Order: trimethoprim/sulfamethexazole (Septra) 40 mg/200 mg, po, bid.
Drug available:

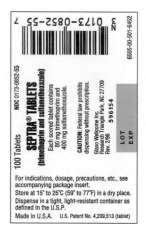

a. The drug label states that each tablet is _____

b. How many tablet(s) would you give? _____

3. Order: digoxin (Lanoxin) 0.5 mg.
Drug available:

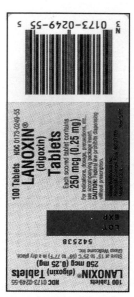

How many tablets should the patient receive? _____

Calculation of Sublingual Medications

EXAMPLES

PROBLEM 1: Order: nitroglycerin (Nitrostat) 0.6 mg, sublingually (SL).
Drug available:

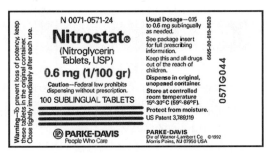

Note: The systems and weights must be the same. See Table 2-1 or Table 5-1.
The label has both systems of measurement.

$$0.6 \text{ mg} = \text{gr } 1/100$$

Methods: BF: $\dfrac{D}{H} \times V = \dfrac{0.6}{0.6} \times 1 = \dfrac{0.6}{0.6} = 1 \text{ SL tablet}$

or

RP: $\quad$ H $\quad$: $\quad$ V $\quad$ :: $\quad$ D $\quad$: $\quad$ X

$\quad \dfrac{1}{100} \text{ gr} : 1 \text{ tab} :: \dfrac{1}{100} \text{ gr} : X \text{ tab}$

$\quad \dfrac{1}{100} X = \dfrac{1}{100}$

$\quad X = \dfrac{1}{100} \times \dfrac{100}{1} = 1 \text{ SL tablet}$

or

DA: no conversion factor

$$\text{SL tab} = \dfrac{1 \text{ tab} \times \overset{1}{\cancel{0.6 \text{ mg}}}}{\underset{1}{\cancel{0.6 \text{ mg}}} \times 1} = 1 \text{ SL tablet}$$

Answer: nitroglycerin (Nitrostat) 0.6 mg = 1 SL tablet

PROBLEM 2: Order: isosorbide dinitrate (Isordil) 5 mg sublingually.
Drug available: Isordil 2.5 mg per tablet.

Methods: BF: $\dfrac{D}{H} \times V = \dfrac{5}{2.5} \times 1 = 2 \text{ SL tablets}$

or

RP: $\quad$ H $\quad$: $\quad$ V $\quad$ :: $\quad$ D $\quad$: $\quad$ X
$\quad$ 2.5 mg : 1 tab :: 5 mg : X tab
$\quad\quad$ 2.5 X = 5
$\quad\quad\quad$ X = 2 SL tablets

or

FE: $\dfrac{H}{V} \times \dfrac{D}{X} = \dfrac{2.5}{1} \times \dfrac{5}{X}$

(Cross multiply) 2.5X = 5
$\quad\quad\quad\quad$ X = 2 tablets

or

DA: no conversion factor

$$\text{SL tablet} = \frac{1\ \text{SL tab} \times \overset{2}{\cancel{5}}\ \cancel{\text{mg}}}{\underset{1}{\cancel{2.5}}\ \cancel{\text{mg}} \times 1} = 2\ \text{SL tablets}$$

Answer: Isordil 5 mg = 2 SL tablets

PRACTICE PROBLEMS: I Oral Medications

Answers can be found on pages 153-157.

For each question, calculate the correct dosage that should be administered.

1. Order: doxycycline hyclate (Vibra-Tabs) 50 mg, po, q12h
   Drug available:

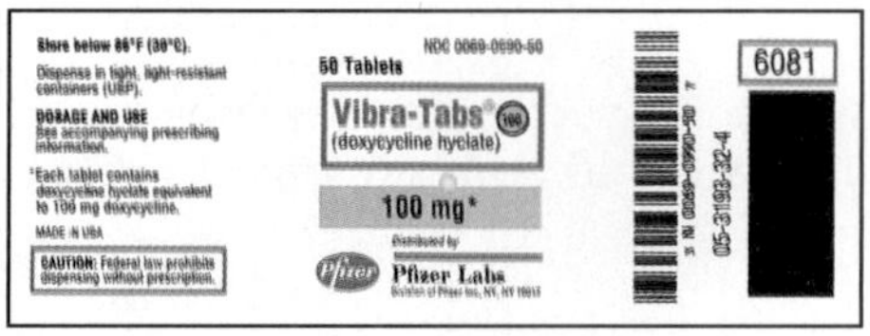

   How many tablets(s) would you give for each dose? ____________________

2. Order: trimethoprim/sulfamethexazole (Septra) 40 mg/200 mg, po, bid.
   Drug available:

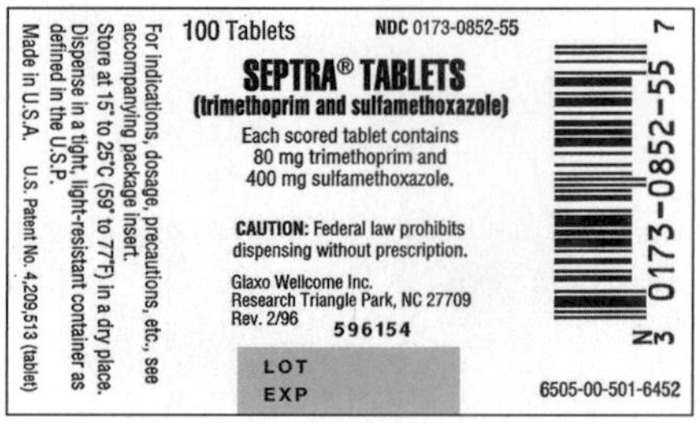

   a. The drug label states that each tablet is ____________________.

   b. How many tablet(s) would you give? ____________________

3. Order: digoxin (Lanoxin) 0.5 mg.
   Drug available:

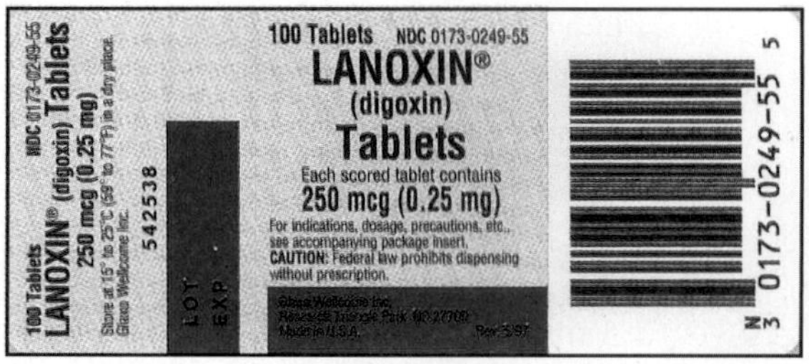

   How many tablets should the patient receive? ____________________

4. Order: codeine gr 1, prn, q4h.
   Drug available:

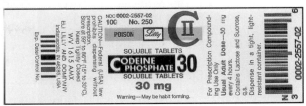

   How many tablet(s) should the patient receive? _____.

5. Order: Diovan HCT (valsartan and hydrochlorothiazide) 160 mg/25 mg, po, daily.
   Drug available:

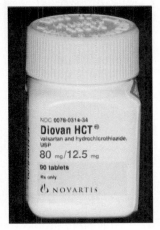

   How many tablets would you give? _____

6. Order: potassium chloride 40 mEq, po.
   Drug available: potassium chloride 20 mEq/15 ml.

   How many milliliters should the patient receive? _____

7. Order: Cefaclor (Ceclor) 250 mg, q8h.
   Drug available:

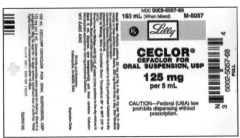

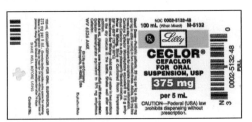

    a. Which Ceclor bottle would you select? Why? _____

    b. How many milliliters per dose should the patient receive? _____

8. Order: ProSom (estazolam) 2 mg, po, at bedtime.
Drug available: 1 mg tablet

How many tablet(s) should be given? _____

9. Order: cefuroxime axetil (Ceftin) 400 mg, po, q12h.
Drug available:

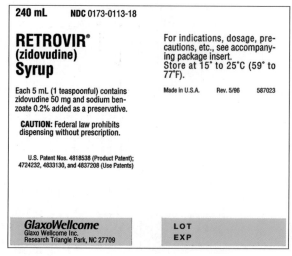

    a. How many milliliters should the patient receive? _____

    b. Which drug bottle would you use? _____

    Why? _____

10. Order: zidovudine (Retrovir) 300 mg, po, q12h.
Drug available:

    a. How many milligrams would you give per day? _____

    b. How many milliliters would you give per dose? _____

11. Order: Dicloxacillin (Dynapen) 100 mg, po, q6h.
    Drug available:

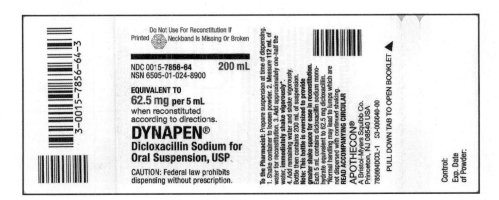

How many milliliters should the client receive? _____

12. Order: HydroDiuril 50 mg, po, daily.
    Drug available:

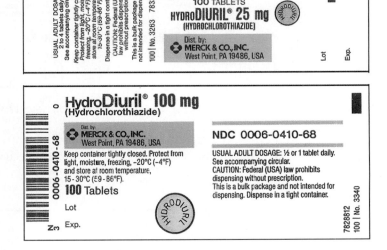

    a. Which drug bottle would you use? _____

    b. How many tablet(s) would you give, if the tablet(s) are not

       scored? _____

       Explain. _____

13. Order: simvastatin (Zocor) 30 mg, po, daily.
Drug available:

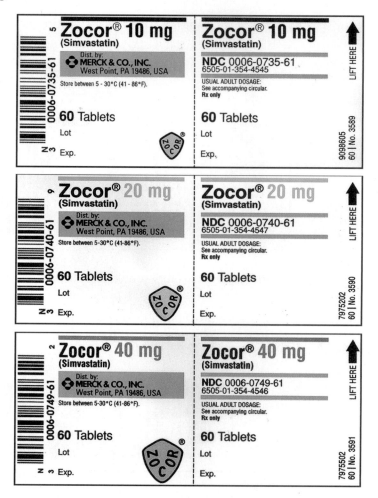

a. Which bottle(s) of Zocor would you select? Why?

_____

b. How many tablet(s) should the patient receive? _____

14. Order: cefadroxil (Duricef) 0.4 g, po, q6h.
Drug available:

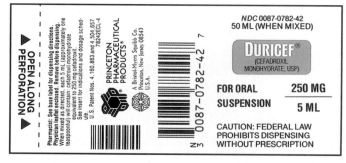

How many milliliters should the patient receive per dose?_____

15. Order: phenobarbital gr ½.
Drug available: phenobarbital 15 mg per tablet.

How many tablet(s) should the patient receive? _____

16. Order: cefprozil (Cefzil) 100 mg, po, q12h.
Drug available:

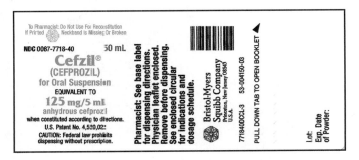

How many milliliters should the patient receive per dose?_____

17. Order: Crestor 20 mg, po, daily.
Drug available:

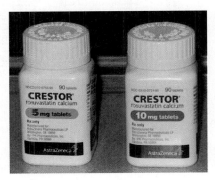

a. Which Crestor bottle(s) would you select?_____

b. How many tablet(s) would you give? _____

18. Order: nitroglycerin gr ¹⁄₁₅₀, SL, STAT.
Drug available:

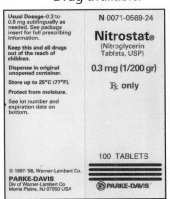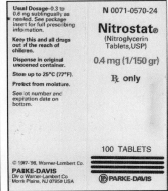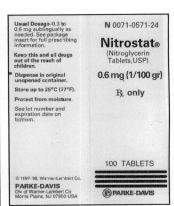

Which Nitrostat SL tablet would you give? (Refer to Table 2-1 or Table 5-1 if

necessary.) _____

19. Order: Mycostatin 250,000 units oral swish and swallow, qid.
    Drug available:

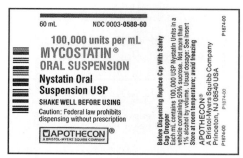

   Calculate the correct dosage. _____

20. Order: Digoxin (Lanoxin) 0.25 mg, po, daily.
    Drug available:

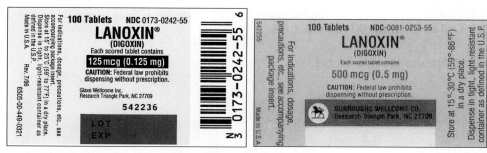

   a. Which Lanoxin bottle would you select? _____

   b. How many tablet(s) would you give? _____

21. Order: diazepam (Valium) 2½ mg.
    Drug available: Valium 5 mg scored tablet.

   Calculate the correct dosage. _____

22. Order: ondansetron HCl (Zofran) 6 mg, po, 30 min before chemotherapy,
    then q8h × 2 more doses.
    Drug available:

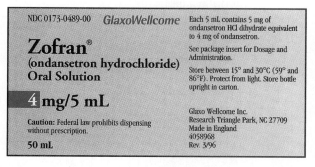

   a. How many milliliters would you give per dose? `

   _____

23. Order: allopurinol 450 mg, po, daily.
Drug available: allopurinol 300 mg scored tablet.

Calculate the correct dosage. _____

24. Order: captopril (Capoten) 25 mg, po, bid, for an elderly patient with heart failure.
Drug available:

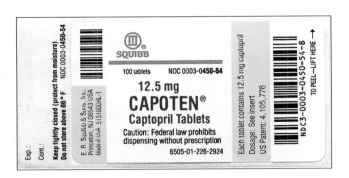

a. How many milligrams should the patient receive per day? _____

b. How many tablet(s) would you give? _____

25. Order: cefadroxil (Duricef) 1 g, po, as a loading dose; then cefadroxil 0.5 g, po, q12h.
Drug available:

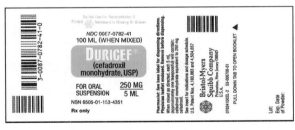

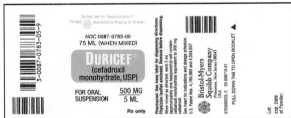

a. Which drug bottle would you select? _____

b. How many milliliters would you give as the loading dose?

_____

c. How many milliliters per 0.5 g? _____

26. Order: amoxicillin/clavulanate potassium (Augmentin) 0.5 g, po, q8h.
Drug available:

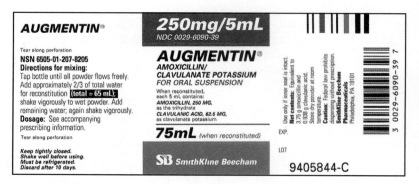

How many milliliters should the patient receive per dose? _____

27. Order: Lorabid (loracarbef) oral suspension, 0.4 g, po, q12h for 10 days.
Drug available:

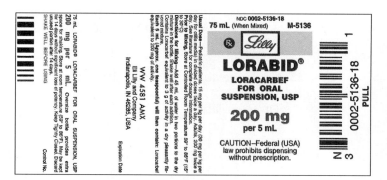

a. Change grams into milligrams. How many milligrams should the patient

receive per dose? _____

b. How many milliliters would you give per dose? _____

Questions 28-32 relate to additional dimensional analysis (factor labeling). Refer
to Chapter 5 as necessary.

28. Order: methyldopa (Aldomet) 0.5 g, po, daily.
Drug available:

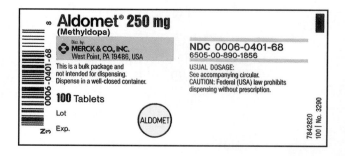

Factors: 250 mg = 1 tablet (drug label)
0.5 g/1 (drug order)
Conversion factor: 1 g = 1000 mg

How many tablet(s) of methyldopa 250 mg would you give? _____

29. Order: Vasotec 5 mg, po, bid.
Drug available:

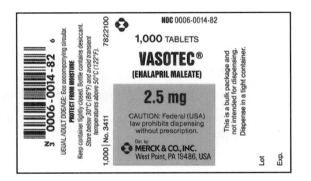

Factors: 2.5 mg = 1 tablet (drug label); 5 mg/1 (drug order)
Conversion factor: none.

How many tablet(s) should the patient receive? _____

30. Order: amoxicillin (Amoxil) 0.4 g, po, q6h.
Drug available:

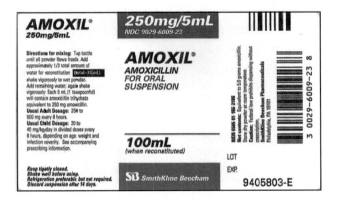

Factors: 250 mg/5 ml (drug label); 0.4 g/1 (drug order)
Conversion factor: 1 g = 1000 mg.

How many milliliters would you give? _____

31. Order: acetaminophen (Tylenol) gr x, po.
Drug available:

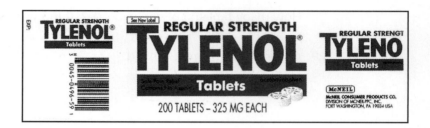

Factors: _____

Conversion factor: _____

How many acetaminophen tablets would you give? _____

32. Order: oxacillin sodium 125 mg, po, q6h.
Drug available:

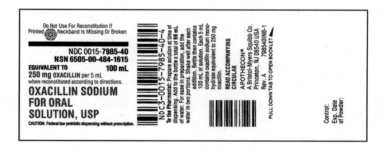

How many milliliters would you give? _____

Questions 33-37 relate to body weight and body surface area. Refer to Chapter 6 as necessary.

33. Order: valproic acid (Depakene) 10 mg/kg/day in three divided doses (tid), po. Patient weighs 165 pounds. How much Depakene should be administered

tid? _____

34. Order: cyclophosphamide (Cytoxan) 4 mg/kg/day, po. Patient weighs 154 pounds. How much Cytoxan would you give per day?

_____

35. Order: mercaptopurine 2.5 mg/kg/day po or 100 mg/m² body surface area po. The patient weighs 132 pounds and is 64 inches tall. The estimated body surface area according to the nomogram is 1.7 m². The amount of drug the

patient should receive according to body weight is _____ and accord-

ing to body surface area is _____.

36. Order: ethosuximide (Zarontin) 20 mg/kg/day in 2 divided doses (q12h). Patient weighs 110 pounds (110 ÷ 2.2 = 50 kg).
Drug available:

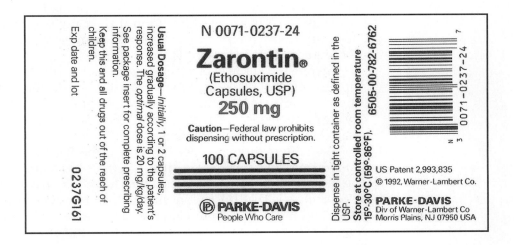

a. How many milligrams should the patient receive per day? _____

b. How many tablet(s) should the patient receive per dose? _____

37. Order: minocycline HCl (Minocin) 4 mg/kg/day in 2 divided doses (q12h).
Patient weighs 132 pounds (132 ÷ 2.2 = 60 kg).
Drug available: Minocin 50 mg/5 ml.

a. How many milligrams should the patient receive per day? _____

b. How many milliliters should the patient receive per dose? _____

ENTERAL NUTRITION AND DRUG ADMINISTRATION

When the patient is unable to take nourishment by mouth, enteral feeding (tube feeding) is usually preferred over intravenous therapy. Candidates for enteral feedings are patients with neurological deficits who have difficulty swallowing, debilitated patients; patients with burns and malnutrition disorders, patients with upper gastric obstructions, and patients who have undergone radical head and neck surgery. The cost of enteral feedings is much less than that of intravenous therapy and there is less risk of infection.

Drugs that can be administered orally can be given via enteral tube. The drug must be in liquid form or dissolved into a liquid. Medications in timed-release, enteric-coated, or sublingual form and bulk-forming laxatives cannot be administered enterally.

Enteral Feedings

Enteral feeding tubes can be identified by their anatomical insertion site and the location of the tip. For example, a nasogastric tube (NG tube) is inserted through the nose, and the end lies in the gastric portion of the gastrointestinal tract. Tubes inserted orally or nasally are primarily for short-term use and cause nasal and pharyngeal irritation if their use is prolonged. Gastrostomy and jejunostomy routes are used for long-term feeding and require a surgical procedure for tube insertion (Figure 7-4).

Enteral feedings may be given as a bolus (intermittent) or as a continuous drip feeding over a specified period. With bolus feedings, the amount of solution administered is approximately 200 ml or less, and feeding times per day are more frequent. Continuous feedings can be given by gravity flow from a bag or by infusion pump (Figure 7-5).

There are two types of feeding tubes: the flexible small bore that has a small diameter (4-8 Fr), and a large bore that has a large diameter (12-18 Fr). The flexible small-bore tube is used on a temporary basis for feeding; the chief disadvantage is that thick, concentrated, and/or fiber-containing enteral formulas and medications can clog the tube. Large-bore tubes are less likely to clog. It is essential to flush the tube before and after feedings and between medication administrations.

Many types of enteral feeding solutions are designed to meet the nutritional needs of patients. Names of common feeding solutions are listed in Table 7-1.

Although enteral feeding solutions are formulated to be given at full strength, this strength may not be tolerated. Solutions that are highly concentrated (hyperosmolar or hypertonic) when given in full strength can cause vomiting, cramping, or excessive diarrhea. When gastrointestinal symptoms occur, the enteral solution can be diluted with water. In many situations, clients have better gastrointestinal tolerance when the strength of the solution is gradually increased. However, in adults, the tube feeding may be started at a rate of 10 to 30 ml/hr if not diluted, depending on the health status of the individual. It may take 3 to 5 days for gastrointestinal tolerance to appear.

If diarrhea continues, changing to a fiber-containing formula may decrease or eliminate it. Any liquid medication should be checked to make sure that it does not contain sorbitol, which has a laxative effect after several doses. Switching from liquid to tablets may be necessary. In some patients, hypoalbuminemia could be a cause of diarrhea, which can lead to malabsorption within the intestines. The prealbumin level is a better indicator of hypoalbuminemia than is the serum albumin test. Other causes of diarrhea may include fecal impaction, *Clostridium difficile,* pseudomembranous colitis, and gut atrophy. A stool specimen should be analyzed for *C. difficile* toxin. If *C. difficile* toxin is detected, antidiarrheal drugs should not be prescribed because diarrhea helps to eliminate the toxin. The cause of diarrhea should be determined.

Blood sugar levels should be monitored during enteral therapy. This is important for patients who are acutely ill, those with septic conditions, those recovering from acute trauma, and those receiving steroids. If hyperglycemia occurs, decreasing the tube feeding rate or concentration may help.

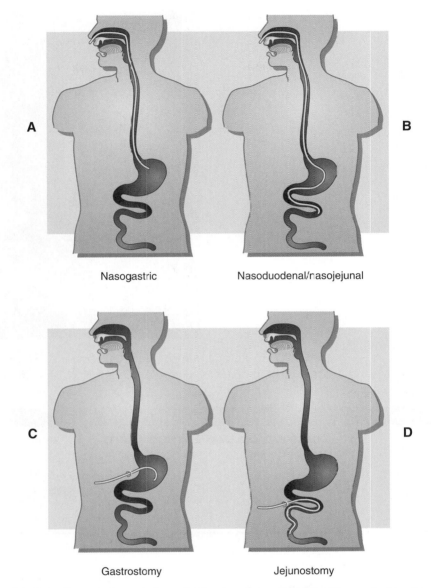

A Nasogastric

B Nasoduodenal/nasojejunal

C Gastrostomy

D Jejunostomy

FIGURE 7-4 Types of gastrointestinal tubes for enteral feedings. **A,** Nasogastric tube is passed from the nose into the stomach. **B,** Weighted nasoduodenal/nasojejunal tube is passed through the nose into duodenum/jejunum. **C,** Gastrostomy tube is introduced through a temporary or permanent opening on the abdominal wall (stoma) into the stomach. **D,** Jejunostomy tube is passed through a stoma directly into the jejunum. (From Kee, J. L., Hayes, E. R., & McCuistion, L. E. [2006]. *Pharmacology: A nursing process approach,* 5th ed. Philadelphia: W. B. Saunders.)

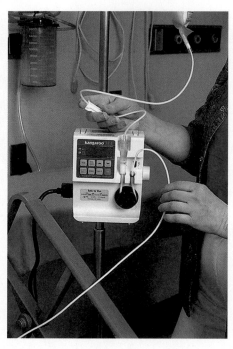

FIGURE 7-5   Enteral pump. (From Lindeman, C. & McAthie, M. [1999]. *Fundamentals of contemporary nursing practice,* Philadelphia: W. B. Saunders.)

TABLE 7-1		
Common Enteral Formulations		
Ensure	Isocal	Nepho
Ensure Plus	Sustacal	Ultracal
Ensure HN	Sustacal HC	Jevity
Osmolite	Vital	Criticare
Osmolite HN	Pulmocare	Promote

When enteral feedings are less than full strength, they are ordered in percent (%). The nurse must calculate the amount of feeding solution and the amount of water that should be given. After enteral feeding, 30 ml of water is given to flush the tube, or the amount as prescribed by the health care professional is given.

Calculation of Percent for Enteral Feeding Solutions

Percent (%) of a solution indicates its strength. Percent is a portion of 100, e.g., 20% is 20 of 100 parts (20/100). The basic formula, ratio and proportion, or a percentage problem can be used to determine percent.

D: desired percent
H: on-hand volume (100)
V: desired total volume
X: unknown amount of solution

METHODS A & B Basic Formula *and* Ratio and Proportion

BF: $\dfrac{D}{H}\left(\dfrac{\text{desired \%}}{\text{on-hand volume}}\right) \times V$ (desired total volume)

or

RP: H   :   V   ::   D   :   X
 on-hand : desired   :: desired : unknown
  volume total volume   %   amount of
                                    solution

or

METHOD C Percentage Problem

Desired total volume × desired % (in hundredths) = amount of tube feeding (TF) solution.

After the tube feeding, 30 ml of water should be given to clear the tubing. The tube is clamped after a bolus feeding.

EXAMPLES

PROBLEM 1: A patient has been receiving intravenous fluids for 5 days. A nasogastric tube was inserted, and 250 ml of 50% Ensure solution was ordered q4h for 1 day. Calculate how much Ensure and water are needed to make 250 ml (50% solution).

Methods: 50% solution is 50 in 100 parts.

BF: $\dfrac{D}{H}\left(\dfrac{\text{desired \%}}{\text{on-hand volume}}\right) \times V$ (desired total volume)

$\dfrac{50}{100} \times 250 = \dfrac{12,500}{100} = 125$ ml of Ensure

or

RP: H : V   :: D : X
       100:250 ml::50:X ml
            100 X = 12,500
                X = 125 ml of Ensure

or

250 ml × 0.50 (50%) = 125 ml of TF solution

How much water should be added?

Total amount − Amount of TF = Amount of water
  250 ml   −   125 ml   =   125 ml

Answer: 125 ml of Ensure + 125 ml of water

PROBLEM 2: Three days later, the patient's tube feeding order is changed. The patient is to receive 250 ml of 70% Osmolite solution q6h.

How much Osmolite solution and water should be mixed to equal 250 ml?

Methods: 70% solution is 70 in 100 parts.

BF: $\dfrac{D}{H} \times V = \dfrac{70}{100} \times 250 = \dfrac{17,500}{100} = 175$ ml of Osmolite

or

RP: H : V :: D : X
100 : 250 ml :: 70 : X ml
100 X = 17,500
X = 175 ml of Osmolite

or

250 ml $\times$ 0.70 (70%) = 175 ml of TF solution

How much water should be added?

Total amount − Amount of TF = Amount of water
250 ml − 175 ml = 75 ml

Answer: 175 ml of Osmolite + 75 ml of water

PROBLEM 3: One week later, the client's tube feeding order is changed to 250 ml of 40% Ensure Plus. How much Ensure Plus and water should be mixed to equal 250 ml?

Methods: 40% solution is 40 in 100 parts.

BF: $\dfrac{D}{H} \times V = \dfrac{40}{100} \times 250 = \dfrac{10,000}{100} = 100$ ml of Ensure Plus

or

RP: H : V :: D : X
100 : 250 ml :: 40 : X ml
100 X = 10,000
X = 100 ml of Ensure Plus

or

250 ml $\times$ 0.40 (40%) = 100 ml of TF solution

How much water should be added?

Total amount − Amount of TF = Amount of water
250 ml − 100 ml = 150 ml

Answer: 100 ml of Ensure Plus + 150 ml of water

PRACTICE PROBLEMS: II Percent of Enteral Solutions

Answers can be found on pages 157-158.

1. Order: 200 ml of 25% Sustacal solution q4h through a nasogastric tube. How much Sustacal solution and water should be mixed to equal

200 ml?_____

2. Order: 300 ml of 75% Pulmocare solution q6h through a nasogastric tube. How much Pulmocare solution and water should be mixed to equal 300 ml?_____

3. Order 500 ml of 60% Ensure Plus solution q8h through a nasogastric tube. How much Ensure Plus solution and water should be mixed to equal 500 ml?_____

4. Order: 400 ml of 30% Osmolite solution q6h through a nasogastric tube. How much Osmolite solution and water should be mixed to equal 400 ml?_____

Enteral Medications

Oral medications in liquid, tablet, or capsule form can be administered through a feeding tube when diluted with 30 to 60 ml of water. Tablets or capsules that can be crushed should be pulverized into a fine powder, then mixed in enough water to form a slurry. The slurry can be given through a large-bore feeding tube with a catheter-tip syringe; 30 to 50 ml of water is flushed through the feeding tube between medications. Some new feeding pumps are designed to include a flush bag that periodically clears the feeding tube and prevents clogging.

NOTE

Enteric-coated tablets and sustained-released or controlled-released tablets/capsules should NOT be crushed.

CAUTION

■ Use caution with crushing devices, such as mortar and pestle, to avoid cross-contamination and possibly an allergic reaction that may occur if the device is not cleaned or if the medication being crushed is not shielded.

All liquid medications greater than 1000 mOsm/kg are hyperosmolar when compared with secretions of the gastrointestinal tract (130 to 350 mOsm/kg). Although the hyperosmolality of fluid medication was once thought to be well tolerated by the gastrointestinal tract, research indicates that cramping, distention, vomiting, and diarrhea can be caused by the administration of undiluted hypertonic liquid medications and electrolyte solutions. Liquid medication should be diluted with water to reduce osmolality to 500 mOsm/kg to decrease gastrointestinal intolerance.

If liquid medications are causing digestive problems and cannot be changed to a tablet, capsule, or IV route, the next option is to schedule the administration of liquid medications at a different time. When scheduling does not lessen gastric symptoms, then the liquid medication should be diluted with more water to reduce the osmolality of the drug.

CAUTION

Excessive dilution of multiple enteral medications could cause fluid overload in the elderly, or for patients who have a cardiac condition. Check with the health care provider about whether this could occur.

Table 7-2 lists the osmolalities of various drug solutions and suspensions.

TABLE 7-2

Osmolalities of Selected Liquid Medications

Medication	Osmolality of Drug (mOsm/kg)
Acetaminophen (Tylenol) elixir, 65 mg/ml	5400
Acetaminophen/Codeine elixir	4700
Aminophylline liquid, 21 mg/ml	450
Amoxicillin suspension, 25 mg	1540
Amoxicillin suspension, 50 mg	2250
Ampicillin suspension, 50 mg/ml	2250
Cephalexin (Keflex) suspension, 50 mg/ml	1950
Cimetidine (Tagamet) solution, 30 mg/ml	2800
Cimetidine (Tagamet) solution, 60 mg/ml	5500
Co-trimoxazole (Bactrim) suspension, SMX 200 mg/TMP 40 mg/5 ml	2200
Dexamethasone solution, 1 mg/ml	3100
Digoxin elixir, 50 mcg/ml	1350
Diphenhydramine HCl (Benadryl) elixir, 2.5 mg/ml	850
Diphenoxylate/atropine suspension	8800
Docusate sodium (Colace) syrup, 3.3 mg/ml	3900
Erythromycin E.S. suspension, 40 mg/ml	1750
Ferrous sulfate liquid, 60 mg/ml	4700
Furosemide (Lasix) solution, 10 mg/ml	2050
Hydroxyzine HCl (Vistaril, Atarax) syrup, 2 mg/ml	4450
Kaolin-pectin suspension	900
Lactulose syrup, 0.67 g/ml	3600
Lithium citrate syrup, 1.6 mEq/ml	6850
Magnesium citrate solution	1000
Milk of magnesia solution/suspension	1250
Multivitamin liquid	5700
Nystatin (Mycostatin) suspension, 100,000 unit/ml	3300
Phenytoin sodium (Dilantin) suspension, 25 mg/ml	1500
Potassium chloride liquid, 10%	3500
Prochlorperazine (Compazine) syrup, 1 mg/ml	3250
Promethazine HCl (Phenergan) syrup, 1.25 mg/ml	3500
Pyridostigmine bromide (Mestinon) syrup, 12 mg/ml	3800
Sodium citrate liquid	2050
Sodium phosphate liquid, 0.5 g/ml	7250
Theophylline solution, 5.33 mg/ml	800
Thiabendazole suspension, 100 mg/ml	2150
Thioridazine (Mellaril) suspension, 20 mg/ml	2050

Adapted from Estoup, M. (1994). Approaches and limitations of medication delivery in patients with enteral feeding tubes. *Critical Care Nurse 1:*70, Table 2; Beckwith C. M., Feddema S. S., Barton R. G., & Graves C. (March 2004). A guide to drug therapy in patients with enteral feeding tubes: Dosage form selection and administration methods. *Hospital Pharmacy 39:*231; and Dickerson R. N. & Melnik G. (April 1988). Osmolality of oral drug solutions and suspensions. *American Journal of Hospital Pharmacy 45:*832-834.

Calculation of Dilution for Enteral Medications

To determine the amount of water needed to dilute a liquid medication, the following information must be obtained:

1. The volume of the drug from the drug order
2. The osmolality of the drug (check drug literature or ask pharmacist)
3. 500 mOsm may be used as a constant for the desired osmolality

METHOD

Step 1 Calculate the volume of drug:

$$\text{BF: } \frac{D}{H} \times V \quad \textbf{or} \quad \text{RP: } H:V::D:X \quad \textbf{or} \quad \text{DA: } V = \frac{V \times C\,(H) \times D}{H \times C\,(D) \times 1}$$

Step 2 Find osmolality (mOsm) of drug mixture

$$\frac{\text{Known mOsm} \times \text{Volume of drug}}{\text{Desired mOsm (500 mOsm)}} = \text{Total volume of liquid}$$

Step 3 Water for dilution:

$$\text{Total volume of liquid} - \text{Volume of drug} = \text{Volume of water for dilution}$$

EXAMPLES

PROBLEM 1: Order: acetaminophen 650 mg, q6h, PRN for pain.
Drug available: acetaminophen elixir 65 mg/ml.
Average mOsm/kg = 5400.

Step 1 Calculate the volume of drug:

$$\text{BF: } \frac{D}{H} \times V = \frac{650}{65} \times 1 = 10 \text{ ml}$$

or
RP: H : V ::   D   : X
       65 mg : 1 ml :: 650 mg : X ml
              65 X = 650
                 X = 10 ml

or
DA: no conversion factor

$$ml = \frac{1 \text{ ml} \times \overset{10}{\cancel{650}} \text{ mg}}{\underset{1}{\cancel{65}} \text{ mg} \times 1} = 10 \text{ ml}$$

Step 2 Find osmolality of drug:

$$\frac{\text{Known mOsm (5400)}}{\text{Desired mOsm (500)}} \times \text{Volume of drug (10)} = \frac{5400}{500} \times 10 = 108 \text{ ml}$$

Step 3 Water for dilution:
Total volume of drug (108 ml) − Volume of drug (10 ml)
= 98 ml volume of water for dilution

PROBLEM 2: Order: Colace 50 mg bid.
Drug available: docusate sodium 3.3 mg/ml.
Average mOsm/kg = 3900.

Step 1: Calculate the volume of drug:

$$\text{BF: } \frac{D}{H} \times V = \frac{50}{3.3} \times 1 = 15.1 \text{ ml}$$

or

$$\text{RP: } \quad H \quad : \quad V \quad :: \quad D \quad :X$$
$$3.3 \text{ mg}:1 \text{ ml} :: 50 \text{ mg}:X$$
$$3.3 \text{ X} = 50$$
$$X = 15.1 \text{ or } 15 \text{ ml}$$

or

DA: no conversion factor

$$\text{ml} = \frac{1 \text{ ml} \times 50 \text{ mg}}{3.3 \text{ mg} \times 1} = \frac{50}{3.3} = 15 \text{ ml}$$

Step 2: Find osmolality of drug:

$$\frac{\text{Known mOsm (3900)}}{\text{Desired mOsm (500)}} \times \text{Volume of drug (15 ml)}$$

$$= \frac{3900}{500} \times 15 = 117 \text{ ml}$$

Step 3: Water for dilution:

Total volume of drug (117 ml) − Volume of drug (15 ml)
= 102 ml volume of water for dilution

PRACTICE PROBLEMS: III Enteral Medications

Answers can be found on pages 158-160.

Calculate the amount of water needed to reduce the osmolality to 500 mOsm for the following medications:

1. Order: amoxicillin suspension 250 mg by tube, qid.
   Drug available: amoxicillin suspension 50 mg/ml.

2. Order: co-trimoxazole (Bactrim) suspension SMX 400 mg/TMP 80 mg, q12h.
   Drug available: Bactrim suspension SMX 200 mg/TMP 40 mg/5 ml.

3. Order: KCl oral solution 40 mEq, daily by tube.
   Drug available: KCl 10% oral solution, 20 mEq/15 ml.

4. Order: thioridazine suspension 50 mg, tid by tube.
   Drug available: thioridazine suspension 20 mg/ml.

ANSWERS

I Oral Medications

1. BF: $\dfrac{D}{H} \times V = \dfrac{50}{100} \times 1$

$$= 100\overline{)50.0}^{.5} = 0.5 = \text{½ tablets}$$

or

RP: H : V :: D : X

100 mg : 1 tab :: 50 mg : X tab

100 X = 50

X = 0.5 or ½ tablets

or

DA: no conversion factor

$$\text{tab} = \frac{1 \text{ tab} \times \overset{1}{\cancel{50}} \text{ m\cancel{g}}}{\underset{2}{\cancel{100}} \text{ m\cancel{g}} \times 1} = \text{½ tablet}$$

2. a. scored

b. ½ tablet

3. 2 tablets

4. Change grains to milligrams (milligram value is on the drug label). Refer to Table 2-1 or Table 5-1: 1 gr = 60 mg.

BF: $\dfrac{D}{H} \times V = \dfrac{60}{30} \times 1 = 2 \text{ tablets}$

or

RP: H : V :: D : X

30 mg : 1 tab :: 60 mg : X tab

30 X = 60

X = 2 tablets

5. 2 tablets daily

6. 30 ml

7. a. Select the 125 mg/5 ml bottle. It is a fractional dosage with the 375 mg/5 ml bottle (3.3 ml).

b. BF: $\dfrac{D}{H} \times V = \dfrac{250}{125} \times 5 \text{ ml} = \dfrac{1250}{125} = 10 \text{ ml of Ceclor}$

or

RP: H : V :: D : X

125 : 5 :: 250 : X

125 X = 1250

X = 10 ml of Ceclor

or

DA: ml = $\dfrac{5 \text{ ml} \times \overset{2}{\cancel{250}} \text{ m\cancel{g}}}{\underset{1}{\cancel{125}} \text{ m\cancel{g}} \times 1} = 10 \text{ ml}$

8. 2 tablets of ProSom

9. **a.** BF: $\dfrac{D}{H} \times V = \dfrac{400}{125} \times 5 = \dfrac{2000}{125} = 16$ ml of Ceftin

  or
  BF: $\dfrac{D}{H} \times V = \dfrac{400}{250} \times 5 = \dfrac{2000}{250} = 8$ ml of Ceftin

  b. Either Ceftin bottle could be used. For fewer milliliters, select the 250 mg/5 ml bottle.

10. **a.** 600 mg per day

  b. BF: $\dfrac{D}{H} \times V = \dfrac{300 \text{ mg}}{50 \text{ mg}} \times 5$ ml
  $= 30$ ml per dose

  or
  RP: H : V :: D : X
  50 mg : 5 ml :: 300 mg : X ml
  50 X = 1500
  X = 30 ml

  or
  FE: $\dfrac{H}{V} \times \dfrac{D}{X} = \dfrac{50 \text{ mg}}{5 \text{ ml}} \times \dfrac{300 \text{ mg}}{X} =$
  (Cross multiply) 50X = 1500
  X = 30 ml per dose

  or
  DA: ml $= \dfrac{5 \text{ ml} \times \overset{6}{\cancel{300 \text{ mg}}}}{\underset{1}{\cancel{50 \text{ mg}}} \times 1} = 30$ ml per dose

11. BF: $\dfrac{D}{H} \times V = \dfrac{100}{62.5} \times 5$ ml $= \dfrac{500}{62.5} = 8$ ml of Dynapen

  or
  RP: H : V :: D : X
  62.5 : 5 :: 100 : X
  62.5 X = 500
  X = 8 ml

12. **a.** The HydroDiuril 25 mg tablet bottle is preferred. A half-tablet from the HydroDiuril 100 mg tablet bottle can be used; however, breaking or cutting the 100 mg tablet can result in an inaccurate dose.

  b. From the HydroDiuril 25 mg bottle, give 2 tablets. From the HydroDiuril 100 mg bottle, give ½ tablet (if the tablet is scored).

13. **a.** Select a 10 mg and 20 mg Zocor bottle.

  b. Give 1 tablet from each bottle.

14. Change grams to milligrams by moving the decimal point three spaces to the right: 0.400 g = 400 mg. Also see Table 2-1 or Table 5-1.

  BF: $\dfrac{D}{H} \times V = \dfrac{400}{250} \times 5$ ml $= \dfrac{2000}{250} = 8$ ml   **or**   RP: H : V :: D : X
  250 mg : 5 ml :: 400 mg : X ml
  250 X = 2000
  X = 8 ml

  or
  FE: $\dfrac{H}{V} \times \dfrac{D}{X} = \dfrac{250 \text{ mg}}{5 \text{ mg}} \times \dfrac{400 \text{ mg}}{X}$
  (Cross multiply) 250 X = 2000
  X = 8 ml

  or
  DA: ml $= \dfrac{5 \text{ ml} \times \overset{4}{\cancel{1000 \text{ mg}}} \times 0.4 \text{ g}}{\underset{1}{\cancel{250 \text{ mg}}} \times 1 \text{ g} \times 1} = 20 \times 0.4 = 8$ ml

15. Use the metric system. According to Table 2-1 or Table 5-1, gr $\overline{ss}$ = 30 mg. Give 2 tablets.

16. BF: $\dfrac{D}{H} \times V = \dfrac{100}{125} \times 5 \text{ ml} = \dfrac{500}{125} = 4 \text{ ml}$

    or

    RP: H : V ::   D :X
        125 mg:5 ml :: 100 mg:X
                125 X = 500
                    X = 4 ml

    or

    FE: $\dfrac{125}{5} \times \dfrac{100}{X} = 125X = 500$

    $\qquad\qquad\qquad X = 4 \text{ ml}$

    or

    DA: no conversion factor

    $ml = \dfrac{5 \text{ ml} \times \overset{4}{\cancel{100}} \text{ m\cancel{g}}}{\underset{5}{\cancel{125}} \text{ m\cancel{g}} \times 1} = \dfrac{20}{5} = 4 \text{ ml}$

17. **a.** Preferred the selection of Crestor 10 mg bottle. Could select Crestor 5 mg bottle; however, the number of tablets given would have to be increased.

    b. 2 tablets from Crestor 10 mg bottle. If Crestor 5 mg bottle was selected, then 4 tablets.

18. Nitrostat 0.4 mg

19. 2½ ml

20. **a.** Preferred the selection of Lanoxin 0.125 mg (125 mcg) bottle. Could select Lanoxin 0.5 mg (500 mcg) bottle because the tablets are scored.

    b. 2 tablets from the Lanoxin 0.125 mg bottle or ½ tablet from the Lanoxin 0.5 mg bottle.

21. ½ tablet

22. BF: $\dfrac{D}{H} \times V = \dfrac{6}{4} \times 5 = \dfrac{30}{4} = 7.5 \text{ ml of Zofran}$

23. 1½ tablets

24. **a.** 50 mg per day

    b. BF: $\dfrac{D}{H} \times V = \dfrac{25 \text{ mg}}{12.5 \text{ mg}} \times 1 \text{ tab} = 2 \text{ tablets}$

    or

    FE: $\dfrac{H}{V} \times \dfrac{D}{X} = \dfrac{12.5 \text{ mg}}{1 \text{ tablet}} \times \dfrac{25 \text{ mg}}{X} =$

    (Cross multiply)   12.5 X = 25

    $\qquad\qquad\qquad X = 2 \text{ tablets}$

    or

    RP: H   : V ::   D : X
        12.5 mg : 1 tab :: 25 mg : X ml
            12.5 mg X = 25 mg
                    X = 2 tablets

    or

    DA: tablets $= \dfrac{1 \text{ tab} \times \overset{2}{\cancel{25}} \text{ m\cancel{g}}}{\underset{1}{\cancel{12.5}} \text{ m\cancel{g}} \times 1} = 2 \text{ tablets}$

25. **a.** For loading dose and maintenance doses, the 500 mg/5 ml is preferred, but either bottle could be used.

    b. Loading dose: change grams to milligrams:
        1.000 g = 1000 mg

Using the 250 mg/5 ml bottle:

BF: $\dfrac{D}{H} \times V = \dfrac{1000}{\underset{50}{\cancel{250}}} \times \cancel{5}^{1} \text{ ml} = \dfrac{1000}{50} = 20 \text{ ml}$

or

FE: $\dfrac{H}{V} \times \dfrac{D}{X} = \dfrac{250 \text{ mg}}{5 \text{ ml}} \times \dfrac{1000 \text{ mg}}{X}$

(Cross multiply) 250 X = 5000

$X = 20 \text{ ml}$

or

RP: H   : V ::   D   : X

250 mg : 5 ml :: 1000 mg : X ml

250 X = 5000

X = 20 ml

or

DA: ml $= \dfrac{5 \text{ ml} \times \overset{2}{\cancel{1000}} \text{ mg} \times \cancel{1} \text{ g}}{\underset{1}{\cancel{500}} \text{ mg} \times \cancel{1} \text{ g} \times 1} = 10 \text{ ml}$ (using 500 mg/5 ml)

Using the 500 mg/5 ml bottle: give 10 ml per dose of Duricef.

c. Maintenance doses per dose, change grams to milligrams

0.500 g = 500 mg

Using the 250 mg/5 ml bottle:

BF: $\dfrac{D}{H} \times V = \dfrac{500}{250} \times 5 \text{ ml} = 10 \text{ ml}$

or

FE: $\dfrac{H}{V} \times \dfrac{D}{X} = \dfrac{250 \text{ mg}}{5 \text{ ml}} \times \dfrac{500 \text{ mg}}{X}$

250 X = 2500

X = 10 ml

or

RP: H   : V ::   D   : X

250 mg : 5 ml :: 500 mg : X

250 X = 2500

X = 10 ml

or

DA: ml $= \dfrac{5 \text{ ml} \times \overset{4}{\cancel{1000}} \text{ mg} \times 0.5 \text{ g}}{\underset{1}{\cancel{250}} \text{ mg} \times 1 \cancel{g} \times 1} = 20 \times 0.5 =$

10 ml (using 250 mg/5 ml)

Using the 500 mg/5 ml: give 5 ml per dose of Duricef.

26. 10 ml

27. a.   0.4 g = 400 mg per dose

b. BF: $\dfrac{D}{H} \times V = \dfrac{\overset{2}{\cancel{400}} \text{ mg}}{\underset{1}{\cancel{200}} \text{ mg}} \times 5 \text{ ml} = 10 \text{ ml}$

or

RP: H   : V ::   D   : X

200 mg : 5 ml :: 400 mg : X ml

200 X = 2000

X = 10 ml

or

FE: $\dfrac{H}{V} \times \dfrac{D}{X} = \dfrac{200}{5} \times \dfrac{400}{X} =$

(Cross multiply)   200 X = 2000

X = 10 ml

or

DA: ml $= \dfrac{5 \text{ ml} \times \overset{5}{\cancel{1000}} \text{ mg} \times 0.4 \cancel{g}}{\underset{1}{\cancel{200}} \text{ mg} \times 1 \cancel{g} \times 1} = 10 \text{ ml}$

Additional Dimensional Analysis

28. Drug label: 250 mg = 1 tablet

tablets $= \dfrac{1 \text{ tab} \times \overset{4}{\cancel{1000}} \text{ mg} \times 0.5 \cancel{g}}{\underset{1}{\cancel{250}} \text{ mg} \times 1 \cancel{g} \times 1} = 0.5 \times 4 = 2 \text{ tablets}$

29. tablets $= \dfrac{1 \times \overset{2}{\cancel{5.0}} \text{ mg}}{\underset{1}{\cancel{2.5}} \text{ mg} \times 1} = 2 \text{ tablets of Vasotec}$

30. $ml = \dfrac{5\ ml \times 1000\ mg \times 0.4\ g}{250\ mg \times 1\ g \times 1} = 8\ ml$

    Give 8 ml per dose of amoxicillin.

31. Drug label: 325 mg = 1 tablet; gr × (10)/1

    Conversion factor: 1 gr = 60 mg

    $tablets = \dfrac{1\ tab \times 60\ mg \times 10\ gr}{325\ mg \times 1\ gr \times 1} = \dfrac{24}{13} = 1.84\ or\ 2\ tablets$

    60 (64) mg = 1 gr (approximate weights). Round off to the nearest whole number.

32. Drug label: 250 mg = 5 ml; 125 mg/1

    Conversion factor: *none*

    $ml = \dfrac{5\ ml \times 125\ mg}{250\ mg \times 1} = \dfrac{5}{2} = 2\frac{1}{2}\ or\ 2.5\ ml$

33. 165 lb = 75 kg (change pounds to kilograms by dividing by 2.2 into 165 pounds, or 165 ÷ 2.2)

    10 mg × 75 = 750 mg

    750 ÷ 3 = 250 mg, tid

34. 154 lb = 70 kg

    4 mg × 70 = 280 mg/day

35. 132 lb = 60 kg

    2.5 mg × 60 = 150 mg **or** 100 × 1.7 = 170 mg

36. **a.** 20 mg/50 kg/day = 20 × 50 = 1000 mg per day

    b. 2 tablets of Zarontin per dose (500 mg per dose)

37. **a.** 4 mg/60 kg/day = 4 × 60 = 240 mg per day **or** 120 mg, q12h

    b. BF: $\dfrac{D}{H} \times V = \dfrac{120}{50} \times 5\ ml = \dfrac{120}{10} = 12\ ml$

    or

    RP: H : V :: D : X

       50 : 5 :: 120 : X

       50 X = 600

          $X = \dfrac{600}{50} = 12\ ml$

    or

    DA: $ml = \dfrac{5\ ml \times 120\ mg}{50\ mg \times 1} = \dfrac{60}{5} = 12\ ml$

    Give 12 ml per dose of minocycline.

II Percent of Enteral Solutions

1. BF: $\dfrac{D}{H} \times V = \dfrac{25}{100} \times 200 = \dfrac{200}{4} = 50\ ml\ of\ Sustacal$

    or

    RP: 100 : 200 :: 25 : X

          100 X = 5000

             X = 50 ml of Sustacal

or

DA: ml = $\dfrac{\overset{2}{\cancel{200}} \text{ ml} \times 25 \text{ } \cancel{\text{mg}}}{\underset{1}{\cancel{100}} \text{ } \cancel{\text{mg}} \times \quad 1} = 50$ ml

or

200 ml × 0.25 (25%) = 50 ml of Sustacal

Total amount − Amount of TF = Amount of water

   200 ml   −   50 ml   =   150 ml

50 ml of Sustacal + 150 ml of water

2. 225 ml of Pulmocare + 75 ml of water

3. BF: $\dfrac{D}{H} \times V = \dfrac{60}{100} \times 500 = \dfrac{30,000}{100} = 300$ ml of Ensure Plus

   or

RP: 100:500 :: 60:X

      100 X = 30,000

          X = 300 ml of Ensure Plus

   or

500 ml × 0.60 (60%) = 300 ml of Ensure Plus

Total amount − Amount of TF = Amount of water

   500 ml   −   300 ml   =   200 ml

300 ml of Ensure Plus + 200 ml of water

4. 120 ml of Osmolite + 280 ml of water

III Enteral Medications

1. *Step 1* BF: $\dfrac{D}{H} \times V = \dfrac{\overset{5}{\cancel{250}}}{\underset{1}{\cancel{50}}} \times 1 = 5$ ml

      or

      RP: H :V:: D :X

          50:1::250:X

        50 X = 250

           X = 5 ml

      or

      DA: no conversion factor

      ml = $\dfrac{1 \text{ ml} \times \overset{5}{\cancel{250}} \text{ } \cancel{\text{mg}}}{\underset{1}{\cancel{50}} \text{ } \cancel{\text{mg}} \times \quad 1} = 5$ ml

Step 2 $\dfrac{\text{Known mOsm (2250)}}{\text{Desired mOsm (500)}} \times$ Volume of drug (5) =

      BF: $\dfrac{2250}{500} \times 5$ ml = 22.5 ml

Step 3 Total volume of liquid (22.5) − Volume of drug (5) = 17.5 ml liquid (water)

      Total: 22.5 ml to be administered (17.5 ml liquid + 5 ml drug = 22.5 ml)

2. *Step 1* BF: $\dfrac{D}{H} \times V = \dfrac{\overset{2}{\cancel{400/80}}}{\underset{1}{\cancel{200/40}}} \times 5 = 10$ ml

   or

   RP: H   : V ::   D   : X

   200\40 : 5 :: 400/80 : X

   200/40 X = 2000/400

   $X = \dfrac{\overset{10}{\cancel{2000/400}}}{\underset{1}{\cancel{200/40}}} = 10$ ml

   or

   DA: ml $= \dfrac{5 \text{ ml} \times 400 \text{ m\cancel{g}}}{80 \text{ m\cancel{g}} \times \quad 1} = 10$ ml

   Step 2 $\dfrac{\text{Known mOsm (2200)}}{\text{Desired mOsm (500)}} \times$ Volume of drug (10)

   $= \dfrac{2200}{500} \times 10 = 44$ ml (liquid and drug)

   Step 3 Total volume of liquid (44 ml) − Volume of drug (10 ml) = 34 ml liquid (water)

3. *Step 1* BF: $\dfrac{D}{H} \times V = \dfrac{\overset{2}{\cancel{40}}}{\underset{1}{\cancel{20}}} \times 15 = 30$ ml

   or

   RP: H   :   V   ::   D   : X

   20 mEq : 15 ml :: 40 mEq : X

   20 X = 600

   X = 30 ml

   or

   DA: ml $= \dfrac{15 \text{ ml} \times \overset{2}{\cancel{40}} \text{ mEq}}{\underset{1}{\cancel{20}} \text{ mEq} \times \quad 1} = 30$ ml

   Step 2 $\dfrac{\text{Known mOsm (3500)}}{\text{Desired mOsm (500)}} \times$ Volume of drug (30)

   $= \dfrac{3500}{500} \times 30 = 210$ ml (liquid and drug)

   Step 3 Total volume of liquid (210) − Volume of drug (30) = 180 ml liquid (water)

4. *Step 1* BF: $\dfrac{D}{H} \times V = \dfrac{\overset{}{\cancel{50}}}{\underset{2}{\cancel{20}}} \times 1 = 2.5$ ml

   or

   RP: H   :   V   ::   D   : X

   20 mg : 1 ml :: 50 mg : X

   20 X = 50

   X = 2.5 ml

   or

   DA: ml $= \dfrac{1 \text{ ml} \times 50 \text{ m\cancel{g}}}{20 \text{ m\cancel{g}} \times \quad 1} = \dfrac{50}{20} = 2.5$ ml

Step 2 $\dfrac{\text{Known mOsm (2050)}}{\text{Desired mOsm (500)}} \times$ Volume of drug (2.5) = 10.25 ml (liquid and drug)

Step 3 Total volume of liquid (10.25 ml) − Volume of drug (2.5 ml) = 7.75 ml liquid (water)

Additional practice problems are available on the enclosed CD-ROM in the "Basic Calculations" section.

Injectable Preparations With Clinical Applications

OBJECTIVES

- Select the correct syringe and needle for a prescribed injectable drug.
- Calculate dosages of drugs for subcutaneous and intramuscular routes from solutions in vials and ampules.
- Explain the procedure for preparing and calculating medications in powder form for injectable use.
- Determine prescribed insulin dosage in units using an insulin syringe.
- Explain the methods for mixing two insulin solutions in one insulin syringe and for mixing two injectable drugs in one syringe.
- Explain the various methods of insulin administration.
- State the various sites for intramuscular injection.
- Explain how to administer intradermal, subcutaneous, and intramuscular injections.

OUTLINE

Medications administered by injection can be given intradermally (under the skin), subcutaneously (SubQ, into fatty tissue), intramuscularly (IM, into the muscle), and intravenously (IV, into the vein). Intravenous injectables are discussed in Chapter 9. Injectable drugs are ordered in grams, milligrams, micrograms, grains, or units. Preparations of injectable drugs may be packaged in a solvent (diluent or solution) or in a powdered form.

This chapter is divided into five sections: (1) injectable preparations, such as vials, ampules, syringes, needles, and pre-filled cartridges; (2) intradermal injections; (3) subcutaneous injections, including heparin; (4) insulin injections; and (5) intramuscular injections from prepared liquid and reconstituted powder in vials and ampules and the mixing of drugs in a syringe. Examples and practice problems follow each section, and the answers to the practice problems are located at the end of the chapter.

NOTE: Answers should be rounded off in tenths or whole numbers.

INJECTABLE PREPARATIONS

Vials and Ampules

Drugs are packaged in vials (sealed rubber-top containers) for single and multiple doses and in ampules (sealed glass containers) for a single dose. Multiple-dose vials can be used more than once because of their self-sealing rubber top; however, ampules are used only once after the glass-necked container is opened. The drug is available in either liquid or powder form in vials and ampules. When drugs in solution deteriorate rapidly, they are packaged in dry form and solvent (diluent) is added before administration. If the drug is in powdered form, mixing instructions and dose equivalents such as milligrams (mg) per milliliter (ml) are usually given; if not, check the drug information insert. After the dry form of the drug is reconstituted with sterile water, bacteriostatic water, or saline solution, the drug must be used immediately or refrigerated. Usually, the reconstituted drug in the vial is used within 48 hours to 1 week; check the drug information insert. A vial and an ampule are shown in Figure 8-1.

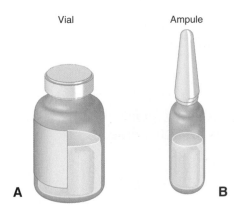

Vial   Ampule

A   B

FIGURE 8-1 A, Vial. **B,** Ampule. (From Kee, J. L., Hayes, E. R., & McCuistion, L. E. [2006]. *Pharmacology: A nursing process approach.* 5th ed. Philadelphia: W. B. Saunders.)

The route by which the injectable drug can be given, such as SubQ, IM, or IV, is printed on the drug label.

Syringes

Types of syringes used for injection include 3-ml and 5-ml calibrated syringes, metal and plastic syringes for pre-filled cartridges, tuberculin syringes, and insulin syringes. There are 10-ml, 20-ml, and 50-ml syringes that are used mostly for drug preparations. A syringe is composed of a barrel (outer shell), a plunger (inner part), and the tip, where the needle joins the syringe (Figure 8-2).

Three-Milliliter Syringe

The 3-ml syringe is calibrated in tenths (0.1 ml). The amount of fluid in the syringe is determined by the rubber end of the plunger that is closer to the tip of the syringe (Figure 8-3). An advance in safety needle technology is

FIGURE 8-2 Parts of a syringe.

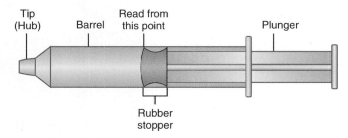

FIGURE 8-3 Three-milliliter syringes: **A**, 3-ml syringe with 0.1-ml markings. **B**, 3-ml syringe with a needle cover. **C**, 3-ml syringe with a protective cover over the needle after injection. (**B** and **C**, from Kee, J. L., Hayes, E. R., & McCuistion, L. E. [2006]. *Pharmacology: A nursing process approach.* 5th ed. Philadelphia: W. B. Saunders.)

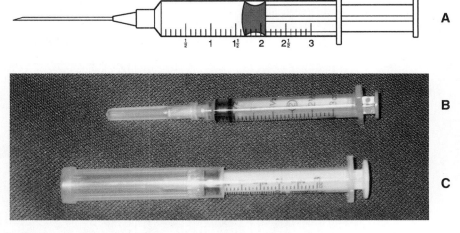

the SafetyGlide shielding hypodermic needle (Figure 8-4). The purpose of this type of needle is to reduce needlestick injuries.

Five-Milliliter Syringe

The 5-ml syringe is calibrated in 0.2 ml. A 5-ml syringe usually is used when the fluid needed is more than 2½ ml. This syringe is frequently used to reconstitute a dry drug form with sterile water, bacteriostatic water, or saline solution. Figure 8-5 shows the 5-ml syringe and its markings and the 5-ml needleless syringe.

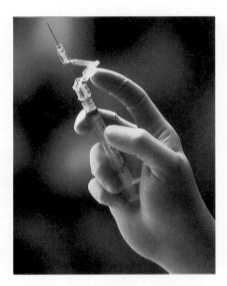

FIGURE 8-4 BD-SafetyGlide™ needle. (From Becton, Dickinson and Company, Franklin Lakes, NJ.)

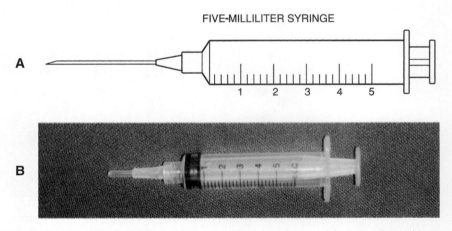

FIGURE 8-5 Five-milliliter syringes. **A,** 5-ml syringe with 0.2-ml markings. **B,** Needleless 5-ml syringe that can penetrate a rubber-top vial. (**B,** from Kee, J. L., Hayes, E. R., & McCuistion, L. E. [2006]. *Pharmacology: A nursing process approach.* 5th ed. Philadelphia: W. B. Saunders.)

Tuberculin Syringe

The tuberculin syringe is a 1-ml slender syringe that is calibrated in tenths (0.1 ml), hundredths (0.01 ml), and minims (Figure 8-6). This syringe is used when the amount of drug solution to be administered is less than 1 ml and for pediatric and heparin dosages. The tuberculin syringe is also available in a $^1/_2$-milliliter (ml) syringe. Figure 8-7 shows the ½-ml and the 1-ml tuberculin syringes.

Insulin Syringe

The insulin syringe has a capacity of 1 ml. Insulin is measured in units, and insulin dosage *must NOT* be calculated in milliliters. Insulin syringes are calibrated as 2 units per mark, and 100 units equal 1 ml (Figure 8-8). *Insulin syringes, NOT tuberculin syringes, must be used for administering insulin.* Insulin syringes are available in $^3/_{10}$-ml, ½-ml, and 1-ml sizes. The 1-ml insulin syringe may be purchased with a permanently attached needle or detachable needle (Figure 8-9).

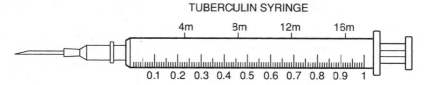

FIGURE 8-6 Tuberculin syringe.

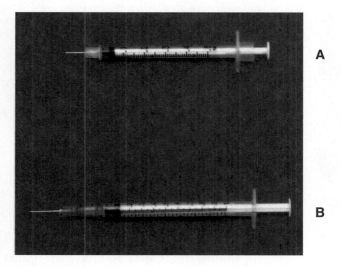

FIGURE 8-7 Two types of tuberculin syringes: **A,** ½-ml tuberculin syringe with a permanently attached needle. **B,** 1-ml tuberculin syringe with a detachable needle. (From Becton, Dickinson and Company, Franklin Lakes, NJ.)

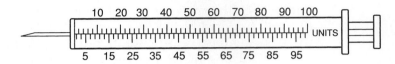

FIGURE 8-8 Insulin syringe.

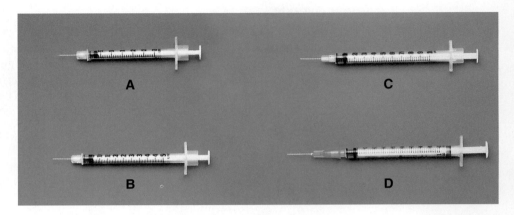

FIGURE 8-9 Four types of insulin syringes: **A,** ³⁄₁₀-ml insulin syringe with a permanently attached needle. **B,** ½-ml insulin syringe with a permanently attached needle. **C,** 1-ml insulin syringe with a permanently attached needle. **D,** 1-ml insulin syringe with a detachable needle. (From Becton, Dickinson and Company, Franklin Lakes, NJ.)

Pre-Filled Drug Cartridge and Syringe

Many injectable drugs are packaged in pre-filled disposable cartridges. The disposable cartridge is placed into a reusable metal or plastic holder. A pre-filled cartridge usually contains 0.1 to 0.2 ml of excess drug solution. On the basis of the amount of drug to be administered, the excess solution must be expelled before administration. Injectables are also supplied by pharmaceutical companies in ready-to-use pre-filled syringes that do not require a holder. Figure 8-10, *A,* shows a Carpuject syringe. Figure 8-10, *B,* shows a Tubex syringe.

Needles

A needle consists of (1) a hub (large metal or plastic part attached to the tip of the syringe), (2) a shaft (thin needle length), and (3) a bevel (end of the needle). Figure 8-11 shows the parts of a needle.

Needle size is determined by gauge (diameter of the lumen) and by length. The larger the gauge number, the smaller the diameter of the lumen. The smaller the gauge number, the larger the diameter of the lumen. The usual range of needle gauges is from 18 to 26. Needle length varies from ³⁄₈ inch to 2 inches. Table 8-1 lists the sizes and lengths of needles used in intradermal, subcutaneous, and intramuscular injections.

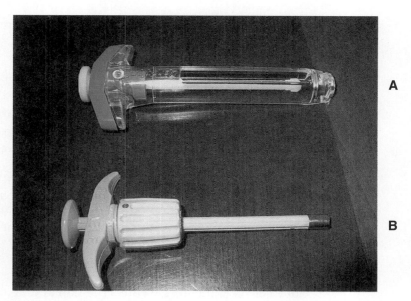

FIGURE 8-10 **A,** Carpuject syringe. **B,** Tubex syringe. (From Kee, J. L., Hayes, E. R., & McCuistion, L. E. [2006]. *Pharmacology: A nursing process approach.* 5th ed. Philadelphia: W. B. Saunders.)

PARTS OF A NEEDLE

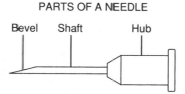

FIGURE 8-11 Parts of a needle. (From Kee, J. L., Hayes, E. R., & McCuistion, L. E. [2006]. *Pharmacology: A nursing process approach.* 5th ed. Philadelphia: W. B. Saunders.)

When choosing the needle length for an intramuscular injection, the nurse must consider the size of the patient and the amount of fatty tissue. A patient with minimal fatty tissue may need a needle length of 1 inch. For an obese patient, the length of the needle for an intramuscular injection may be 1½ to 2 inches.

Insulin syringes and pre-filled cartridges have permanently attached needles. With other syringes, needle sizes can be changed. Needle gauge and

TABLE 8-1

Needle Size and Length

Type of Injection	Needle Gauge	Needle Lengths (inch)
Intradermal	25, 26	⅜, ½, ⅝
Subcutaneous	23, 25, 26	⅜, ½, ⅝
Intramuscular	19, 20, 21, 22	1, 1½, 2

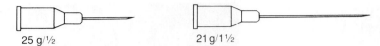

25 g/½   21 g/1½

FIGURE 8-12 Two combinations of needle gauge and length.

length are indicated on the syringe package or on the top cover of the syringe. These values appear as gauge/length, such as 21 g/1½ inch. Figure 8-12 shows two types of needle gauge and length.

Research has shown that after an injection, medication remains in the hub of the syringe, where the needle joins the syringe. This volume can be as much as 0.2 ml. There is controversy as to whether air should be added to the syringe before administration to ensure that the total volume is given. The best practice is to follow the institution's policy.

Angles for Injection

For injections, the needle enters the skin at different angles. Intradermal injections are given at a 10- to 15-degree angle; subcutaneous injections, at a 45- to 90-degree angle; and intramuscular injections, at a 90-degree angle. Figure 8-13 shows the angles for intradermal, subcutaneous, and intramuscular injections.

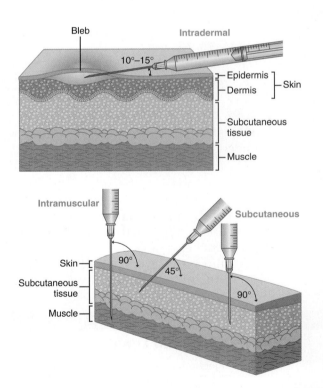

FIGURE 8-13 Angles of injection. (From Kee, J. L., Hayes, E. R., & McCuistion, L. E. [2006]. *Pharmacology: A nursing process approach.* 5th ed. Philadelphia: W. B. Saunders.)

PRACTICE PROBLEMS: I Needles

Answers can be found on pages 202 to 203.

1. Which would have the larger needle lumen: a 21-gauge needle or a 25-gauge needle? _____

2. Which would have the smaller needle lumen: an 18-gauge needle or a 26-gauge needle? _____

3. Which needle would have a length of 1½ inches: a 20-gauge needle or a 25-gauge needle? _____

4. Which needle would have a length of ⅝ inch: a 21-gauge needle or a 25-gauge needle? _____

5. Which needle would be used for an intramuscular injection: a 21-gauge needle with a 1½-inch length or a 25-gauge needle with a ⅝-inch length? _____

INTRADERMAL INJECTIONS

Usually, an intradermal injection is used for skin testing. Primary uses are for tuberculin and allergy testing. The tuberculin syringe (25 g/½ inch) holds 1 ml (16 minims) and is calibrated in 0.1 to 0.01 ml.

The inner aspect of the forearm is often used for diagnostic testing because there is less hair in the area and the test results are easily seen. The upper back can also be used as a testing site. The needle is inserted with the bevel upward at a 10- to 15-degree angle. Do not aspirate. Test results are read 48 to 72 hours after the intradermal injection. A reddened or raised area indicates a positive reaction.

SUBCUTANEOUS INJECTIONS

Drugs injected into the subcutaneous (fatty) tissue are absorbed slowly because there are fewer blood vessels in the fatty tissue. The amount of drug solution administered subcutaneously is generally 0.5 to 1 ml at a 45-, 60-, or 90-degree angle. Irritating drug solutions are given intramuscularly because they could cause sloughing of the subcutaneous tissue.

The two types of syringes used for subcutaneous injection are the tuberculin syringe (1 ml), which is calibrated in 0.1 and 0.01 ml, and the 3-ml syringe, which is calibrated in 0.1 ml (Fig. 8-14). The needle gauge commonly used is 25 or 26 gauge, and the length is usually ⅜ to ⅝ inch. Insulin is also administered subcutaneously and is discussed later in this chapter.

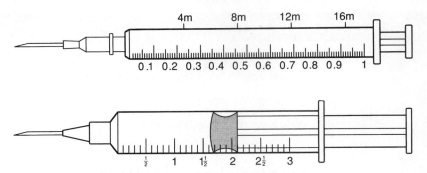

FIGURE 8-14 Syringes used for subcutaneous injections.

Calculations for Subcutaneous Injections

Formulas for solving problems of subcutaneous injections are the basic formula, ratio and proportion, fractional equation, and dimensional analysis (see Chapter 5). The following problems are examples of injections that can be given subcutaneously.

EXAMPLES

PROBLEM 1: Order: heparin 5000 units, subQ.
Drug available:

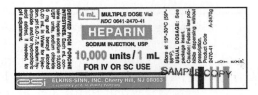

Methods:

Basic formula (BF)

$$\frac{D}{H} \times V = \frac{5000}{10,000} \times 1 = \frac{5}{10} = 0.5 \text{ ml}$$

or

Ratio and proportion (RP)

$$H \quad : \quad V \quad :: \quad D \quad : \quad X$$
$$10,000 \text{ units}:1 \text{ ml} :: 5000 \text{ units}:X \text{ ml}$$

$$10,000 \text{ X} = 5000$$

$$X = \frac{5000}{10,000} = \frac{5}{10} = 0.5 \text{ ml}$$

or

Fractional equation (FE)

$$FE: \frac{H}{V} \times \frac{D}{X} = \frac{10,000}{1} \times \frac{5000}{x} =$$
(Cross multiply) $10,000 \text{ X} = 5,000$
$$X = 0.5 \text{ ml}$$

Dimensional analysis (DA)

$$V = \frac{V \times C(H) \times D}{H \times C(D) \times 1}$$

$$ml = \frac{1\ ml \times \overset{1}{\cancel{5,000}}\ units}{\underset{2}{\cancel{10,000}}\ units \times 1} = \frac{1}{2}\ or\ 0.5\ ml$$

Answer: Heparin 5000 units = 0.5 ml

PROBLEM 2: Order: morphine 10 mg, subQ.
Drug available:

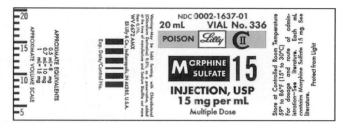

See label with approximate equivalents.

Methods: BF: $\dfrac{D}{H} \times V = \dfrac{10}{15} \times 1 = \dfrac{2}{3} = 0.67$ ml or 0.7 ml (round off in tenths)

or
RP: H : V :: D : X
15 mg : 1 ml :: 10 mg : X ml

15 X = 10

$$X = \frac{\overset{2}{\cancel{10}}}{\underset{3}{\cancel{15}}} = \frac{2}{3} = 0.67\ ml\ or\ 0.7\ ml$$

or
FE: $\dfrac{H}{V} \times \dfrac{D}{X} = \dfrac{15}{1} \times \dfrac{10}{X} =$

(Cross multiply) 15X = 10

$$X = \frac{10}{15} = \frac{2}{3} =$$
0.67 or 0.7

or
DA: no conversion factor

$$ml = \frac{1\ ml \times \overset{2}{\cancel{10}}\ mg}{\underset{3}{\cancel{15}}\ mg \times 1} = \frac{2}{3}\ or\ 0.7\ ml$$

Answer: Morphine 10 mg = 0.67 or 0.7 ml (use a tuberculin syringe or a 3-ml syringe) (Round off in tenths.)

PRACTICE PROBLEMS: II Subcutaneous Injections

Answers can be found on pages 203 to 204.

Use the formula you chose for calculating oral drug dosages in Chapter 7.

1. Which needle gauge and length should be used for a subcutaneous injection:

   a. 25 g/⅝ inch or 26 g/⅜ inch? _____

2. Order: heparin 4000 units, subQ.
   Drug available:

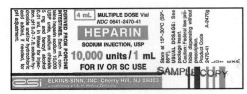

   a. How many milliliters of heparin would you give? _____

   b. At what angle would you administer the drug? _____

3. Order: heparin 7500 units, subQ.
   Drug available:

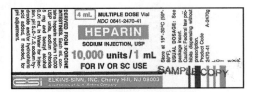

How many milliliters of heparin would you give? _____

4. Order: Lovenox (enoxaparin sodium) 30 mg, subQ, q12h. Lovenox is a low-molecular-weight heparin (LMWH).

   Drug available:

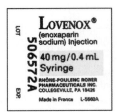

How many milliliters would you give? _____

5. Order: atropine sulfate gr $\frac{1}{100}$, subQ.
   Drug available:

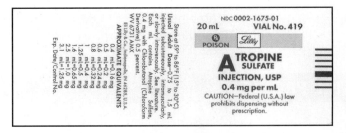

How many milliliters of atropine would you give? _____

6. Order: epoetin alfa (Epogen) 50 units/kg subQ.
   Drug available: Epogen 10,000 units/ml.
   Patient weighs 65 kg.

   a. What is the correct dosage? _____

   b. How many milliliters would you give?_____

7. Order: filgrastim (Neupogen) 6 mcg/kg subQ bid.
   Drug available: Neupogen 300 mcg/ml.
   Patient weighs 198 pounds.

   a. How many kilograms does the patient weigh? _____

   b. How many micrograms (mcg) would you give? _____

   c. How many milliliters would you give?_____

   d. Explain how the drug should be drawn up. _____

INSULIN INJECTIONS

Insulin is prescribed and measured in USP units. Most insulins are manufactured in concentrations of 100 units per milliliter. Insulin should be administered with an insulin syringe, which is calculated to correspond with the units 100 insulin. Insulin bottles and syringes are color-coded. The units 100 insulin bottle and the units 100 syringe are color-coded orange.

The insulin syringe may be marked on one side in even units (10, 20, 30) and on the other side in odd units (5, 15, 25, etc.).

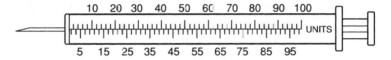

Insulin is easy to prepare and administer as long as the nurse uses the *same insulin concentration with the same calibrated insulin syringe,* e.g., a units 100 insulin bottle and a units 100 insulin syringe. For example, if the prescribed insulin dosage is 30 units, withdraw 30 units from a bottle of units 100 insulin using a units 100–calibrated insulin syringe.

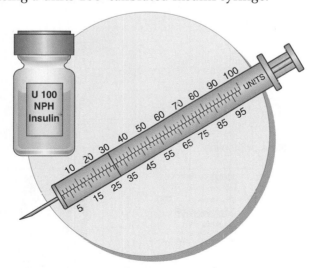

AVOID administering insulin with a tuberculin syringe.

TYPES OF INSULIN

Insulin is categorized as fast-acting, intermediate-acting, long-acting, and commercial premixed insulin. The following drug labels are arranged according to insulin action.

A, Fast-acting insulins

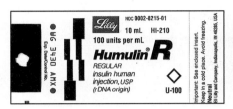
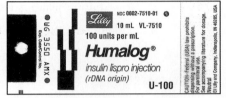

B, Intermediate-acting insulins

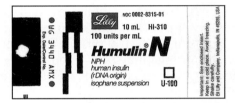

C, Long-acting insulin

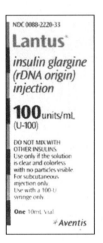

D, Selected combinations of insulins

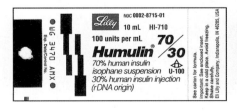
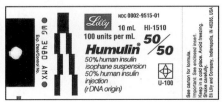

E, Selected insulins for pen injections

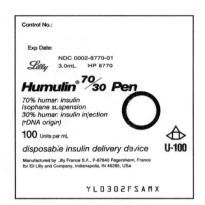
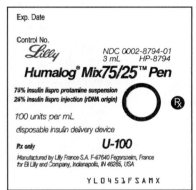

Insulins are clear (regular or crystalline insulin) or cloudy (NPH) because of the substances (protamine and zinc) used to prolong the action of insulin in the body. Only regular insulin can be given intravenously as well as subcutaneously. Insulin that contains protamine and zinc can be administered only subcutaneously.

A fast-acting insulin that was approved for use in 1996 is lispro insulin (Humalog). Lispro insulin acts faster than regular insulin and thus can be administered 5 minutes before mealtime, whereas regular insulin is given 30 minutes before meals. Lispro insulin is formed by reversing two amino acids in human regular insulin (Humulin).

The new long-acting insulin is Lantus, an insulin glargine that is an analog of human insulin. Lantus is the first long-acting recombinant DNA (rDNA) human insulin for clients with type 1 and 2 diabetes mellitus. It is a clear, colorless insulin that is to be given subcutaneously only and NOT intravenously. It CANNOT be mixed with other insulins. The Lantus vial is taller and narrower than the other types of insulin. It has a purple top and purple writing on the label (Figure 8-15, Lantus vial). It is usually administered at bedtime; incidence of noctural hypoglycemia is not as common as

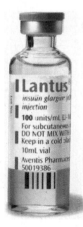

FIGURE 8-15 Lantus (insulin glargine) vial. (From Sanofi-Aventis U. S. Inc., Bridgewater, N. J.)

with other insulins. Some patients report more pain at the site when Lantus is used as compared with Humulin N insulin.

The use of commercially premixed combination insulins has become popular for the patient with diabetes who mixes fast-acting and intermediate-acting insulins. Examples of combination insulins are Humulin 70/30, Novolin 70/30, and Humulin 50/50. The Humulin 70/30 vial contains 70% human insulin isophane and 30% human (regular) insulin; the Humulin 50/50 vial contains 50% human insulin isophane and 50% human (regular) insulin. Humulin 70/30 may come in vials or pre-filled cartridge pens (Figure 8-16). The exterior of the insulin pen resembles a fountain pen (Figure 8-17). Some people need less than 30% regular (Humulin R) insulin and more isophane (Humulin N) insulin; they will need to mix the two insulins together.

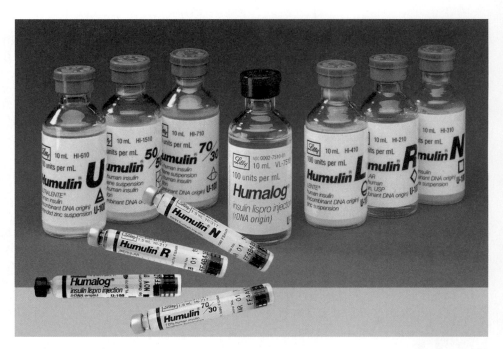

FIGURE 8-16 Insulin vials and cartridges used in insulin pens. Humulin® L Lente® and Humulin® U Ultralente® have been discontinued and are no longer available. Please see *www.lillydiabetes.com* for more information. Humulin® is a registered trademark of Eli Lilly and Company. Lente® and Ultralente® are registered trademarks of Novo Nordisk Pharmaceuticals. (Copyright Eli Lilly and Company. All rights reserved. Used with permission.)

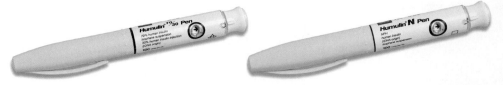

FIGURE 8-17 Insulin pens. (Copyright Eli Lilly and Company. All rights reserved. Used with permission.)

Many individuals have been allergic to beef insulin, so in 1998, beef insulin was no longer manufactured. Pork insulin was more frequently prescribed because it has biologic properties similar to those of human insulin. Since December 2005, pork insulin is no longer available in the United States. Some patients may be importing it. Today, the types of insulin used are Humulin R and N. Also, combinations of Humulin R and N (isophane) may be prescribed for use with an insulin syringe or an insulin pen.

Table 8-2 lists the insulins according to categories of insulin action.

TABLE 8-2
Insulin

Generic (Brand)	Route and Dosage	Pregnancy Category	Half-Life	Protein-Binding	Action		
					Onset	Peak	Duration
Rapid-Acting							
Lispro (Humalog)	A: subQ: 5-10 units; dose individualized	B	<13 hr	UK	5 min	0.5-1 hr	2-4 hr
Short-Acting							
Humulin R	A & C: subQ/IV: 100 units/ml; dose is individualized according to blood sugar	B	10 min-1 hr	UK	0.5-1 hr	2-4 hr	6-8 hr
Intermediate-Acting							
Humulin N insulin	A & C: subQ: 100 units/ml; dose is individualized according to blood sugar	B	13 hr	UK	1-2 hr	8-12 hr	18-24 hr
Long-Acting							
Lantus (insulin glargine)	Dose individualized	C	UK	UK	UK	UK	24 hr
Combinations							
Humulin 70/30 (70% human insulin isophane; 30% human insulin)	Dose individualized	B	13 hr	UK	0.5 hr	4-8 hr	22-24 hr
Humulin 50/50 (50% human insulin isophane; 50% human insulin)	Dose individualized	B	13 hr	UK	0.5 hr	4-8 hr	24 hr
Exubera (human insulin)	Inhalation powder	B	UK	UK	10 min	30-90 min	varies

A, Adult; C, child; hr, hour; IV, intravenous; min, minute; subQ, subcutaneous; UK, unknown; <, less than.
Modified from Kee, J. L., Hayes, E. R., & McCuistion, L. E. (2006). *Pharmacology: A nursing process approach.* 5th ed. Philadelphia: W. B. Saunders.

Insulin is administered subcutaneously at a 45-, 60-, or 90-degree angle into the subcutaneous tissue. The angle for administering insulin depends on the amount of fatty tissue in the patient. For a very thin person, a 45-degree angle is suggested. A 90-degree angle should be used on obese or average-sized persons. When a 90-degree angle is used, the skin should be pinched upward so the insulin is deposited into the fatty tissue.

MIXING INSULINS

Regular insulin is frequently mixed with insulins containing protamine, such as Humulin N.

EXAMPLES

Problem and method for mixing insulin.

PROBLEM 1: Order: Humulin R insulin units 10 and Humulin N insulin units 40, subQ.
Drug available: Humulin R insulin units 100 and Humulin N insulin units 100, both in multidose vials. The insulin syringe is marked units 100.

Methods:

1. Cleanse the rubber tops with alcohol. Gently roll insulin bottles between palms to evenly distribute the insulin solution.

2. Draw up 40 units of air* and inject into the Humulin N insulin bottle. Do not allow the needle to come into contact with the Humulin R insulin solution. Withdraw the needle.

3. Draw up 10 units of air and inject into the Humulin R insulin bottle.

4. Withdraw 10 units of Humulin R insulin. Humulin R insulin is withdrawn before Humulin N insulin.

5. Withdraw 40 units of Humulin N insulin.

6. Administer the two insulins immediately after mixing. Do not allow the insulin mixture to stand, because unpredicted physical changes might occur.

PRACTICE PROBLEMS: III Insulin

Answers can be found on page 204.

1. Order: Humulin N insulin 35 units, subQ.
   Drug available: Humulin N insulin units 100 and units 100 insulin syringe.
   Indicate on the insulin syringe the amount of insulin that should be withdrawn.

---

*You may draw up 50 units of air; inject 40 units into the NPH bottle and 10 units into the regular insulin bottle.

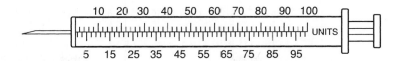

2. Order: Humulin L insulin 50 units, subQ.
Drug available: Humulin L insulin units 100 and units 100 insulin syringe.
Indicate on the insulin syringe the amount of insulin that should be withdrawn.

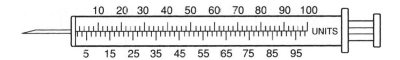

3. Order: Humulin R insulin units 8 and Humulin N insulin units 52.
Drug available: Humulin R insulin units 100 and Humulin N insulin units 100.
The insulin syringe is units 100.
Explain the method for mixing the two insulins.

_____

Indicate on the units 100 insulin syringe how much Humulin R insulin should be withdrawn and how much Humulin N insulin should be withdrawn.

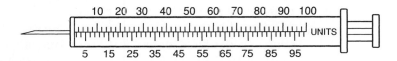

4. Order: Humulin R insulin units 15 and Humulin N insulin units 45.
Drug available: Humulin R insulin units 100 and Humulin N insulin units 100.
The insulin syringe is units 100.
Explain the method for mixing the two insulins.

_____

Indicate on the units 100 insulin syringe how much Humulin R insulin and how much Humulin N insulin should be withdrawn.

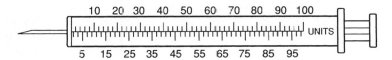

Insulin Pen Injectors

As was stated before, an insulin pen resembles a fountain pen. The pen contains disposable needles and an insulin-filled cartridge. Pens come in two types: pre-filled and reusable. Actually, the purpose of the insulin pen is to deliver an insulin dose more accurately than the traditional units 100 syringe and vial. Insulin pen injectors have been used in Europe and now are frequently used in the United States.

When the insulin pen is used, the amount of insulin that is desired is obtained by turning the dial to the number of insulin units needed. The capacity of the pre-filled or reusable insulin pen is 150 to 300 units or 1.5 to 3 ml of the combination of insulins. The new long-acting insulin product, Lantus, can be administered with the insulin pen injector. However, both Humalog and Lantus are more expensive.

The use of insulin pens may enhance the patient's compliance with the insulin regimen. For work or travel, the patient may find use of the insulin pen more convenient. With insulin pens, many patients state that there is less injection pain than with the traditional insulin syringe.

Insulin Inhalation (Exubera)

Exubera® is the first inhaled insulin that has been approved by the FDA to help in the control of diabetes mellitus. This type of insulin should be used by nonsmokers, those who have stopped smoking for 6 months, and those who do not have an unstable or poorly controlled lung disease, such as COPD.

The patient inhales the insulin powder 10 minutes before meals. The Exubera® kit contains the inhaler, chamber, two (2) release units, and blister packs of 1 mg and 3 mg insulin powder. The blue handle is on the side of the inhaler (Figures 8-18 and 8-19). Follow these steps when using the inhaler:
1. Pull the handle out of the chamber using the black pull ring at the bottom of the base and listen for the "click."
2. Place the blister pack into the inhaler with the packet containing the insulin powder faced down. Load only one blister pack.
3. Pull out the blue handle from the bottom of the handle.
4. Squeeze the handle firmly until it snaps shut; this will put pressure on the system.
5. Press the blue button until it clicks. A cloud of insulin powder will fill the chamber. The mouthpiece should have been closed.
6. Open the mouthpiece and inhale immediately, taking a normal deep breath and holding your breath for 5 seconds.
7. Turn the mouthpiece to its closed position.
8. Press the gray button to release the used blister pack.
9. Squeeze the chamber release buttons located on both sides of the base at the same time; then push the base back into the chamber.

The blister packets come in 1-mg and 3-mg sizes. Three 1-mg blister packs do NOT equal a 3-mg blister pack; otherwise the patient would receive too much insulin. The Exubera® blisters should be stored at room temperature. Do NOT expose the blisters to excess heat or put the blisters into the freezer. No batteries are required for this device. The inhaler should be cleaned at least once a week, and the device should *never* be put into the dishwasher.

See Figure 8-20 as an example of how Exubera is used.

Insulin Jet Injectors

Insulin jet injectors administer insulin without a needle; the insulin goes directly through the skin into the fatty tissue. Because the insulin is given un-

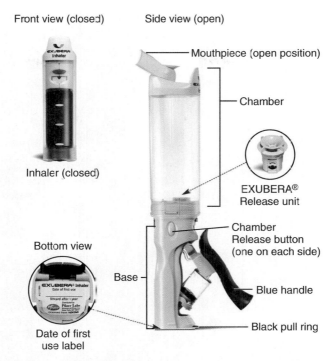

FIGURE 8-18 Exubera® insulin inhaler. (Used with permission from Pfizer, Inc.)

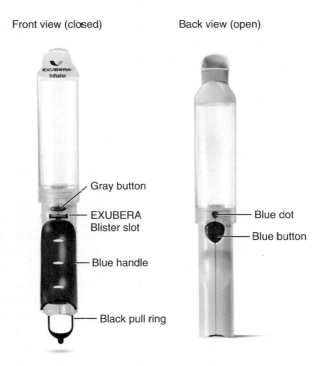

FIGURE 8-19 Front and back view of Exubera® insulin inhaler. (Used with permission from Pfizer, Inc.)

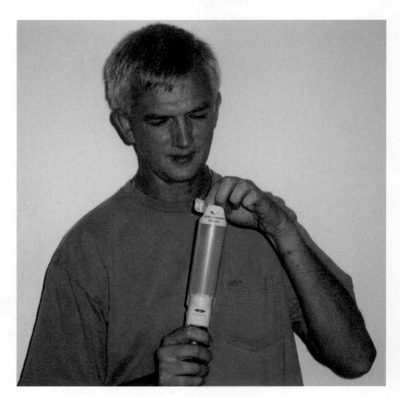

FIGURE 8-20 Patient using Exubera®, taking a deep breath.

der high pressure, stinging, burning, pain, and bruising may occur. This method of insulin administration is not recommended for children or older adults. Also, this method is more expensive than the subcutaneous technique.

Insulin Pumps

There are two types of insulin pumps: the implantable and the portable. The implantable insulin pump is surgically implanted in the abdomen and delivers a basal insulin infusion and bolus doses with meals either intravenously or intraperitoneally. With implantable insulin pumps, there are fewer hypoglycemic reactions, and blood glucose levels are mostly controlled.

Portable (external) insulin pumps, also called *continuous subcutaneous insulin infusion (CSII)*, have been available since 1983. The portable (external) insulin pump keeps blood glucose (sugar) levels as close to normal as possible. The insulin pump is a battery-operated device that administers regular insulin, which is stored in a reservoir syringe placed inside the device. The device is the size of a "cell phone" and weighs about 3.5 ounces. Infusions are programmed by the patient to (1) infuse insulin at a set basal rate of units per hour, (2) deliver bolus infusions to cover meals (the patient pushes a button to deliver a bolus dose at meals), (3) change delivery rates at specific times of the day (e.g., from 3:00 AM to 9:00 AM) to avoid early morning hyperglycemia, and (4) override the set basal rate to allow for unexpected changes in activity, such as early morning exercise.

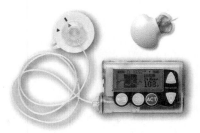

FIGURE 8-21 Medtronic Paradigm REAL-Time System. (From Medtronic, Inc., Minneapolis, MN.)

Insulin is delivered from the device through plastic tubing that is attached to a metal or plastic needle and placed subcutaneously by the patient. The needle can be inserted into the abdomen, upper thigh, or upper arm. Only regular insulin is used; protamine insulin such as Humulin N is not used because of unpredictable control of blood sugars. The pump can deliver small amounts of insulin such as 0.1 or 0.2 units much more accurately than a traditional insulin syringe.

The ongoing insulin delivery system helps to decrease the risk of a severe hypoglycemic reaction and maintains glucose control. However, glucose levels should still be monitored at least daily with or without an insulin pump. The person with type 1 diabetes mellitus receives the greatest benefit from the use of the insulin pump. This method should reduce the number of long-term diabetic complications compared with the use of multiple injections of regular and modified types of insulins. Portable (external) insulin pumps are expensive.

Figure 8-21 shows an example of an insulin pump.

INTRAMUSCULAR INJECTIONS

The IM injection is a common method of administering injectable drugs. The muscle has many blood vessels (more than fatty tissue), so medications given by intramuscular injection are absorbed more rapidly than those given by subQ injection. The volume of solution for an IM injection is 0.5 to 3.0 ml, with the average being 1 to 2 ml. A volume of drug solution greater than 3 ml causes increased muscle tissue displacement and possible tissue damage. Occasionally, 5 ml of certain drugs, such as magnesium sulfate, may be injected into a large muscle, such as the dorsogluteal. Dosages greater than 3 ml are usually divided and are given at two different sites.

Needle gauges for IM injections containing thick solutions are 19 gauge and 20 gauge, and for thin solutions, 20 gauge to 21 gauge. IM injections are administered at a 90-degree angle. The needle length depends on the amount of adipose (fat) and muscle tissue; the average needle length is 1½ inches.

Common sites for IM injections are the deltoid, dorsogluteal, ventrogluteal, and vastus lateralis muscles. Figure 8-22 displays the sites for each muscle used with IM injection. Table 8-3 gives the volume for drug administration, common needle size, patient's position, and angle of injection for the four IM injection sites.

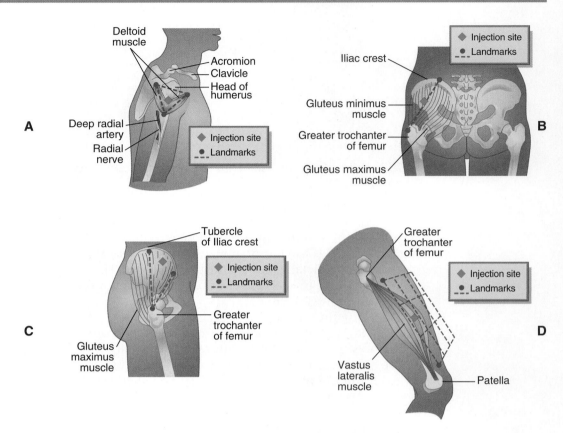

FIGURE 8-22 Intramuscular injection sites. **A**, Deltoid. **B**, Dorsogluteal. **C**, Ventrogluteal. **D**, Vastus lateralis. (From Kee, J. L., Hayes, E. R., & McCuistion, L. E. [2006]. *Pharmacology: A nursing process approach.* 5th ed. Philadelphia: W. B. Saunders.)

The discussion on intramuscular injection is divided into three subsections: (1) drug solutions for injection, (2) reconstitution of powdered drugs, and (3) mixing of injectable drugs. An example is given for each type, and practice problems follow.

Drug Solutions for Injection

Commercially premixed drug solutions are stored in vials and ampules for immediate use. At times, enough drug solution may be left in a vial for another dose, and the vial may be saved. The balance of a drug solution in an ampule is *always* discarded after the ampule has been opened and used.

EXAMPLES

Two problems are given as examples for calculating IM dosage. Choose one of the four methods for calculating drug dosage.

TABLE 8-3

Intramuscular Injection Sites in the Adult

	Deltoid	Dorsogluteal	Ventrogluteal	Vastus Lateralis
Volume for drug administration	*Usual:* 0.5-1 ml *Maximum:* 2.0 ml	*Usual:* 1.0-3 ml *Maximum:* 3 ml; 5 ml gamma globulin	*Usual:* 1-3 ml *Maximum:* 3-4 ml	*Usual:* 1-3 ml *Maximum:* 3-4 ml
Common needle size	23-25 gauge; ⅝-1½ inches	18-23 gauge; 1¼-3 inches	20-23 gauge; 1¼-2½ inches	20-23 gauge; 1¼-1½ inches
Patient's position	Sitting; supine; prone	Prone	Supine; lateral	Sitting (dorsiflex foot); supine
Angle of injection	90-degree angle, angled slightly toward the acromion	90-degree angle to flat surface; upper outer quadrant of the buttock *or* outer aspect of line from the posterior iliac crest to the greater trochanter of the femur	80-degree–90-degree angle; angle the needle slightly toward the iliac crest	80-degree–90-degree angle For thin person: 60-degree–75-degree angle

PROBLEM 1: Order: gentamycin (Garamycin) 60 mg, IM, q12h. Drug available:

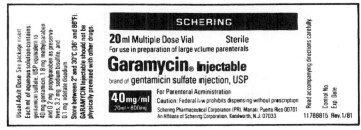

Methods: BF: $\dfrac{D}{H} \times V = \dfrac{60 \text{ mg}}{40 \text{ mg}} \times 1 \text{ ml} = \dfrac{3}{2}$

= 1.5 ml of gentamycin

or

RP: H : V :: D : X
40 mg:1 ml :: 60 mg:X ml
40X = 60
X = 1.5 ml

or

FE: $\dfrac{H}{V} = \dfrac{D}{X} = \dfrac{40 \text{ mg}}{1 \text{ ml}} \times \dfrac{60 \text{ mg}}{X} =$

(Cross multiply) 40 X = 60
X = 1.5 ml of gentamycin

or

DA: ml $= \dfrac{1 \text{ ml} \times \overset{3}{\cancel{60}} \text{ mg}}{\underset{2}{\cancel{40}} \text{ mg} \times 1} = \dfrac{3}{2}$

= 1.5 ml of gentamycin

Answer: gentamycin 60 mg = 1.5 ml

PROBLEM 2: Order: Naloxone 0.5 mg, IM, STAT.
Drug available:

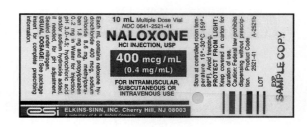

Methods: BF: $\dfrac{D}{H} \times V = \dfrac{0.5}{0.4} \times 1 = \dfrac{1.25 \text{ ml}}{0.4 \overline{)0.5\,00}}$

or

RP: H :V :: D :X

0.4 : 1 :: 0.5 : X

0.4 X = 0.5

X = 1.25 ml

or

DA: ml = $\dfrac{1 \text{ ml} \times \overset{10}{\cancel{1000}} \text{ mcg} \times 0.5 \text{ mg}}{\underset{4}{\cancel{400}} \text{ mcg} \times 1 \text{ mg} \times 1} = \dfrac{10 \times 0.5}{4} = \dfrac{5}{4} = 1.25$ ml

Answer: Naloxone 0.5 mg = 1.25 ml

Reconstitution of Powdered Drugs

Certain drugs lose their potency in liquid form. Therefore, manufacturers package these drugs in powdered form, and they are reconstituted before administration. To reconstitute a drug, look on the drug label or in the drug information insert (circular or pamphlet) for the type and amount of diluent to use. Sterile water, bacteriostatic water, and normal saline solution are the primary diluents. If the type and amount of diluent are not specified on the drug label or in the drug information insert, call the pharmacy.

The powdered drug occupies space and therefore increases the volume of drug solution. Usually, manufacturers determine the amount of diluent to mix with the drug powder to yield 1 to 2 ml per desired dose. After the powdered drug has been reconstituted, the unused drug solution should be dated, initialed, and refrigerated. Most drugs retain their potency for 48 hours to 1 week when refrigerated. Check the drug information insert or drug label to see how long the reconstituted drug may be used.

EXAMPLES

PROBLEM 1: Order: oxacillin sodium 500 mg, IM, q6h.
Drug available:

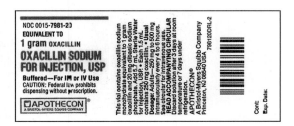

According to the label on the bottle, the amount of powdered drug in the vial is 1 g. The drug label states:

Add 5.7 ml of sterile water (diluent) to the vial. Each 250 mg = 1.5 ml or 1 g = 6 ml.

Methods: Change grams to milligrams or change milligrams to grams (see Table 5-1). 1 gram = 1000 mg *or* 500 mg = 0.500 g (0.5 g).

Move the decimal point three spaces to the left.

Milligrams

$$\text{BF:} \frac{D}{H} \times V = \frac{500}{1000} \times 6 \text{ ml} = \frac{3000}{1000} = 3 \text{ ml}$$

or
Grams
RP: H : V :: D : V
   1 g : 6 ml :: 0.5 g : X
        X = 3.0
        X = 3.0 ml

or
$$\text{FE:} \frac{H}{V} \times \frac{D}{X} = \frac{1 \text{ g}}{6 \text{ ml}} \times \frac{0.5 \text{ g}}{X}$$
$$X = 3.0 \text{ ml}$$

or
$$\text{DA: ml} = \frac{6 \text{ ml} \times \quad 1\,\cancel{g} \quad \times \overset{1}{\cancel{500}} \text{ mg}}{1\,\cancel{g} \times \underset{2}{\cancel{1000}} \text{ mg} \times \quad 1} = \frac{6}{2} = 3 \text{ ml}$$

Answer: oxacillin sodium 500 mg = 3 ml

PROBLEM 2: Order: nafcillin sodium 250 mg, IM, q6h.
Drug available:

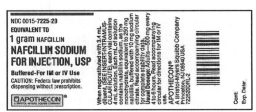

The drug label says to add 3.4 ml of sterile or bacteriostatic water. Each 4 ml contains 1 gram (1000 mg) of nafcillin.

Methods: BF: $\dfrac{D}{H} \times V = \dfrac{250}{1000} \times 4 \text{ ml} = \dfrac{1000}{1000} = 1 \text{ ml nafcillin}$

or

RP: H   : V   ::   D   : X
     1000 mg : 4 ml :: 250 mg : X
            $1000 X = 1000$
                 $X = \dfrac{1000}{1000}$
                 $= 1 \text{ ml of nafcillin}$

or

DA: $\text{ml} = \dfrac{4 \text{ ml} \times \quad 1 \cancel{g} \quad \times \cancel{250}^{1} \text{ mg}}{1 \cancel{g} \times \underset{4}{1000} \cancel{mg} \times \quad 1} = \dfrac{4}{4} = 1 \text{ ml of nafcillin}$

Answer: nafcillin 250 mg = 1 ml

MIXING OF INJECTABLE DRUGS

Drugs mixed together in the same syringe must be compatible to prevent precipitation. To determine drug compatibility, check drug references or check with a pharmacist. When in doubt about compatibility, do *not* mix drugs.

The three methods of drug mixing are (1) mixing two drugs in the same syringe from two vials, (2) mixing two drugs in the same syringe from one vial and one ampule, and (3) mixing two drugs in a pre-filled cartridge from a vial.

METHOD 1

Mixing Two Drugs in the Same Syringe From Two Vials

1. Draw air into the syringe to equal the amount of solution to be withdrawn from the first vial, and inject the air into the first vial. Do *not* allow the needle to come into contact with the solution. Remove the needle.
2. Draw air into the syringe to equal the amount of solution to be withdrawn from the second vial. Invert the second vial and inject the air.
3. Withdraw the desired amount of solution from the second vial.
4. Change the needle unless you will use the entire volume in the first vial.
5. Invert the first vial and withdraw the desired amount of solution.

or

1. Draw air into the syringe to equal the amount of solution to be withdrawn, and inject the air into the first vial. Withdraw the desired drug dose.
2. Insert a 25-g needle into the rubber top (not in the center) of the second vial. This acts as an air vent. Injecting air into the second vial is *not* necessary.
3. Insert the needle in the center of the rubber-top vial (beside the 25-g needle–air vent), invert the second vial, and withdraw the desired drug dose.

METHOD 2

Mixing Two Drugs in the Same Syringe From One Vial and One Ampule

1. Remove the amount of desired solution from the vial.
2. Aspirate the amount of desired solution from the ampule.

METHOD 3

Mixing Two Drugs in a Pre-filled Cartridge From a Vial

1. Check the drug dose and the amount of solution in the pre-filled cartridge. If a smaller dose is needed, expel the excess solution.
2. Draw air into the cartridge to equal the amount of solution to be withdrawn from the vial. Invert the vial and inject the air.
3. Withdraw the desired amount of solution from the vial. Make sure the needle remains in the fluid and do *not* take more solution than needed.

EXAMPLES

Mixing drugs in the same syringe.

PROBLEM 1: Order: meperidine (Demerol) 60 mg and atropine sulfate gr $\frac{1}{150}$, IM.
The two drugs are compatible.
Drugs available:

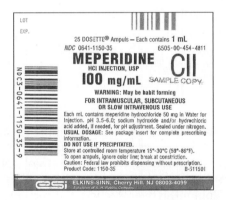

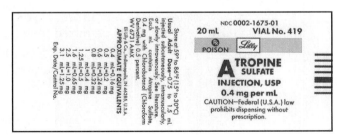

Note: Meperidine is in an ampule, and atropine sulfate is in a vial.

How many milliliters of each drug would you give? Explain how to mix the two drugs.

Methods: meperidine

$$BF: \frac{D}{H} \times V = \frac{60}{100} \times 1 = 0.6 \text{ ml}$$

or

RP: H : V :: D : X
     100 mg : 1 ml :: 60 mg : X ml
              100 X = 60
                   X = 0.6 ml

or

$$FE: \frac{H}{V} \times \frac{D}{X} = \frac{100 \text{ mg}}{1 \text{ ml}} \times \frac{60 \text{ mg}}{X}$$

(Cross multiply) 100 X = 60
                       X = 0.6 ml

or

DA: no conversion factor

$$ml = \frac{1 \text{ ml} \times 60 \text{ mg}}{100 \text{ mg} \times 1} = \frac{60}{100} = 0.6 \text{ ml}$$

atropine SO_4
gr $\frac{1}{150}$ = 0.4 mg (see Tables 2-1 and 5-1).

Answer: meperidine (Demerol) 60 mg = 0.6 ml
         atropine gr $\frac{1}{150}$ = 1 ml

Procedure: Mix two drugs in a syringe for IM injection:

1. Remove 1 ml of atropine solution from the vial.

2. Withdraw 0.6 ml of meperidine (Demerol) from the ampule into the syringe containing atropine solution.

3. Syringe contains atropine 1 ml and meperidine 0.6 ml = total 1.6 ml.

PROBLEM 2: Order: meperidine 25 mg, Vistaril 25 mg, and Robinul 0.1 mg, IM. All three drugs are compatible.
Drugs available: meperidine (Demerol) is in a 2-ml Tubex cartridge labeled 50 mg/ml. Hydroxyzine (Vistaril) is in a 50-mg/ml ampule. Glycopyrrolate (Robinul) is available in a 0.2-mg/ml vial.

How many milliliters of each drug would you give?
Explain how the drugs could be mixed together.

Methods:

a. meperidine 25 mg. Label: 50 mg/ml

$$BF: \frac{D}{H} \times V = \frac{25}{50} \times 1 = 0.5 \text{ ml}$$

or

RP: H : V :: D : X
     50 mg : 1 ml :: 25 mg : X ml
              50 X = 25
                  X = ½ ml or 0.5 ml

or

$$FE: \frac{H}{V} \times \frac{D}{X} = \frac{50 \text{ mg}}{1 \text{ ml}} \times \frac{25 \text{ mg}}{X}$$

(Cross multiply) 50 X = 25
                      X = 0.5 ml

or

$$DA: ml = \frac{1 \; ml \; \times \; \overset{1}{\cancel{25} \; \cancel{mg}}}{\underset{2}{\cancel{50}} \; \cancel{mg} \times \; 1} = \frac{1}{2} \; ml \text{ or } 0.5 \; ml \text{ meperidine}$$

b. Vistaril 25 mg. Label: 50 mg/ml ampule.

$$BF: \frac{D}{H} \times V = \frac{25}{50} \times 1 = 0.5 \; ml$$

or

$$FE: \frac{H}{V} \times \frac{D}{X} = \frac{50 \; mg}{1 \; ml} \times \frac{25 \; mg}{X}$$

$$50X = 25$$
$$X = 0.5 \; ml$$

or

RP: H : V ::   D : X
     50 mg : 1 ml :: 25 mg : X ml
              50 X = 25
                 X = ½ ml or 0.5 ml

or

DA: same as above 0.5 ml Vistaril

c. Robinul 0.1 mg. Label: 0.2 mg/ml.

$$BF: \frac{D}{H} \times V = \frac{0.1}{0.2} \times 1 = 0.5 \; ml$$

or

$$FE: \frac{H}{V} \times \frac{D}{X} = \frac{0.2 \; mg}{1 \; ml} \times \frac{0.1 \; ml}{X}$$

$$0.2 \; X = 0.1$$
$$X = 0.5 \; ml$$

or

RP: H : V ::   D : X
     0.2 mg : 1 ml :: 0.1 mg : X ml
              0.2 X = 0.1
                  X = 0.5 ml

or

$$DA: ml = \frac{1 \; ml \; \times \; 0.1 \; \cancel{mg}}{0.2 \; \cancel{mg} \times \; 1} = \frac{0.1}{0.2} = \frac{1}{2} \text{ or } 0.5 \; ml \text{ Robinul}$$

Answer: meperidine (Demerol) 25 mg = 0.5 ml; Vistaril 25 mg = 0.5 ml; Robinul 0.1 mg = 0.5 ml

Procedure: Mix three drugs in the cartridge:

1. Check drug dose and volume on pre-filled cartridge. Expel 0.5 ml of meperidine and any excess of drug solution from cartridge.

2. Draw 0.5 ml of air into the cartridge and inject into the vial containing the Robinul.

3. Withdraw 0.5 ml of Robinul from the vial into the pre-filled cartridge containing meperidine.

4. Withdraw 0.5 ml of Vistaril from the ampule into the cartridge.

PRACTICE PROBLEMS: IV Intramuscular Injections

Answers can be found on pages 205 to 210.

Round off to the nearest tenths.

1. Order: tobramycin (Nebcin) 50 mg, IM, q8h.
   Drug available:

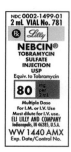

   How many milliliters of tobramycin would you give? _____

2. Order: methylprednisolone (Solu-Medrol) 75 mg, IM, daily.
   Drug available: 125 mg/2 ml in vial.

   How many milliliters would you give? _____

3. Order: vitamin B$_{12}$ (cyanocobalamin) 30 mcg, IM, daily.
   Drug available:

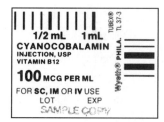

   How many milliliters of cyanocobalamin would you give?_____

4. Order: naloxone 0.2 mg, IM, STAT.
   Drug available:

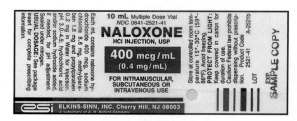

   How many milliliters would you give? _____

5. Order: cefepime HCl (Maxipime) 500 mg, IM, q12h.
   Drug available:

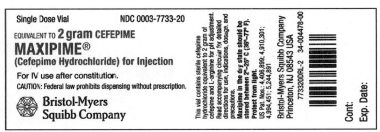

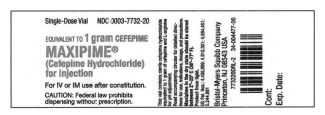

   a. Which single-dose vial of Maxipime would you select? _____

      Explain. _____

   b. How many milliliters (ml) of diluent should you use for reconstitution of

      the drug? _____

      Note: The drug label does not indicate the amount of diluent to use.
      This may be found in the drug information insert. Usually, if you inject
      2.6 ml of diluent, the amount of drug solution may be 3.0 ml. If you
      inject 3.4 or 3.5 ml of diluent, the amount of drug solution should be
      4.0 ml.

   c. How many milliliters of drug solution should the client receive? _____

6. Order: prochlorperazine (Compazine) 4 mg, IM, q8h, as needed.
   Drug available:

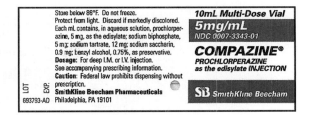

   How many milliliters should the patient receive? _____

7. Order: secobarbital (Seconal) 125 mg, IM, 1 hour before surgery.
   Drug available: Seconal 50 mg/ml.

   How many milliliters would you give? _____

8. Order: Thiamine HCl 75 mg, IM, daily.
   Drug available: 100 and 200 mg/ml vials.

   a. Which vial would you use? _____

   b. How many milliliters would you give?_____

9. Order: hydroxyzine (Vistaril) 25 mg, deep IM, STAT.
   Drug available: Vistaril 100 mg/2 ml in a vial.

   How many milliliters would you give? _____

10. Order: cefonicid (Monocid) 750 mg, IM, daily.
    Drug available:

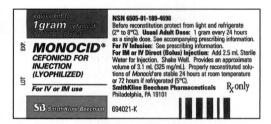

Change grams to milligrams (3 spaces to the right) or milligrams to gram (3 spaces to the left).

$$1.000 \text{ g} = 1000 \text{ mg or } 1000 \text{ mg} = 1 \text{ g}$$

   a. How many gram(s) is 750 mg, IM, daily? _____

   b. How many milliliters of diluent should be injected into the vial (see drug

      label)? _____

   c. How many milliliters of cefonicid (Monocid) should the patient receive per

      day? _____

11. Order: meperidine (Demerol) 35 mg and promethazine (Phenergan) 10 mg,
    IM.
    Drugs available: meperidine 50 mg/ml in an ampule; promethazine 25 mg/ml
    in an ampule.

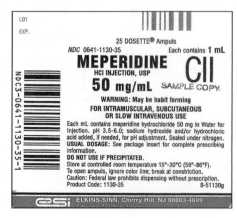

a. How many milliliters of meperidine would you give?_____

b. How many milliliters of promethazine would you give? _____

c. Explain how the two drugs should be mixed.

_____

12. Order: meperidine (Demerol) 50 mg and atropine sulfate 0.3 mg, IM.
Drugs available:

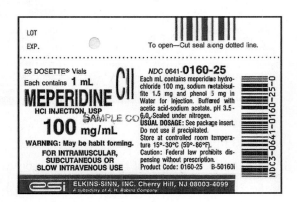
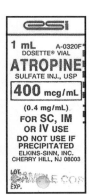

a. How many milliliters of meperidine would you give?_____

b. How many milliliters of atropine would you give? _____

c. Explain how the two drugs should be mixed.

_____

13. Order: tobramycin 50 mg, IM, q8h.
Drug available:

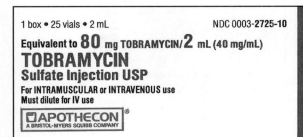

How many milliliters of tobramycin would you withdraw? _____

14. Order: heparin 2500 units, subQ, q6h.
Drug available:

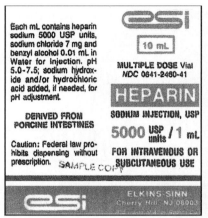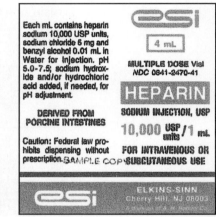

a. Which drug vial would you use? _____

b. How many milliliters of heparin would you give? _____

15. Order: chlordiazepoxide HCl (Librium) 50 mg, IM, STAT.
Drug available: 5 ml of dry Librium (100 mg) powder in ampule.
Add 2 ml of special intramuscular diluent to the ampule. When diluted, the powder content may increase the volume.

How many milliliters would be equivalent to 50 mg? _____

Explain. _____

16. Order: cefamandole (Mandol) 500 mg, IM, q6h.
Drug available:

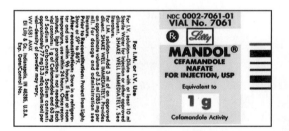

a. Change milligrams to grams (see Chapter 1).

_____

b. How many milliliters of diluent would you add (see drug label)?

_____

c. What size syringe would you use? _____

d. How many milliliters = 1 g; how many milliliters = 500 mg? _____

17. Order: ticarcillin (Ticar), 400 mg, IM, q6h.
Drug available:

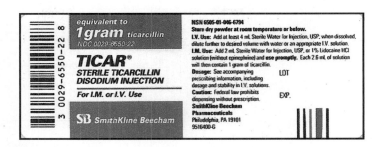

a. Drug label reads to add 2 ml of diluent. Total volume of solution is

_____

b. How many milliliters of ticarcillin should be withdrawn?_____

18. Order: morphine gr ⅙, IM, STAT.
Drug available:

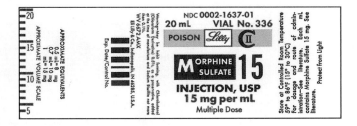

a. Change grains to milligrams (see Chapter 1 or Tables 2-1 and 5-1).

_____

b. How many milliliters of morphine would you give? _____

19. Order: Vistaril (hydroxyzine) 25 mg, deep IM, q4–6h, PRN for nausea.

Drug available:

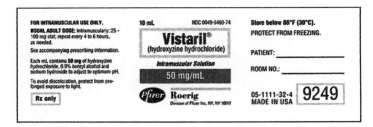

How many milliliters should the patient receive per dose? _____

20. Order: Decadron (dexamethasone) 2 mg, IM, q6h.

Adult Parameters: 0.75–9 mg/day in 2 to 4 divided doses.

Drug available:

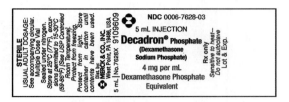

  a. Is the dose according to adult parameters? _____

  b. How many milliliters would you give? _____

  c. What type of syringe could be used? _____

  d. Can the Decadron vial be used again? _____

  Explain. _____

21. Order: ceftazidime (Fortaz) 500 mg, IM, q8h.
Add 2 ml of diluent = 2.6 ml drug solution. Check the drug information insert.
Drug available:

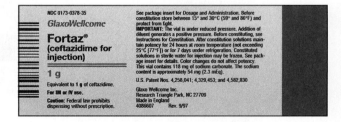

  a. How many gram(s) of ceftazidime (Fortaz) should the patient receive per

  day? _____

  b. How many milliliters of ceftazidime would you give per dose?

  _____

22. Order: ampicillin 0.25 g, IM, q6h.
Drug available:

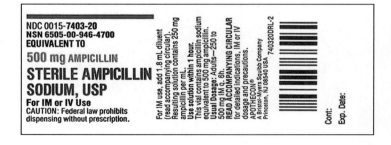

    a. To change grams to milligrams, move the decimal point 3 spaces to the

    _____ .

    b. How many milliliters of diluent would you add to the vial? _____

    c. How many milliliters should the patient receive per dose? _____

23. Order: diazepam 8 mg, IM, STAT and repeat in 4 hours if necessary.
Drug available:

    a. Which ampule or vial of diazepam would you select? _____

    b. How many milliliters (ml) of diazepam should the patient receive?

    _____

24. Order: benztropine mesylate (Cogentin) 1.5 mg, IM, daily.
Drug available:

How many milliliters (ml) of Cogentin should the patient receive?

_____

25. Order: interferon alfa-2b (Intron A) 10 million international units IM 3 × week.
Drug available: interferon alfa-2b (Intron A) 25 million international units/
5 ml vials.

How many milliliters would you give per dose? _____

26. Order: vitamin K (AquaMEPHYTON) 2.5 mg IM × 1.
Drug available:

How many milliliters would you give? _____

27. Order: Unasyn (ampicillin/sulbactam) 1 g, IM, q8h.
Drug available:
(add 3.6 ml of diluent to the vial; drug and diluent equals 4 ml)

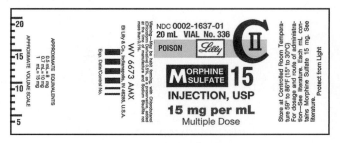

   a. Unasyn 3 g vial equals _____.

   b. How many milliliters of Unasyn would you give every 8 hours? _____

Questions 28 through 32 relate to additional dimensional analysis. Refer to Chapter 5.

28. Order: droperidol 2 mg, IM, STAT.
Drug available: droperidol 5 mg/2 ml.
Factors: 5 mg/2 ml; 2 mg/1
Conversion factor: *none;* order and drug are both available in milligrams.

How many milliliters of droperidol should be given?_____

29. Order: morphine sulfate ⅙ gr, IM, PRN.
Drug available:

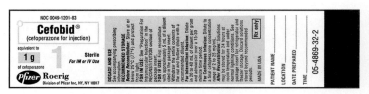

Conversion factor: 1 gr = 60 mg

How many milliliters of morphine would you give?_____

30. Order: cefobid 500 mg, IM, q6h.
Add 2 ml of diluent to equal 2.4 ml solution.
Drug available:

a. How many milliliters of diluent would you add?_____

      b. Cefobid 1 g = _____ ml; 500 mg = _____ ml

      Conversion factor: 1 g = 1000 mg

      c. How many milliliters of Cefobid would you give? _____

31. Order: oxacillin 300 mg, IM, q8h.
      Drug available:

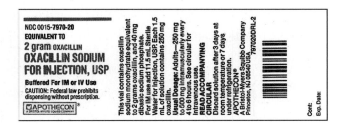

      a. Drug label and drug order: _____

      b. Conversion factor: _____

      c. How many milliliters of oxacillin would you give? _____

32. Order: cefazolin (Ancef) 0.25 g, IM, q12h.
      Drug available:

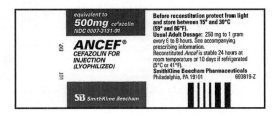

      Note: Change grams to milligrams; drug label is in milligrams.

      a. Label states to add _____ ml or _____ diluent.

      b. How many milliliters of Ancef would you give? _____

Questions 33 through 35 relate to drug dosage per body weight.

33. Order: amikacin (Amikin) 15 mg/kg/day, q8h, IM.
      Drug available:

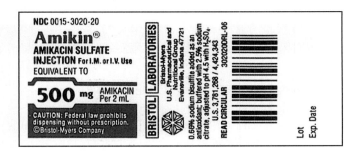

Patient weighs 140 pounds.

   a. How many kilograms does the patient weigh? _____

   b. How many milligrams should the patient receive daily? _____

   c. How many milligrams should the patient receive q8h (three divided

      doses)? _____

   d. How many milliliters should the patient receive q8h? _____

34. Order: netilmicin sulfate (Netromycin) 2 mg/kg, q8h, IM.
Patient weighs 174 pounds.
Drug available: netilmicin 100 mg/ml.

   a. How many kilograms does the patient weigh? _____

   b. How many milligrams should the patient receive daily? _____

   c. How many milligrams should the patient receive q8h?_____

   d. How many milliliters should the patient receive q8h? _____

35. Order: kanamycin (Kantrex) 15 mg/kg/day, q12h.
Drug available (drug is also available in 1 g = 3 ml vial):

Patient weighs 67 kg.

   a. How many milligrams should the patient receive per day?_____

   b. How many milligrams should the patient receive every 12 hours?

     _____

   c. How many milliliters should the patient receive per dose? _____

   d. How many milliliters from the 1 g = 3 ml vial should the patient receive

      per dose? _____

ANSWERS

I Needles

1. The 21-gauge needle because it is the smaller gauge number.

2. The 26-gauge needle because it is the larger gauge number.

3. The 20-gauge needle because it has the larger lumen (small gauge). A needle with a 20 gauge and 1½-inch length is used for IM injection.

4. The 25-gauge needle, because it has the smaller lumen (larger gauge). It is used for subQ injections. The needle is not long enough for an IM injection.

5. The 21-gauge needle with 1½-inch length (21 g/1½ inch). Muscle is under subcutaneous or fatty tissue, so a longer needle is needed.

II Subcutaneous Injections

1. *Both* needle gauge and length combinations could be used.

2. a. 0.4 ml

   b. 45- to 60-degree angle. The angle depends on the amount of fatty tissue in the patient.

3. ¾ ml or 0.75 ml

4. BF: $\dfrac{D}{H} \times V = \dfrac{\overset{3}{\cancel{30}} \text{ mg}}{\underset{4}{\cancel{40}} \text{ mg}} \times 0.4 \text{ ml} = \dfrac{1.2}{4}$

$= 0.3 \text{ ml of Lovenox}$

FE: $\dfrac{H}{V} \times \dfrac{D}{X} = \dfrac{40}{0.4} \times \dfrac{30}{X} =$

(Cross multiply) 40X = 12

$X = 0.3 \text{ ml of Lovenox}$

or

RP: H : V :: D : X

40 mg : 0.4 ml :: 30 mg : X ml

40 X = 12

X = 0.3 ml

or

DA ml $= \dfrac{0.4 \text{ ml} \times 30 \cancel{\text{mg}}}{40 \cancel{\text{mg}} \times 1} = \dfrac{12}{40} = 0.3 \text{ ml}$

5. Change grains (apothecary system) to milligrams (metric system). See Table 2-1. gr $\frac{1}{100} = 0.6$ mg.

BF: $\dfrac{D}{H} \times V = \dfrac{0.6}{0.4} \times 1 = \dfrac{0.6}{0.4} = 1.5 \text{ ml}$

or

RP: H : V :: D : X

0.4 mg : 1 ml :: 0.6 mg : X ml

0.4 X = 0.6

$X = \dfrac{0.6}{0.4} = 1.5 \text{ ml}$

or

DA: ml $= \dfrac{1 \text{ ml} \times 0.6 \cancel{\text{mg}}}{0.4 \cancel{\text{mg}} \times 1} = \dfrac{0.6}{0.4} = 1.5 \text{ ml}$

6. a. 50 units/kg × 65 kg = 3250 units

   b. $\dfrac{D}{H} \times V = \dfrac{3250}{10,000} \times 1 = 0.325 \text{ ml}$

   or

   H   :   V ::   D   : X

   10,000 units : 1 ml :: 3250 units : X

   10,000 X = 3250

   X = 0.325 ml

   Answer: Epogen 3250 units = 0.325 ml

   X = 0.325 ml or 0.33 ml

7. a. 198 lb ÷ 2.2 kg = 90 kg

   b. 90 kg × 6 mcg/kg = 540 mcg

c. $\dfrac{D}{H} \times V = \dfrac{540 \text{ mcg}}{300 \text{ mcg}} \times 1 \text{ ml} = 1.8 \text{ ml}$

Answer: Neupogen 540 mcg = 1.8 ml

d. Drug can be prepared in two syringes, one with 1 ml, and the other with 0.8 ml. With subcutaneous injections, one (1) ml is given per site unless the person weighs more than 200 lb, or the dose has been approved by the health care provider.

III Insulin

1. Withdraw 35 units of Humulin N insulin to the 35 mark on the insulin syringe. Both the insulin and the syringe have the same concentration: units 100.

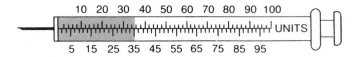

2. Withdraw 50 units of Humulin L insulin to the 50 mark on the insulin syringe. Both the insulin and the syringe have the same concentration: units 100.

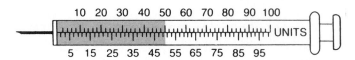

3. Inject 52 units of air into the Humulin N insulin bottle. Do not allow the needle to touch the insulin solution. Inject 8 units of air into the Humulin R insulin bottle and withdraw 8 units of Humulin R insulin. Withdraw 52 units of Humulin N insulin. Total amount of insulin should be 60 units. Do *not* allow the insulin mixture to stand. Administer immediately because Humulin N contains protamine, and unpredicted physical changes could occur with a delay in administration.

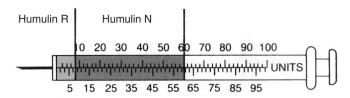

4. Inject 45 units of air into the Humulin N insulin bottle. Inject 15 units of air into the Humulin R insulin bottle and withdraw 15 units of Humulin R insulin. Withdraw 45 units of Humulin N insulin. Total amount of insulin should be 60 units.

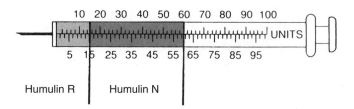

IV Intramuscular Injections

1. BF: $\dfrac{D}{H} \times V = \dfrac{50}{80} \times 2 \text{ ml} = \dfrac{100}{80} = 1.25 \text{ ml or } 1.3 \text{ ml}$

or

RP: H : V :: D : X
80 mg : 2 ml :: 50 mg : X ml

$$80 \text{ X} = 100$$

$$\text{X} = \dfrac{100}{80} = 1.25 \text{ ml or } 1.3 \text{ ml}$$

or

FE: $\dfrac{H}{V} \times \dfrac{D}{X} = \dfrac{80 \text{ mg}}{2 \text{ ml}} \times \dfrac{50 \text{ mg}}{X} =$

(Cross multiply) 80 X = 100

$$\text{X} = 1.25 \text{ or } 1.3 \text{ ml}$$

or

DA: no conversion factor

$$\text{ml} = \dfrac{2 \text{ ml} \times \overset{5}{\cancel{50}} \text{ mg}}{\underset{8}{\cancel{80}} \text{ mg} \times 1} = \dfrac{10}{8} = 1.25 \text{ ml or } 1.3 \text{ ml}$$

Answer: tobramycin 50 mg = 1.25 ml or 1.3 ml

2. $\dfrac{D}{H} \times V = \dfrac{\overset{3}{\cancel{75}}}{\underset{5}{\cancel{125}}} \times 2 \text{ ml} = \dfrac{6}{5} = 1.2 \text{ ml}$

or

    H : V :: D : X
125 mg : 2 ml :: 75 mg : X ml

$$125 \text{ X} = 150$$

$$\text{X} = 1.2 \text{ ml}$$

Answer: methylprednisolone 75 mg = 1.2 ml

3. 0.3 ml of vitamin B_{12} (cyanocobalamin)

4. 0.5 ml of naloxone (Narcan)

5. a. Select the Maxipime 1-gram vial. The Maxipime 2-gram vial is for intravenous use according to the drug label and cannot be used for intramuscular injection.

  b. Using 2.6 ml diluent = 3.0 ml of solution

  c. Change 500 mg to 0.5 g or 1 g to 1000 mg

$$\dfrac{D}{H} \times V = \dfrac{0.5 \text{ g}}{1 \text{ g}} \times 3 \text{ ml} = 1.5 \text{ ml of cefepime twice a day}$$

6. BF: $\dfrac{D}{H} \times V = \dfrac{4}{5} \times 1 \text{ ml} = \dfrac{4}{5} \; 0.8 \text{ ml of compazine}$

or

RP: H : V :: D : X
5 mg : 1 ml :: 4 mg : X

$$5 \text{ X} = 4$$

$$\text{X} = 0.8 \text{ ml}$$

or

FE: $\dfrac{H}{V} \times \dfrac{D}{X} = \dfrac{5 \text{ mg}}{1 \text{ ml}} \times \dfrac{4 \text{ mg}}{X} = 5X = 4$

$$\text{X} = 0.8 \text{ ml}$$

or

DA: ml $= \dfrac{1 \text{ ml} \times 4 \text{ mg}}{5 \text{ mg} \times 1} = \dfrac{4}{5} = 0.8 \text{ ml}$

7. 2.5 ml of secobarbital
8. **a.** 100-mg vial
   b. 0.75 ml of thiamine
9. ½ or 0.5 ml of hydroxyzine
10. **a.** 750 mg of cefonicid (Monocid) is equivalent to 0.75 g.
    b. Drug label indicates that 2.5 ml of diluent should be added to the drug powder, which yields 3.1 ml of drug solution.
    c. $\dfrac{D}{H} \times V = \dfrac{0.75\ g}{1\ g} \times 3.1\ ml$

    $\quad\quad = 2.33\ ml\ or\ 2.3\ ml\ of\ cefonicid\ solution$
11. **a.** meperidine 35 mg = 0.7 ml
    b. promethazine 10 mg = 0.4 ml
    c. Procedure: 1. Obtain 0.7 ml of meperidine from the ampule and 0.4 ml of promethazine from the ampule.
    2. Discard the remaining solutions within the ampules.
12. **a.** meperidine 50 mg = ½ or 0.5 ml
    b. atropine 0.3 mg = 0.75 or 0.8 ml (Round off in tenths)
       Atropine

       BF: $\dfrac{D}{H} \times V = \dfrac{0.3}{0.4} \times 1\ ml = 0.75\ or\ 0.8\ ml$

       or
       Atropine
       RP: H : V :: D : X
       0.4 mg : 1 ml :: 0.3 mg : X ml
       0.4 X = 0.3
       $X = \dfrac{0.3}{0.4} = 0.75\ or\ 0.8\ ml$

       or
       Atropine
       FE: $\dfrac{H}{V} \times \dfrac{D}{X} = \dfrac{0.4\ mg}{1\ ml} \times \dfrac{0.3\ mg}{X} =$
       0.4X = 0.3
       X = 0.75 or 0.8 ml

       or
       Meperidine
       DA: ml $= \dfrac{1\ ml\ \times\ \overset{1}{\cancel{50}}\ \cancel{mg}}{\underset{2}{\cancel{100}}\ \cancel{mg}\ \times\ 1} = \dfrac{1}{2}\ or\ 0.5\ ml$

    c. 1. The two drugs are compatible.
    2. Inject 0.75 (0.8) ml of air into the atropine vial.
    3. Inject 0.5 ml of air into the meperidine vial and withdraw 0.5 ml of meperidine.
    4. Withdraw 0.8 ml of atropine from the atropine vial. Discard both vials.

13. BF: $\dfrac{D}{H} \times V = \dfrac{\overset{5}{\cancel{50}}\ \cancel{mg}}{\underset{8}{\cancel{80}}\ \cancel{mg}} \times 2\ ml = \dfrac{10}{8} = 1.25\ ml\ or\ 1.3\ ml$

    or
    RP: H : V :: D : X
    80 mg : 2 ml :: 50 mg : X ml
    80 X = 100
    X = 1.25 ml or 1.3 ml

    Answer: tobramycin 50 mg = 1.25 ml or 1.3 ml

14. **a.** Use either heparin vial; 5000 units/ml or 10,000 units/ml
   b. 0.5 ml of heparin (units 5000); 0.25 ml of heparin (units 10,000)
15. Librium 50 mg = 1 ml (100 mg = 2 ml)
   After adding 2 ml of diluent, withdraw the entire drug solution to determine the total volume of drug solution. Expel half of the solution; the remaining drug solution is equivalent to chlordiazepoxide (Librium) 50 mg.
16. **a.** Change milligrams to grams (smaller to larger number) by moving the decimal point three spaces to the *left.* 500. mg = 0.5 g.

   Because the drug weight on the label is in grams, the conversion is to grams. However, the drug can be converted to milligrams by changing grams to milligrams (moving the decimal point three spaces to the *right*): 1 g = 1.000 mg = 1000 mg.

   b. Drug label states to add 3 ml of diluent and, after it is reconstituted, the drug solution will be 3.5 ml. Mandol 1 g = 3.5 ml.
   c. A 5-ml syringe is preferred: however, a 3-ml syringe can be used because less than 3 ml of the drug solution is needed.

   d. BF: $\dfrac{D}{H} \times V = \dfrac{0.5}{1} \times 3.5$ ml = 1.75 or 1.8 ml

   or

   RP: H : V :: D : X
   1000 mg : 3.5 ml :: 500 mg : X ml
   1000 X = 1750
   X = 1.75 or 1.8 ml

   or

   DA: ml = $\dfrac{3.5 \text{ ml} \times 0.5 \text{ g}}{1 \text{ g} \times 1}$ = 1.75 or 1.8 ml

   Answer: cefamandole (Mandol) 500 mg = 1.8 ml
17. Change 400 milligrams to grams
   400 mg = 0.400 g or 0.4 g

   a. Total volume of drug solution is 2.6 ml, see drug label.

   b. BF: $\dfrac{D}{H} \times V = \dfrac{0.4}{1} \times 2.6 = 1$ ml

   or

   RP:H : V :: D : X
   1 g : 2.6 ml :: 0.4 g : X ml
   X = 2.6 × 0.4
   X = 1 ml
   ticarcillin 400 mg or 0.4 g = 1 ml

   or

   FE: $\dfrac{H}{V} \times \dfrac{D}{X} = \dfrac{1 \text{ g}}{2.6 \text{ ml}} \times \dfrac{0.4 \text{ g}}{X} =$
   (Cross multiply) X = 1.04 ml or 1 ml

   or

   DA = $\dfrac{2.6 \text{ ml} \times 0.4 \text{ g}}{1 \text{ g} \times 1}$ = 1.04 ml or 1 ml

18. **a.** 1 gr = 60 mg; gr ⅙ = 10 mg

   b. $\dfrac{D}{H} \times V = \dfrac{\overset{2}{10}}{\underset{3}{15}} \times 1$ ml $= \dfrac{2}{3} = 0.66$ or 0.7 ml

or

H : V :: D : X

15 mg : 1 ml :: 10 mg : X ml

$\qquad$ 15 X = 10

$\qquad$ X = 0.66 or 0.7 ml

19. 0.5 ml of Vistaril

20. **a.** Yes, 8 mg per day

$$\textbf{b. } BF: \frac{D}{H} \times V = \frac{\overset{1}{\cancel{2}}\ mg}{\underset{2}{\cancel{4}}\ mg} \times 1\ ml = \text{½ or 0.5 ml} \qquad DA: ml = \frac{1\ ml \times \overset{1}{\cancel{2}}\ mg}{\underset{2}{\cancel{4}}\ mg \times 1} = \text{½ or 0.5 ml}$$

c. 3-ml syringe

d. Yes, the vial has a rubber top that is self-sealing.

21. **a.** Change milligrams to grams; move the decimal point three spaces to the left: 500. mg = 0.5 g

$\qquad$ 0.5 g × 3 (q8h) = 1.5 g per day

b. Add 2 ml of diluent to yield 2.6 ml (check drug information insert):

$$BF: \frac{D}{H} \times V = \frac{0.5\ g}{1\ g} \times 2.6\ ml = 1.3\ ml\ \text{per dose}$$

22. **a.** right, 0.25 g = 250 mg

b. 1.8 ml (after dilution, 2 ml)

c. 1 ml = 250 mg of ampicillin

23. **a.** Either the ampule or the vial could be used. The diazepam 5 mg/ml is a multiple-dose vial that contains 10 ml of drug solution.

$$\textbf{b. } BF: \text{Ampule: } \frac{8\ mg}{10\ mg} \times 2\ ml = 1.6\ ml\ \text{of diazepam}$$

$$BF: \text{Vial: } \frac{8\ mg}{5\ mg} \times 1\ ml = 1.6\ ml\ \text{of diazepam}$$

or

$$DA: \text{Ampule: } ml = \frac{2\ ml \times \overset{4}{\cancel{8}}\ mg}{\underset{5}{\cancel{10}}\ mg \times 1} = \frac{8}{5} = 1.6\ ml$$

or

$$DA: \text{Vial: } ml = \frac{1\ ml \times 8\ mg}{5\ mg \times 1} = \frac{8}{5} = 1.6\ ml$$

$$\textbf{24. } \frac{D}{H} \times V = \frac{1.5\ mg}{\underset{1}{\cancel{2}}\ mg} \times \overset{1}{\cancel{2}}\ ml = 1.5\ ml\ \text{of Cogentin}$$

$$\textbf{25. } BF: \frac{D}{H} \times V = \frac{10}{25} \times 5 = 0.4 \times 5 = 2\ ml$$

or

RP: $\qquad$ H : V :: D : X

$\qquad$ 25 million units : 5 ml :: 10 million units : X ml

$\qquad\qquad$ 25 X = 50

$\qquad\qquad$ X = 2 ml

Answer: Intron A 2 ml three times a week

26. BF: $\dfrac{D}{H} \times V = \dfrac{2.5}{10} \times 1 = 0.25$ ml or 0.3 ml

or

RP: H : V :: D : X

  10 mg : 1 ml :: 2.5 mg : X

      10 X = 2.5

        X = 0.25 ml or 0.3 ml

or

DA: no conversion factor

$$ml = \dfrac{1\ ml\ \times\ \overset{1}{\cancel{2.5}}\ \cancel{mg}}{\underset{4}{\cancel{10}}\ \cancel{mg}\ \times\ 1} = \dfrac{1}{4}\ or\ 0.25\ ml$$

Answer: AquaMEPHYTON 2.5 mg = 0.25 ml

or

FE: $\dfrac{H}{V} \times \dfrac{D}{X} = \dfrac{10\ mg}{1\ ml} \times \dfrac{2.5\ mg}{X} =$

      10X = 2.5

        X = 0.25 ml or 0.3 ml

27. a. 4 ml equal 3 g

b. BF: $\dfrac{D}{H} \times V = \dfrac{1\ g}{3\ g} \times 4\ g = \dfrac{4}{3} = 1.3$ ml of Unasyn

or

RP: H : V :: D : X

    3 g : 4 ml :: 1 g : Xml

        3 X = 4

          X = 1.3 ml of Unasyn

28. $ml = \dfrac{2\ ml \times 2\ \cancel{mg}}{5\ \cancel{mg} \times 1} = \dfrac{4}{5} = 0.8$ ml

0.8 ml of droperidol

29. $ml = \dfrac{1\ ml\ \times\ \overset{4}{\cancel{60}}\ \cancel{mg} \times \frac{1}{6}\ \cancel{gr}}{\underset{1}{\cancel{15}}\ \cancel{mg} \times 1\ \cancel{gr}\ \times\ 1} = \dfrac{4}{6} = \dfrac{2}{3}$ ml or 0.66 ml or 0.7 ml

30. a. 2 ml of diluent (sterile or bacteriostatic water)

b. 1 g = 2.4; 500 mg = 1.2 ml

c. $ml = \dfrac{2.4\ ml \times\ 1\ \cancel{g}\ \times\ \overset{1}{\cancel{500}}\ \cancel{mg}}{1\ \cancel{g}\ \times\ \underset{2}{\cancel{1000}}\ \cancel{mg} \times\ 1} = \dfrac{2.4}{2} = 1.2$ ml

Give 1.2 ml of Cefobid

31. a. Factors: drug label: 2 g = 12 ml (add 11.5 ml) **or** 250 mg = 1.5 ml **or** 0.25 g = 1.5 ml

       drug order: 300 mg/1

b. Conversion factor: 1 g = 1000 mg

c. $ml = \dfrac{1.5\ ml \times\ 1\ \cancel{g}\ \times\ \overset{3}{\cancel{300}}\ \cancel{mg}}{0.25\ \cancel{g} \times \underset{10}{\cancel{1000}}\ \cancel{mg} \times\ 1} = \dfrac{4.5}{2.5} = 1.8$ ml of oxacillin per dose

or

$ml = \dfrac{\overset{6}{\cancel{12}}\ ml \times\ 1\ \cancel{g}\ \times\ \overset{3}{\cancel{300}}\ \cancel{mg}}{2\ \cancel{g}\ \times\ \underset{10}{\cancel{1000}}\ \cancel{mg} \times\ 1} = \dfrac{18}{10} = 1.8$ ml of oxacillin

32. 0.25 g = 0.0$\underset{5}{\underset{\frown}{25}}$ mg (250 mg)

a. Drug label: add 2 ml diluent = 2.2 ml of drug solution.

b. Give 1.1 ml of Ancef.

33. a. $140 \div 2.2 = 63.6$ kg

   b. $15 \text{ mg} \times 63.6 \times 1 = 954$ mg daily

   c. $954 \div 3 = 318$ mg of amikacin q8h

   d. BF: $\dfrac{D}{H} \times V = \dfrac{318}{500} \times 2 = \dfrac{636}{500} = 1.27$ or 1.3 ml

   or

   RP: H   :   V   ::   D   :   X

   500 mg : 2 ml :: 318 mg : X ml

   500 X = 636

   X = 1.27 or 1.3 ml (tenths)

   or

   DA: ml $= \dfrac{2 \text{ ml} \times 318 \text{ mg}}{500 \text{ mg} \times 1} = \dfrac{636}{500} = 1.3$ ml per dose

   Answer: give 1.27 or 1.3 ml of amikacin q8h (three times a day)

   or

   FE: $\dfrac{H}{V} \times \dfrac{D}{X} = \dfrac{500 \text{ mg}}{2 \text{ ml}} \times \dfrac{318 \text{ mg}}{X \text{ ml}} =$

   (Cross multiply) 500X = 636

   X = 1.27 or 1.3 ml

34. a. $174 \div 2.2 = 79.1$ kg

   b. $2 \text{ mg} \times 79.1 = 158$ mg daily

   c. $158 \div 3 = 52$ mg or 50 mg q8h

   d. BF: $\dfrac{D}{H} \times V = \dfrac{\overset{5}{\cancel{50}}}{\underset{10}{\cancel{100}}} \times 1 \text{ ml} = \dfrac{5}{10} = 0.5$ ml

   or

   RP: H   :   V   ::   D   :   X

   100 mg : 1 ml :: 50 mg : X ml

   100 X = 50

   X = 0.5 ml

   or

   DA: ml $= \dfrac{1 \text{ ml} \times \overset{1}{\cancel{50}} \text{ mg}}{\underset{2}{\cancel{100}} \text{ mg} \times 1} = \dfrac{1}{2}$ or 0.5 ml

   Answer: netilmicin 50 mg = 0.5 ml

   or

   FE: $\dfrac{H}{V} \times \dfrac{D}{X} = \dfrac{100 \text{ mg}}{1 \text{ ml}} \times \dfrac{50 \text{ mg}}{X \text{ ml}} =$

   100X = 50

   X = 0.5 ml

35. a. 15 mg/67 kg/day = $15 \times 67 = 1005$ mg/day.

   b. 500 mg (1005 mg $\div$ 2 = 500 mg)

   c. $\dfrac{\overset{1}{\cancel{500}}}{\underset{1}{\cancel{500}}} \times 2 = 2$ ml per dose of Kantrex

   d. 1 g = 1000 mg $\dfrac{D}{H} \times V = \dfrac{\overset{1}{\cancel{500}}}{\underset{2}{\cancel{1000}}} \times 3 = \dfrac{3}{2} = 1.5$ ml

 Additional practice problems are available on the enclosed CD-ROM in the "Basic Calculations" and "Advanced Calculations" sections.

Intravenous Preparations With Clinical Applications

OBJECTIVES

- Name catheter sites for intravenous access.
- Examine the three methods for calculating intravenous (IV) flow rate and select one of the methods for IV calculation.
- Calculate drops per minute of prescribed IV solutions for IV therapy.
- Determine the drop factor according to the manufacturer's product specification.
- Calculate the drug dosage for IV medications.
- Calculate the flow rate for IV drugs being administered in a prescribed amount of solution.
- Explain the types and uses of electronic IV infusion devices.
- Calculate the rate of direct IV injection.

OUTLINE

Intravenous (IV) therapy is used for administering fluids containing water, dextrose, fat emulsions, vitamins, electrolytes, and drugs. Approximately 90% of all hospitalized patients, some outpatients, and some home-care patients receive IV therapy. Drugs are administered intravenously for direct absorption and fast action. Many drugs cannot be absorbed through the gastrointestinal tract, and the IV route provides bioavailability. Certain drugs that need to be absorbed immediately are administered by direct intravenous injection—often diluted, over several minutes. However, many drugs administered intravenously are irritating to the veins because of the drug's pH or osmolality and must be diluted and administered slowly.

Advantages of IV drug therapy are (1) rapid drug distribution into the bloodstream, (2) rapid onset of action, and (3) no drug loss to tissues. There are many complications of IV therapy, some of which are sepsis, thrombosis, phlebitis, air emboli, infiltration, and extravasation. The nurse must monitor for signs of these complications during the course of IV therapy.

Three methods are used to administer IV fluid and drugs: (1) direct IV drug injection, (2) continuous IV infusion, and (3) intermittent IV infusion. Continuous IV administration replaces fluid loss, maintains fluid balance, and is a vehicle for drug administration. Intermittent IV administration is primarily used for giving IV drugs.

Nurses play an important role in preparing and administering IV solutions and drugs. Nursing functions and responsibilities include (1) knowledge of IV sets and their drop factors, (2) calculating IV flow rates, (3) verifying compatibility of the IV solution and the drug, (4) mixing drugs and diluting in IV solution, (5) regulating IV infusion devices, and (6) maintaining patency of IV accesses.

INTRAVENOUS ACCESS SITES

The successful administration of IV drugs and fluids depends on a patent vascular access. The most common site for short term (less than 1 week) intravenous therapy is the peripheral short site, which uses the dorsal and ventral surfaces of the upper extremities. Catheter length is normally 1 to 3 inches.

The peripheral midline site for intravenous therapy that may last 2 to 4 weeks uses the veins in the area of the anticubital fossa—the basilic, brachial, cephalic, cubital, or medial. Midline peripheral catheters are between 3 and 8 inches in length.

The peripherally inserted central catheter (PICC) can be used for intravenous therapy up to 1 year. Catheter length is 21 inches. The insertion site is the region of the antecubital fossa that uses the same veins as the peripheral midline. The catheter is advanced through the vein in the upper arm until the tip rests in the lower third of the superior vena cava. In some states, registered nurses certified in intravenous therapy also can be certified to insert PICC catheters.

The central venous site is used for patients who need long-term continuous infusions of fluids, medication, or nutritional support that cannot be sustained with a peripheral site. Central venous catheter (CVC) sites are the superior vena cava and the inferior vena cava. The superior vena cava is accessed from the internal jugular vein and the right or left subclavian vein, whereas the inferior vena cava is accessed from the femoral vein. Length of the CVC can vary from 6 to 28 inches. Insertion requires a minor surgical procedure—a percutaneous vein cannulation with the introduction of a single or multi-lumen catheter; the tip of the catheter rests in the superior vena cava just above the right atrium.

Patients who need vascular access for long-term use, such as chemotherapy, antibiotic therapy, or nutritional support, are given much longer catheters, which are tunneled under the skin after the vein is cannulated. The catheter and its drug infusion port exit from the subcutaneous tissue to a site on the chest. Examples of these devices are the Hickman, Groshong, Neostar, and Cook catheters.

Another type of catheter for long-term use has an implantable infusion port that is inserted in the subcutaneous tissue under the skin. These devices are called *vascular access ports* and they have a larger drug port or septum than other catheters. Care must be taken to use a non-coring needle that slices the port instead of making holes, so that the septum will close instead of leaking after the needle has been removed (Figure 9-1).

Intermittent Infusion Add-On Devices

When IV access sites are used for intermittent therapy instead of continuous infusion, they must be irrigated periodically to maintain patency. An intermittent infusion add-on device can be attached to the end of the vascular access device, catheter, or needle, to close the connection that was attached to the IV tubing. There are many types of add-on devices, such as extension loops, solid cannula caps, and injection access caps. All add-on devices should use Luer-Lok design as a safety measure. Use of add-on devices should be included as part of the protocol of the institution (Figure 9-2). These devices have ports (stoppers) where needleless syringes can be inserted when drug therapy is resumed. This practice can eliminate the need for a constant low-rate infusion to keep the vein open (KVO) and reduce excessive fluid intake. The use of intermittent infusion devices can allow the patient greater mobility and can be cost-effective because less IV tubing, IV solution, and regulating equipment are needed.

IV sites should be irrigated every 8 to 12 hours or before and after each drug infusion, depending on institutional policy, to maintain patency. Table 9-1 gives suggested flushing/irrigation times. Pre-filled single-use syringes of saline solution are available to flush infusion devices. The intent of pre-filled single-use syringes is to prevent the cross-contamination that can occur with a multidose vial. The volume of the flush used for vascular access devices is twice the volume of the catheter plus any connected devices such as a three-way stopcock or an extension set. Heparinized saline solution flushes are generally used for venous access devices that are tunneled or implanted.

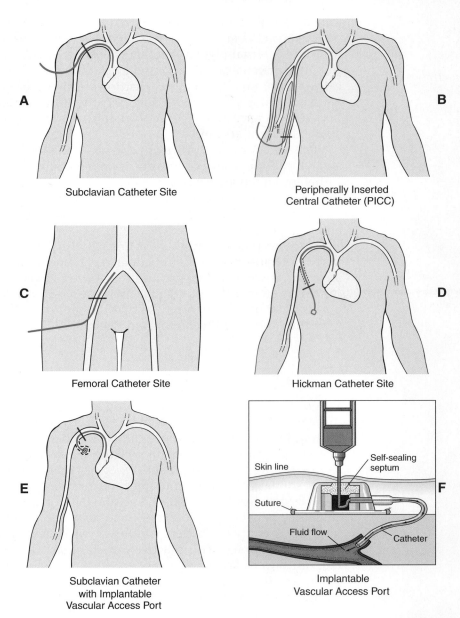

FIGURE 9-1 Central venous access sites. **A,** Subclavian catheter. **B,** Peripherally inserted central catheter (PICC). **C,** Femoral catheter. **D,** Hickman catheter. **E,** Subclavian catheter with implantable vascular access port. **F,** Implantable vascular access port. (**F,** from Perry, A. G., & Potter, P. A. [2006]. *Clinical nursing skills and techniques.* 6th ed. St. Louis: Mosby.)

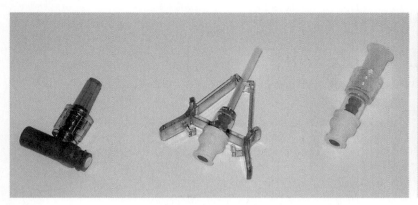
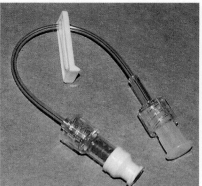

FIGURE 9-2 Needleless infusion devices. Medication in a needleless syringe can be inserted into a needleless infusion device.

TABLE 9-1				

Venous Access Devices: Flushing for Peripheral and Central Venous*

Type	Length (inches)	Flush Before Drug Use	Flush After Drug Use	Volume/ml
Peripheral	1-2	NSS	NSS	1-3
Central venous				
Single-lumen	8	NSS	HSS	1-3
Multilumen	8	NSS	HSS	1-3
External tunneled	35	NSS	HSS or NSS	10
Hickman, Cook,			Flush q12h if not used	
or Groshong				
Peripherally inserted	20	NSS	NSS	10
central catheter (PICC)			Flush q12h if not used	
Implanted vascular	35	NSS	HSS or NSS	10
access device			Flush q12h if not used	

*If the adapter/cap is pressurized, then normal saline solution is used, not a heparin solution. Follow the institution policy procedure and manufacturer's guidelines.
HSS, Heparinized saline solution; *NSS*, normal saline solution.

DIRECT INTRAVENOUS INJECTIONS

Medications that are given by the IV injection route are calculated in the same manner as medications for intramuscular (IM) injection. This route is often referred to as *IV push*. Clinically, it is the preferred route for patients with poor muscle mass or decreased circulation, or for a drug that is poorly absorbed from the tissues. Medications administered by this route have a rapid onset of action, and calculation errors can have serious, even fatal, consequences. Drug information inserts must be read carefully, and attention must be paid to the amount of drug that can be given per minute. If the drug is pushed into the bloodstream at a faster rate than is specified in the drug literature, adverse reactions to the medication are likely to occur.

Calculating the amount of time needed to infuse a drug given by direct IV infusion can be done with the use of ratio and proportion.

REMEMBER

When giving drugs by direct IV infusion, always verify the compatibility of the IV solution and the drug, or precipitation may result. Incompatibility can be avoided if the IV tubing is flushed with a compatible solution of normal saline before and after administration.

EXAMPLES

Set up a ratio and proportion using the recommended amount of drug per minute on one side of the equation; these are the known variables. On the other side of the equation are the desired amount of drug and unknown desired minutes: a. amount in milliliters (ml); b. number of minutes.

PROBLEM 1: Order: Dilantin 200 mg, IV, STAT.
Drug available: Dilantin 250 mg/5 ml. IV infusion not to exceed 50 mg/min.

a. BF: $\dfrac{D}{H} \times V = \dfrac{\overset{4}{\cancel{200}}}{\underset{5}{\cancel{250}}} \times 5 = \dfrac{20}{5} = 4$ ml

or

RP: H : V ::   D   : X
250 mg : 5 ml :: 200 mg : X ml
250 X = 1000
X = 4 ml

or

FE: $\dfrac{H}{V} \times \dfrac{D}{X} = \dfrac{250 \text{ mg}}{5 \text{ ml}} = \dfrac{200 \text{ mg}}{X} =$

(Cross multiply)   250 X = 1000
X = 4 ml

or
DA: ml = $\dfrac{5 \text{ ml} \times \overset{4}{\cancel{200 \text{ mg}}}}{\underset{5}{\cancel{250 \text{ mg}}} \times 1} = \dfrac{20}{5} = 4$ ml

200 mg = 4 ml (discard 1 ml of the 5 ml).

b. known drug : known minutes :: desired drug : desired minutes
50 mg   :   1 min   ::   200 mg   :   X
50 X = 200
X = 4 min

PROBLEM 2: Order: Lasix 120 mg, IV, STAT.
Drug available: Lasix 10 mg/ml. IV infusion not to exceed 40 mg/min.

a. RP: H : V ::   D   : X
10 mg : 1 ml :: 120 mg : X
10 X = 120
X = 12 ml of Lasix

or

DA: ml = $\dfrac{1 \text{ ml} \times \cancel{120}^{\,12} \text{ mg}}{\cancel{10}_{1} \text{ mg} \times 1}$ = 12 ml of Lasix

b. known drug : known minutes :: desired drug : desired minutes

$$40 \text{ mg} \quad : \quad 1 \text{ min} \quad :: \quad 120 \text{ mg} \quad : \quad X$$
$$40\,X = 120$$
$$X = 3 \text{ min}$$

When dosing instructions give the amount of drug and specify infusion time, the amount of drug can be divided by the number of minutes to attain the per minute amount to be infused.

EXAMPLE

PROBLEM 3: Order: Amrinone (Inocor) 65 mg, IV bolus over 3 minutes.
Drug available: Inocor 100 mg/20 ml

a. H : V :: D : X

$$100 \text{ mg} : 20 \text{ ml} :: 65 \text{ mg} : X$$
$$100\,X = 1300$$
$$X = 13 \text{ ml}$$

or

DA: ml = $\dfrac{\cancel{20}^{\,1} \text{ ml} \times 65 \text{ mg}}{\cancel{100}_{5} \text{ mg} \times 1} = \dfrac{65}{5}$ = 13 ml

b. $\dfrac{13 \text{ ml}}{3 \text{ min}}$ = 4.3 ml/min

PRACTICE PROBLEMS: I Direct IV Injection

Answers can be found on page 246.

a. Determine the amount in milliliters of drug solution to administer.

b. Determine the number of minutes that is required for the direct IV drug dose to be administered for each of the practice problems.

1. Order: protamine sulfate 50 mg, IV, STAT.
    Drug available:

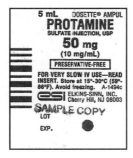

IV infusion not to exceed 5 mg/min.

    a. Amount in milliliters _____

    b. Number of minutes to administer _____

2. Order: dextrose 50% in 50 ml, IV, STAT.
Drug available: dextrose 50% in 50 ml.
IV infusion not to exceed 10 ml/min.

Number of minutes to administer 50% of 50 ml _____

3. Order: calcium gluconate 4.5 mEq, IV, STAT.
Drug available:

CALCIUM GLUCONATE	NDC 0517-3910-25
INJECTION, USP 10% 4.65mEq/10mL Calcium (0.465mEq/mL)	Each mL contains: Calcium Gluconate (Monohydrate) 98mg, Calcium Saccharate (Tetrahydrate) 4.6mg, Water for Injection q.s. pH adjusted with Sodium Hydroxide and/or Hydrochloric Acid. Calcium Saccharate provides 6.2% of the total Calcium content. 0.68mOsmol/mL. Sterile, nonpyrogenic.
FOR SLOW INTRAVENOUS USE 10mL SINGLE DOSE VIAL AMERICAN REGENT LABORATORIES, INC SUBSIDIARY OF LUITPOLD PHARMACEUTICALS, INC SHIRLEY, NY 11967 REV. 1/91	CAUTION: Federal Law (USA) Prohibits Dispensing Without Prescription. WARNING: DISCARD UNUSED PORTION IF CRYSTALLIZATION OCCURS, WARMING MAY DISSOLVE THE PRECIPITATE (See Insert). THE INJECTION MUST BE CLEAR AT THE TIME OF USE. Directions for Use: See Insert

IV infusion not to exceed 1.5 ml/min. **Note:** 4.65 mEq/10 ml.

    a. Amount in milliliters _____

    b. Number of minutes _____

4. Order: prednisolone 50 mg, IV, q12h.
Drug available: prednisolone 50 mg in 5 ml.
IV infusion not to exceed 10 mg/min.

    a. Amount in milliliters _____

    b. Number of minutes _____

5. Order: morphine sulfate 6 mg, IV, q3h, PRN.
Drug available:

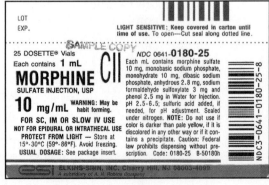

Infusion not to exceed 10 mg/4 min.

    a. Amount in milliliters _____

    b. Number of minutes _____

6. Order: digoxin 0.25 mg, IV, daily.
   Drug available:

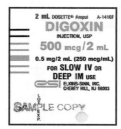

   Infuse slowly over 5 minutes.

   a. Amount in milliliters _____

   b. How many ml/min should be infused? _____

7. Order: Haldol 2 mg, IV, q4h, PRN.
   Drug available: Haldol 5 mg/ml.
   IV infusion not to exceed 1 mg/min.

   a. Amount in milliliters _____

   b. Number of minutes _____

8. Order: Ativan 6 mg, IV, q6h, PRN.
   Drug available: Ativan 4 mg/ml.
   IV infusion not to exceed 2 mg/min.

   a. Amount in milliliters _____

   b. Number of minutes _____

9. Order: diltiazem (Cardizem) 20 mg IV over 2 minutes.
   Drug available:

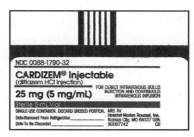

   a. How many milliliters (ml) would you give? _____

   b. How many milliliters (ml) would you infuse per minute? _____

10. Order: granisetron (Kytril) 10 mcg/kg, 30 minutes before chemotherapy.
    Infuse 1 mg over 60 seconds.
    Patient weighs 140 pounds.
    Drug available:

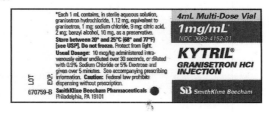

    a. How many kilograms (kg) does the patient weigh? _____

    b. How many milligrams (mg) should the patient receive? _____

    c. For how many seconds should the drug dose be infused? _____

REMEMBER

Consider the length of the injection port on the tubing from the patient's IV site. If the IV rate is very low, like 30 ml/hr, the IV medication may take a long time to reach the patient. The drug dose is not complete until the drug has entered the patient. Therefore, the tubing will have to be flushed to ensure that the dose reaches the patient in a timely manner.

CONTINUOUS INTRAVENOUS ADMINISTRATION

When IV solutions are required, the health care provider orders the amount of solution per liter or milliliter to be administered for a specific time, such as for 24 hours. The nurse calculates the IV flow rate according to the drop factor, the amount of fluid to be administered, and the infusion time.

Intravenous Infusion Sets

All infusion sets have the same components: a sterile spike for entry into the IV bag or bottle, a drip chamber for counting drops and managing flow, a roller clamp that controls flow through the tubing, tubing length from drip chamber to IV site, Y-site for adding a secondary set or giving drugs IV, a filter (which removes bacteria, particles, and air), and the adapter (which attaches to the needle or catheter) (Figure 9-3). Figure 9-4 shows the IV containers, bag, and bottle.

    If the IV infusion is not placed on a flow control device, but instead is delivered by gravity, then the hourly rate will have to be adjusted manually. It is necessary to know the drop factor of the IV set to calculate the hourly infusion rate. The drop factor, or the number of drops per milliliter (ml), is printed on the package of the infusion set and found on top of the drip chamber. Sets that deliver large drops per milliliter (10-20 gtt/ml) are referred to as macrodrip sets, and those that deliver small drops per milliliter (60 gtt/ml) are called microdrip or minidrip sets (Table 9-2, Figure 9-5).

TABLE 9-2

Intravenous Sets

	Drops (gtt) per Milliliter	
	Macrodrip Sets	**Microdrip Sets**
	10 gtt/ml	60 gtt/ml
	15 gtt/ml	
	20 gtt/ml	

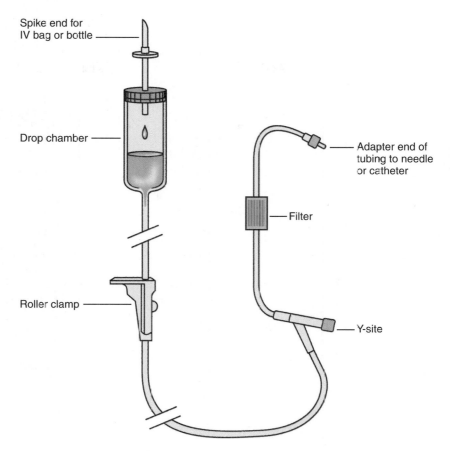

Spike end for
IV bag or bottle

Drop chamber

Adapter end of
tubing to needle
or catheter

Filter

Roller clamp

Y-site

FIGURE 9-3 Intravenous tubing.

Drip rates are adjusted by counting the drops coming through the spike into the drip chamber. While looking at the second hand of your watch, adjust the roller clamp to determine the correct number of drops in one minute. It is more difficult to count when the drops are smaller and the drop rate is faster. One advantage of the microdrip set is that the number of milliliters per hour is the same as the drops per minute (e.g., if the infusion rate is 50 ml/hr, the drip rate is 50 gtt/min). When the IV rate is 100 ml/hr or higher, the macrodrip set generally is used. Slow drip rates (less than 100 ml/hr) make macrodrip adjustments too difficult (e.g., at 50 ml/hr, the macrodrip rate would be 8 gtt/min). Therefore, if the IV rate is 100 ml/hr or lower, the microdrip is preferred.

When the manual process is used to adjust the infusion rate, the IV drip rate should be monitored every half-hour to hour, so that IV fluids are infused as prescribed.

At times, IV fluids are given at a slow rate to *keep vein open* (KVO), also called *to keep open* (TKO). Reasons for ordering KVO include (1) a suspected or potential emergency situation requiring rapid administration of fluids and drugs, and (2) the need to maintain an open line to give IV drugs at specified hours. For KVO, a microdrip set (60 gtt/ml) and a 250-ml IV bag can be used.

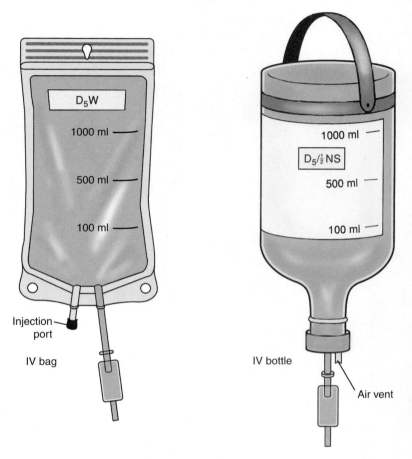

FIGURE 9-4 Intravenous containers.

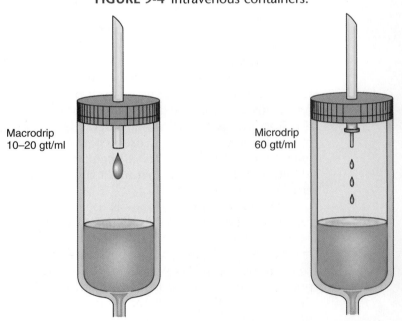

FIGURE 9-5 Macrodrop and microdrip sizes.

KVO should have a specific infusion rate, such as 10 to 20 ml/hr, or should be given according to the institution's protocol.

CALCULATION OF INTRAVENOUS FLOW RATE

Three different methods can be used to calculate IV flow rate (drops per minute or gtt/min). The nurse should select one of these methods, memorize it, and use it to calculate dosages.*

THREE-STEP METHOD

a. $\dfrac{\text{Amount of solution}}{\text{Hours to administer}} = \text{ml/hr}$

b. $\dfrac{\text{ml per hour}}{\text{60 minutes}} = \text{ml/min}$

c. ml per minute $\times$ gtt per ml of IV set $=$ gtt/min

TWO-STEP METHOD

a. Amount of fluid $\div$ Hours to administer $=$ ml/hr

b. $\dfrac{\text{ml per hour} \times \text{gtt/ml (IV set)}}{\text{60 minutes}} = \text{gtt/min}$

ONE-STEP METHOD

$\dfrac{\text{Amount of fluid} \times \text{gtt/ml (IV set)}}{\text{Hours to administer} \times \text{minutes per hour (60)}} = \text{gtt/min}$

Safety Considerations

All IV infusions should be checked every half-hour or hour, according to the policy of the institution, to ensure the appropriate rate of infusion and to assess for potential problems. Common problems associated with IV infusions are kinked tubing, infiltration, and "free flow" IV rates. If IV tubing kinks, and the flow is interrupted, the prescribed amount of fluid will not be given, and the access site can clot. When infiltration occurs, IV fluid extravasates into the tissues, not into the vascular space, and trauma occurs to tissues at the IV site. Again, in this situation, the prescribed amount of IV fluid is not infused. "Free flow" IV rate refers to a rapid infusion of IV fluids—much faster than prescribed—causing fluid overload, which occurs as too much fluid in the vascular space or medication is administered faster than prescribed, resulting in a

---

*The two-step method is the most commonly used method of calculating IV flow rate.

toxic reaction. This is the most prevalent drug error and has led to the use of electronic infusion devices. Electronic infusion devices are not without flaws; mechanical problems occur and these devices can be incorrectly programmed, resulting in the wrong infusion rate. Fluid overload, thrombus formation, and infiltration are complications of IV therapy that can be avoided with frequent monitoring of IV infusions. See Appendix A for more detailed information on safe practice for IV drug administration.

Adding Drugs Used for Continuous Intravenous Administration

Drugs such as multiple vitamins and potassium chloride can be added to the IV solution bag for continuous infusion. This process of mixing or compounding an IV solution should be completed before the IV bag or bottle is hung. The medication is prepared using sterile technique and is added through the injection port to the bag or bottle that is to be rotated, to ensure that the drug is dispersed. Medication labels must be placed on the IV bag or bottle, clearly stating the patient's name and any other identifiers as specified by policy, such as name of the drug, amount, concentration, and strength of all ingredients without abbreviation; also, date, time, and time IV should be completed should be provided. It is important to follow institutional policies and procedures when adding medication to continuous intravenous fluid.

NOTE

DO NOT add the drug while the infusion is running unless the bag is rotated. A drug solution injected into an upright infusing IV solution causes the drug to concentrate into the lower portion of the IV bag and not be dispersed. The patient will receive a concentrated drug solution, and this can be harmful (e.g., if the drug is potassium chloride).

Types of Solutions

All intravenous solutions contain various solutes and electrolytes that are added for specific therapies. Common solutes include dextrose (D) and sodium chloride (NaCl). The strength of the solution is expressed in percent (%), such as 0.45%, which means 0.45 g in 100 ml. Common commercially prepared IV solutions are dextrose in water (D_5W), dextrose with one-half normal saline solution (D_5 0.45%), normal saline solution (0.9% NaCl), one-half normal saline solution (0.45% NaCl), and lactated Ringer's solution (LRS). Lactated Ringer's solution contains sodium, chloride, potassium, calcium, and lactate.

Tonicity of IV Solutions

The terms *tonicity* and *osmolality* have been used interchangeably, but *tonicity* refers to the concentration of intravenous (IV) solution, whereas *osmolality* is the concentration of body fluids (e.g., blood, serum). Intravenous solutions produce tonicity in the cells of the body; this is the movement of water molecules into and out of the cells because of their surrounding fluid environment. IV solutions are divided into three categories: hypertonic, hypotonic, and isotonic. The range of tonicity is measured in milliosmoles, and the normal range is 240 to 340 mOsm: a + 50 mOsm and/or −50 mOsm of 290 mOsm. Hypertonic solutions cause water molecules to diffuse out of the cells and exert a hyperosmolar effect. For example, a hypertonic solution is D_5 0.9% normal saline (NaCl) because it has an osmolarity of 560 mOsm. Hypotonic solutions cause water molecules to diffuse into the cells and exert a hypo-osmolar effect. A solution of 0.45% normal saline (NaCl) is hypo-osmolar and has an osmolarity of 154 mOsm. D_5W is iso-osmolar with an osmolality of 250 mOsm; however, the dextrose is metabolized quickly leaving only water, thus making the solution hypotonic. Isotonic solutions maintain the same concentration of water molecules on both sides of the cell, so no net movement occurs. The osmolarity of isotonic solutions is 240 to 340 mOsm, similar to blood, and lactated Ringer's solution and 0.9% normal saline solution (NaCl) are the best examples. Table 9-3 lists the names of selected IV solutions, their tonicity, and their mOsm, as well as the abbreviations for these solutions.

EXAMPLES

Two problems in determining IV flow rate are given. Each problem is solved with each of the three methods for calculating IV flow rate.

PROBLEM 1: Order: 1000 ml of $D_5\frac{1}{2}$ NSS (5% dextrose in $\frac{1}{2}$ normal saline solution) in 6 hours.
Available: 1 L (1000 ml) of $D_5\frac{1}{2}$ NSS solution bag: IV set labeled 10 gtt/ml. How many drops per minute (gtt/min) should the patient receive?

Three-Step Method: **a.** $\dfrac{1000 \text{ ml}}{6 \text{ hr}}$ = 166.6 or 167 ml/hr

TABLE 9-3			
Abbreviations for IV Solutions With Tonicity and Osmolarity			
IV Solution	**Tonicity**	**mOsm**	**Abbreviation(s)**
5% dextrose in water	Iso	250	D_5W, 5% D/W
10% dextrose in water	Hyper	500	$D_{10}W$, 10% D/W
0.9% sodium chloride, normal saline solution	Iso	310	0.9% NaCl, NSS, PSS
0.45% sodium chloride, $\frac{1}{2}$ normal saline solution	Hypo	154	0.45% NaCl, $\frac{1}{2}$ NSS, $\frac{1}{2}$ PSS
5% dextrose in 0.9% sodium chloride	Hyper	560	D_5NSS, 5% D/NSS, 5% D/0.9% NaCl, D_5 PSS
Dextrose 5%/0.2% sodium chloride	Iso	326	D_5/0.2% NaCl
5% dextrose in 0.45% sodium chloride, 5% Dextrose in $\frac{1}{2}$ normal saline solution	Hyper	410	$D_5\frac{1}{2}$ NSS, 5% D/$\frac{1}{2}$ NSS, D_5 PSS, $\frac{1}{2}$ PSS
Lactated Ringer's solution	Iso	274	LRS

b. $\dfrac{167 \text{ ml}}{60 \text{ min}} = 2.7 \text{ or } 2.8 \text{ ml/min}$

c. $2.8 \text{ ml/min} \times 10 \text{ gtt/ml} = 28 \text{ gtt/min}$

Two-Step Method: **a.** $1000 \text{ ml} \div 6 \text{ hr} = 167 \text{ ml/hr}$

b. $\dfrac{167 \text{ ml/hr} \times \overset{1}{\cancel{10}} \text{ gtt/ml}}{\underset{6}{\cancel{60}} \text{ min}} = \dfrac{167}{6} = 28 \text{ gtt/min}$

10 and 60 cancel to 1 and 6.
If ml/hr is given, use only part **b** of the two-step method for calculating IV flow rate.

One-Step Method: $\dfrac{1000 \text{ ml} \times \overset{1}{\cancel{10}} \text{ gtt/ml}}{6 \text{ hr} \times \underset{6}{\cancel{60}} \text{ min}} = \dfrac{1000}{36} = 27\text{–}28 \text{ gtt/min}$

10 and 60 cancel to 1 and 6.
For the purpose of avoiding errors, the use of a hand calculator is strongly suggested.

Answer: 28 gtt/min.

PROBLEM 2: Order: 1000 ml of D_5W (5% dextrose in water), 1 vial of MVI (multiple vitamin), and 20 mEq of KCl (potassium chloride) every 8 hours.
Available: 1000 ml D_5W solution bag
      1 vial of MVI = 5 ml
      40 mEq/20 ml of KCl in an ampule
      IV set labeled 15 gtt/ml
How many milliliters (ml) of KCl would you withdraw as equivalent to 20 mEq of KCl?
How would you mix KCl in the IV bag?
How many drops per minute should the patient receive?

Procedure: MVI: Inject 5 ml of MVI into the rubber stopper on the IV bag.
      KCl: Calculate the prescribed dosage for KCl by using the basic formula, ratio and proportion, or dimensional analysis.

BF: $\dfrac{D}{H} \times V = \dfrac{20}{40} \times 20 = \dfrac{400}{40} = 10 \text{ ml}$

or

RP: H : V ::   D : X
     40 mEq: 20 ml :: 20 mEq: X ml
             40 X = 400
                X = 10 ml

or

FE: $\dfrac{H}{V} \times \dfrac{D}{X} = \dfrac{40 \text{ mEq}}{20 \text{ ml}} \times \dfrac{20 \text{ mEq}}{X}$

(Cross multiply)   40 X = 400
                   X = 10 ml

or

DA: $ml = \dfrac{V \times D}{H \times 1}$

$ml = \dfrac{20 \text{ ml} \times \overset{1}{\cancel{20} \text{ mEq}}}{\underset{2}{\cancel{40} \text{ mEq}} \times 1} = \dfrac{20}{2} = 10 \text{ ml}$

Withdraw 10 ml of KCl and inject it into the rubber stopper on the IV bag. Make sure the KCl solution and MVI additives are dispersed throughout the IV solution by rotating the IV bag.

Three-Step Method: **a.** $\dfrac{1000 \text{ ml}}{8 \text{ hr}} = 125 \text{ ml/hr}$

b. $\dfrac{125 \text{ ml}}{60 \text{ min}} = 2.0\text{–}2.1 \text{ ml/min}$

c. $2.1 \times 15 = 31\text{–}32 \text{ gtt/min}$

Two-Step Method: **a.** $1000 \div 8 = 125 \text{ ml/hr}$

b. $\dfrac{125 \text{ ml/hr} \times \overset{1}{\cancel{15}} \text{ gtt/ml}}{\underset{4}{\cancel{60}} \text{ min}} = \dfrac{125}{4} = 31\text{–}32 \text{ gtt/min}$

15 and 60 cancel to 1 and 4.
IV flow rate should be 31 to 32 gtt/min.

One-Step Method: $\dfrac{1000 \text{ ml} \times \overset{1}{\cancel{15}} \text{ gtt/ml}}{8 \text{ hr} \times \underset{4}{\cancel{60}} \text{ min}} = \dfrac{1000}{32} = 32 \text{ gtt/min}$

15 and 60 cancel to 1 and 4.
IV flow rate should be 31 to 32 gtt/min.

NOTE

Medication volume can be added to the total volume if strict intake and output are recorded. In general, an IV bag contains more fluid than is labeled on the bag; some estimates are as high as 50 ml. If an electronic infusion device is used, the patient will receive the amount programmed into the device. When the volume of the medication exceeds 20 ml, the amount should be added to the total volume to be infused. If the volume is less than 20 ml, this will not greatly change the hourly rate.

PRACTICE PROBLEMS: II Continuous Intravenous Administration

Answers can be found on page 248.

Select *one* of the three methods for calculating IV flow rate. The two-step method is preferred by most nurses.

1. Order: 1000 ml of D₅W to run for 12 hours.

    a. Would you use a macrodrip or microdrip IV set? _____

    b. Calculate the drops per minute (gtt/min) using one of the three methods.

    _____

2. Order: 3 L of IV solutions for 24 hours: 2 L of 5% D/½ NSS and 1 L of D₅W.

    a. One liter is equal to _____ ml.

   b. Each liter should run for _____ hours.

   c. The institution uses an IV set with a drop factor of 15 gtt/ml. How many drops per minute (gtt/min) should the patient receive? _____

3. Order: 250 ml of D₅W for KVO.

   a. What type of IV set would you use? _____
   Why? _____

   b. How many drops per minute should the patient receive? _____

4. Order: 1000 ml of 5% D/0.2% NaCl with 10 mEq of KCl for 10 hours.
   Available: Macrodrip IV set with a drop factor of 20 gtt/ml and microdrip set;
   KCl 20 mEq/20 ml vial.

   a. How many milliliters (ml) of KCl should be injected into the IV bag?

   _____

   b. How is KCl mixed in the IV solution? _____

   c. How many drops per minute (gtt/min) should the patient receive with both the macrodrip set and the microdrip set? _____

5. A liter (1000 ml) of IV fluid was started at 9 ᴀᴍ and was to run for 8 hours. The IV set delivers 15 gtt/ml. Four hours later, only 300 ml has been absorbed.

   a. How much IV fluid is left? _____

   b. Recalculate the flow rate for the remaining IV fluids. _____

6. The patient is to receive D₅W, 100 ml/hr.
   Available: Microdrip set (60 gtt/ml).

   How many drops per minute should the patient receive? _____

7. Order: 1000 D₅W with 40 mEq KCl at 125 ml/hr.
   Drug available:

   a. Which concentration of KCl would you choose? _____

   b. How many milliliters of KCl should be injected into the IV bag?

   _____

   c. How many hours will the IV last? _____

8. Order: 1000 D_5/½ NSS with 20 mEq KCl at 100 ml/hr.
Available: Macrodrip set (10 gtt/ml)
Drug available:

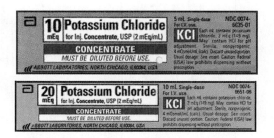

a. Which concentration of KCl would you choose?_____

b. How many milliliters of KCl should be injected into the IV bag?

_____

c. How many hours will the IV last? _____

d. How many drops per minute should the patient receive?

_____

INTERMITTENT INTRAVENOUS ADMINISTRATION

Giving drugs via the intermittent IV route has many advantages. The IV route allows for rapid therapeutic concentration of the drug and control over the onset of action and peak concentrations. Blood serum concentrations can be achieved via the IV route if the oral route is unavailable because of the patient's condition, such as gastrointestinal malabsorption or neurological deficits that prevent swallowing. The intermittent IV route can be used on an outpatient basis and can ensure compliance with drug therapy. The IV route also allows for the rapid correction of electrolyte imbalances. IV medications can be given at intervals within a 24-hour period for days or weeks. These medications are administered in a small volume of fluid (50 to 250 ml of D_5W or saline solution). The drug solution usually is delivered to the patient in 15 minutes to 1 hour, depending on the medication. A separate delivery set or secondary set is used for intermittent therapy if the patient is also receiving continuous infusion through the same IV site.

Secondary Intravenous Sets

Two sets available for administering IV drugs are (1) the calibrated cylinder (chamber) with tubing, such as Buretrol, Volutrol, and Soluset, and (2) the secondary set, which is similar to a regular IV set except that the tubing is shorter (Figure 9-6). The secondary set is used primarily for infusing small volumes, such as 50-, 100-, and 250-ml bags or bottles. The chambers of the Buretrol, Volutrol, and Soluset devices each hold 150 ml of solution. Medication

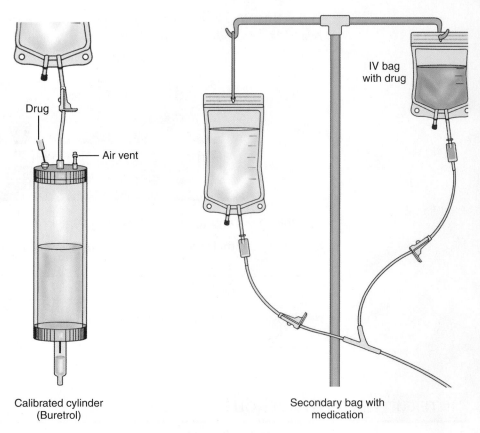

FIGURE 9-6 Secondary intravenous sets.

is injected into the chamber and is diluted with solution. These methods for administering IV drugs are referred to as *IV piggyback* (IVPB).

When IV drugs are administered with the secondary set, the Buretrol or the bag is raised higher than the primary set, which allows gravity to aid in the infusion. The chamber must be flushed with 15 ml after medication is given to make sure all of the drug is cleared from the cylinder and the tubing.

Adding Drugs Used for Intermittent Intravenous Administration

Usually, drugs for IV infusion are diluted and administered over time. Clinical agencies frequently have their own protocols for dilutions; if not, the drug information insert should provide infusion guidelines. If the information is not available, the hospital pharmacy should be contacted. Guidelines and protocols help prevent drug and fluid incompatibilities.

Drugs administered by Buretrol, Volutrol, or Soluset are prepared by the nurse. Powdered drugs must be reconstituted with sterile water or normal saline. Once the medication is added to the Buretrol, then the appropriate amount and type of IV fluid is added to the medication, and the infusion rate is adjusted. For medication diluted in bags or bottles, the powdered drug can be reconstituted the same way, or a spike adaptor can be used that can be at-

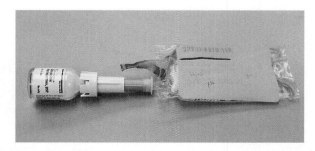

FIGURE 9-7 Medication mixed and attached to an IV bag.

tached to the vial and the bag. Fluid from the IV bag is flushed into the vial, reconstituting the powder, and then is flushed back into the bag. This process decreases contamination and is cost-effective. Mixing can be done by the pharmacy or by the nurse (Figure 9-7).

The current trend in IV medication administration is the use of premixed IV drugs in 50- to 500-ml bags. These premixed IV medications can be prepared by the manufacturer or by the hospital pharmacy. Problems of contamination and drug errors are decreased with the use of premixed IV medication. Each IV drug bag has separate tubing to prevent admixture. Cost is higher but risk is lower with the use of premixed IV drug bags. Because not all medication can be premixed in the solution, nurses will continue to prepare some drugs for IV administration.

NOTE

Sometimes the medication volume that is added to a bag or bottle adds a significant amount of volume. In those situations the 10% guideline applies. If the volume of medication for IV infusion exceeds 10% of the IV solution volume in the bag or bottle, then the amount of the medication volume should be withdrawn from the IV bag/bottle and replaced with the medication. For example, if the medication volume is 10 ml and a 100 ml bag is used, 10 ml should be aspirated from the IV bag and replaced with the medication so the total volume will still be 100 ml. If the amount of medication volume is less than 10%, then add the volume of medication to the volume of the bag or bottle. For example, 7 ml of medication is less than 10% of a 100 ml bag, so the total volume will be 107 ml.

Add-Vantage System

This system is similar to a secondary IV with medication, or a piggyback system in which the nurse or pharmacist prepares the IV drugs. Figure 9-8 shows steps that the nurse takes in preparing the Add-Vantage drug for IV administration.

Electronic Intravenous Infusion Devices

IV Infusion Pumps

An IV infusion pump pushes with positive pressure to infuse the fluid. The two types of IV infusion pumps are the linear peristaltic pump and the volu-

ADD-Vantage® System
As Easy as 1, 2, 3

1 Assemble
——— Use Aseptic Technique

Swing the pull ring over the top of the vial and pull down far enough to start the opening. Then pull straight up to remove the cap. Avoid touching the rubber stopper and vial threads.

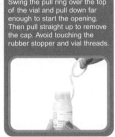

Hold diluent container and gently grasp the tab on the pull ring. Pull up to break the tie membrane. Pull back to remove the cover. Avoid touching the inside of the vial port.

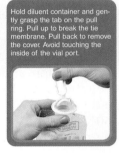

Screw the vial into the vial port until it will go no further. Recheck the vial to assure that it is tight. Label appropriately.

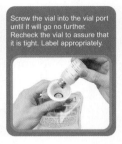

2 Activate
— Pull Plug/Stopper to Mix Drug with Diluent

Hold the vial as shown. Push the drug vial down into container and grasp the inner cap of the vial through the walls of the container.

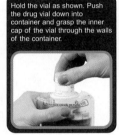
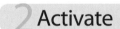

Pull the inner plug from the drug vial: allow drug to fall into diluent container for fast mixing. Do not force stopper by pushing on one side of inner cap at a time.

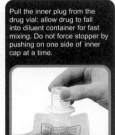

Verify that the plug and rubber stopper have been removed from the vial. The floating stopper is an indication that the system has been activated.

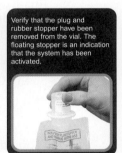

3 Mix and Administer
— Within Specified Time

Mix container contents thoroughly to assure complete dissolution. Look through bottom of vial to verify complete mixing. Check for leaks by squeezing container firmly. If leaks are found, discard unit.

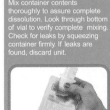
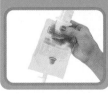

Pull up hanger on the vial.

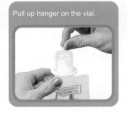

Remove the white administration port cover and spike (pierce) the container with the piercing pin. Administer within the specified time.

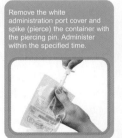

For more information on Advancing Wellness with ADD-Vantage® family of devices, contact your Hospira representative at 1-877-9467(1-877-9Hospira) or visit www.Hospira.com

©Hospira, Inc. - 275 North Field Drive, Lake Forest, IL 60045   6-131-1-Nov. 04

FIGURE 9-8 Hospira ADD-Vantage® System. (From Hospita, Inc., Lake Forest, IL.)

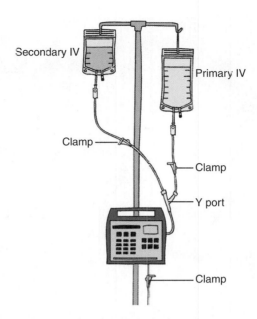

FIGURE 9-9 Infusion pump.

metric pump (Figure 9-9). The linear peristaltic pump and the volumetric pump have different pushing mechanisms. With the peristaltic pump, ridges move in wavelike motion against the IV tubing. The pressure on the IV tubing moves the fluid along.

The volumetric pump is more accurate. It requires a specific administration set that functions as a reservoir. The pump fills the reservoir and empties every cycle to deliver the programmed fluid rate. The increments of fluid delivered with micropumps can be as low as one tenth to one hundredth of a milliliter.

Pumps have safety features such as *air-in-line, occlusion,* and *infusion complete* alarms, as well as *low battery* or *low power* alerts. The tubing for infusion pumps have a safety feature, called *flow regulator,* to prevent "free flow" when the tubing is removed from the pump. These regulators can be adjusted similarly to the roller clamp, but are only to be used temporarily until the tubing can be placed back in the pump.

IV pumps are recommended for use with all central venous lines, arterial lines, and hyperalimentation. For patients who need multiple infusions, multichanneled pumps are available; these have two or more programmable pumps, each of which can be set for a different infusion rate (Figure 9-10). Every model pump has different features and parameters; nurses must be familiar with the capabilities of the infusion devices they use.

Syringe Pumps

Syringe pumps are used primarily when a small volume of medication is given. The syringe with medication is fitted into the pump, and the plunger is pushed by a piston-controlled mechanism, which delivers the medication at a controlled rate (Figure 9-10, *A*). Some pumps can operate with syringes of various sizes, from 5 ml to 60 ml. Syringe pumps are therapy-specific and are commonly used in pediatrics, oncology, obstetrics, and anesthesia. Syringe pumps

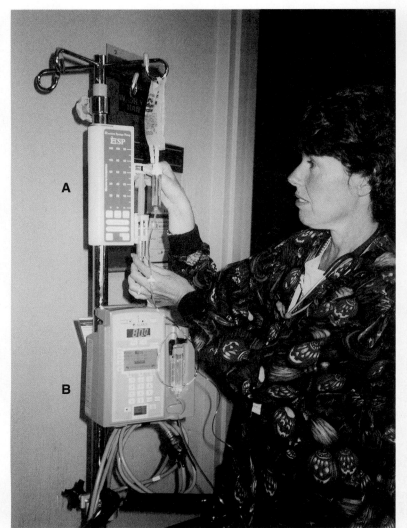

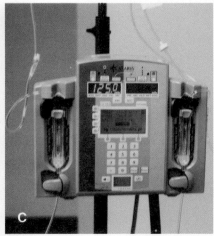

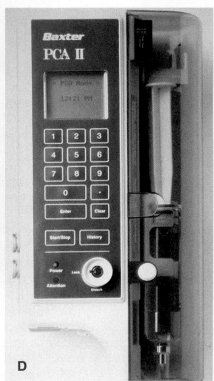

FIGURE 9-10 **A,** Syringe pump. **B,** Single infusion pump.
C, Dual-channel infusion pump. **D,** Patient-controlled analgesia
(PCA) pump.

usually do not have the same alarms as IV delivery pumps and require closer
monitoring.

Patient-Controlled Analgesia (PCA)

Patient-controlled analgesia (PCA) devices enable the patient to self-administer
IV analgesics (Figure 9-10, *D*). These programmable pumps are designed to deliver the analgesic at a loading dose or a continual dose, and they allow a patient to administer a bolus dose at set intervals. The pump can be programmed to lock out bolus doses that are not within the preset time frame to

prevent overdose. Morphine is commonly used as the analgesic with a dilution of 1 mg/ml. Patient's therapy is documented every 2 to 4 hours, with assessments and recordings of the amount of drug infused.

FLOW RATES FOR IV PUMPS

IV pumps are designed to deliver a wide variety of fluids over a broad range of infusion rates from multiple fluid container types. Pumps deliver a specific volume of fluid at a specific rate, measured in milliliters per hour (ml/hr). They deliver general IV fluids and electrolytes, blood and blood products, lipids, cardiovascular drugs, hyperalimentation, anesthetics, antibiotics, and analgesics. The pumps use electronic monitoring to detect partial or full occlusions, especially at low flow rates. In addition, accidental free flow of fluids is eliminated. The pumps are designed to notify the nurse of empty fluid containers and any upstream occlusion, such as a clamp that is not released. Pumps can deliver IV rates from 0.1 to 999.9 ml/hr.

Calculating Flow Rates for Intravenous Drugs and Electrolytes

Drugs that are given by intermittent infusion must be diluted and infused slowly. The pH and the osmolarity determine the dilution. A slower infusion time allows for the medication to be diluted in the blood vessel, thereby preventing phlebitis and high concentrations of the drug in plasma and tissues, which might cause time-related overdose, toxic effects, or allergic reactions. Drug-dosing instructions indicate the amount and type of solution and the length of infusion time. The nurse must calculate the drug dose from the physician's order, then calculate the flow rate from the drug-dosing information.

When calibrated cylinders, such as Voltrol, Buretrol, or Soluset, are used for drug infusion, the tubing must be flushed after each infusion to ensure that the entire drug dose was given. The flush can range from 10 to 25 ml and is added to the IV intake. When a minibag is used, the IV tubing should be drained so the patient receives the complete dose.

Secondary Sets

Secondary sets (calibrated cylinders and 50- to 250-ml IV bags) use drops per minute (gtt/min). The one-step method for calculating drops per minute (gtt/min) is used when IV drugs are administered with secondary sets.

One-Step Method for IV Drug Calculation With Secondary Set

$$\frac{\text{Amount of solution} \times \text{gtt/ml of the set}}{\text{Minutes to administer}} = \text{gtt/min}$$

Infusion Pumps

When secondary sets are used with infusion pumps, the drop factors must be the same on the secondary set and the infusion set for the pump.

Infusion pumps use units of milliliters per hour. Use the following method to calculate milliliters per hour.

$$\text{Amount of solution} \div \frac{\text{Minutes to administer}}{60 \text{ minutes/hour}} = \text{ml/hr}$$

NOTE

Medication volume that exceeds 5 ml should be added to the dilution volume in intermittent drug therapy. Because smaller volumes of fluid are used for IV infusion, drug dosage may be decreased if the volume of medication is not included in the dilution volume. The amount of solution in the formula should include both volumes.

EXAMPLES

PROBLEM 1: Order: Tagamet 200 mg, IV, q6h.
Drug available:

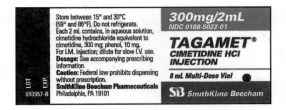

Set and solution: Buretrol set with drop factor of 60 gtt/ml; 500 ml of D_5W.

Instructions: Dilute drug in 100 ml of D_5W and infuse over 20 minutes.

Drug Calculation:

$$\text{BF: } \frac{D}{H} \times V = \frac{200}{300} \times 2 = \frac{400}{300}$$

$$X = 1.3 \text{ ml of Tagamet}$$

or

RP: H   :   V   ::   D   :   X
300 mg : 2 ml :: 200 mg : X ml
$$300 \text{ X} = 400$$

$$X = \frac{400}{300} = 300\overline{)400.0}^{\,1.3}$$

$$X = 1.3 \text{ ml of Tagamet}$$

or
$$\text{FE: } \frac{H}{V} \times \frac{D}{X} = \frac{300 \text{ mg}}{2 \text{ ml}} = \frac{200 \text{ mg}}{X} =$$

(Cross multiply) 300 X = 400
$$X = 1.3 \text{ ml}$$

or

$$\text{DA: ml} = \frac{2 \text{ ml} \times \overset{2}{\cancel{200}} \text{ mg}}{\underset{3}{\cancel{300}} \text{ mg} \times 1} = \frac{4}{3} = 1.3 \text{ ml}$$

Flow Rate Calculation:

$$\frac{\text{Amount of solution} \times \text{gtt/ml}}{\text{Minutes to administer}} = \frac{100 \text{ ml} \times \overset{3}{\cancel{60}} \text{ gtt}}{\underset{1}{\cancel{20}}} = 300 \text{ gtt/min}$$

Answer: Inject 1.3 ml of Tagamet into 100 ml of D₅W in the Buretrol chamber. Regulate IV flow rate to 300 gtt/min.

It would be impossible to count 300 gtt/min. Instead of using the Buretrol, the nurse could use a secondary set with a larger drop factor or a regulator.

PROBLEM 2: Order: Mandol 500 mg, IV, q6h.
Drug available:

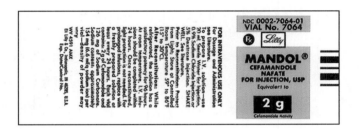

Add 6.6 ml of diluent = 8 ml of drug solution (2 g = 8 ml).
Set and solution: secondary set with 100 ml D₅W and a drop factor of 15 gtt/ml.

Instructions: Dilute in 100 ml of D₅W and infuse over 30 minutes.

Drug Calculation: (2.0 g = 2.000 mg).

$$\text{BF:} \frac{D}{H} \times V = \frac{500}{2000} \times 8 = \frac{4000}{2000} = 2 \text{ ml of Mandol}$$

or

RP: H   : V ::   D   : X
2000 mg : 8 ml :: 500 mg : X ml
        2000 X = 4000
              X = 2 ml of Mandol

or

$$\text{FE:} \frac{H}{V} \times \frac{D}{X} = \frac{2000 \text{ mg}}{8 \text{ ml}} = \frac{500 \text{ mg}}{X} =$$

2000 X = 400
      X = 2 ml

or

$$\text{DA: ml} = \frac{\overset{4}{\cancel{8} \text{ ml}} \times 1 \cancel{g} \times \overset{1}{\cancel{500} \text{ mg}}}{\underset{1}{\cancel{2} \cancel{g}} \times \underset{2}{\cancel{1000} \text{ mg}} \times 1} = \frac{4}{2} = 2 \text{ ml of Mandol}$$

Flow Rate Calculation:

$$\frac{\text{Amount of solution} \times \text{gtt/ml}}{\text{Minutes to administer}} = \frac{100 \text{ ml} \times \overset{1}{\cancel{15}}}{\underset{2}{\cancel{30}}} = \frac{100}{2} = 50 \text{ gtt/min}$$

Answer: Inject 2 ml of Mandol into the 100 ml D₅W bag.
Regulate IV flow rate to 50 gtt/min.

PROBLEM 3: Order: oxacillin 1 g, IV, q6h.
Drug available:

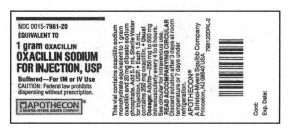

Add 5.7 ml of diluent = 6 ml per 1 g.
Set: Use an infusion pump.

Instructions: Dilute in 50 ml of D_5W and infuse over 15 minutes.

Drug Calculation: oxacillin 1 g = 6 ml of drug solution

Infusion Pump Rate: Amount of solution $\div \dfrac{\text{Minutes to administer}}{60 \text{ minutes}} = \text{ml/hr}$

$$56 \text{ ml} \div \frac{15 \text{ min}}{60 \text{ min}} = 56 \times \frac{\overset{4}{\cancel{60}}}{\underset{1}{\cancel{15}}} = 224 \text{ ml/hr}$$

Note: Amount of solution is 50 ml of D_5W + 6 ml of medication = 56 ml.

Answer: Rate on infusion pump should be set at 224 ml/hr to deliver oxacillin 1 g in 15 minutes.

PROBLEM 4: Order: albumin 25 g, IV.
Available: albumin 25 g in 50 ml.
Set: Use an infusion pump.

Instructions: Administer over 25 minutes, or 2 ml/min.

Drug Calculation: Not applicable.

Infusion Pump Rate:

$$50 \text{ ml} \div \frac{25 \text{ min}}{60 \text{ min}} = 50 \times \frac{60}{25} = \frac{3000}{25} = 120 \text{ ml/hr}$$

Answer: Infusion rate should be set at 120 ml/hr.

PROBLEM 5: Order: potassium phosphate 10 mM IV in 100 ml NSS over 90 minutes.
Drug available:

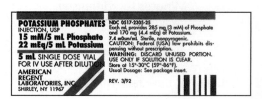

Set: Use infusion pump.

Drug Calculation:

BF: $\dfrac{D}{H} \times V = \dfrac{10}{15} \times 5 = \dfrac{50}{15} = 3.3$ ml of potassium phosphate

or

RP: H   :   V   ::   D   :   X
     15 mM : 5 ml :: 10 mM : X ml
                15 X = 50
                    X = 3.3 ml or
                       potassium phosphate

or

FE: $\dfrac{H}{V} \times \dfrac{D}{X} = \dfrac{15 \text{ mM}}{5 \text{ ml}} = \dfrac{10 \text{ mM}}{X} =$
                15 X = 50
                    X = 3.3 ml of
                       potassium phosphate

or

DA: ml $= \dfrac{5 \text{ ml} \times \overset{2}{\cancel{10}} \text{ mM}}{\underset{3}{\cancel{15}} \text{ mM} \times 1} = \dfrac{10}{3} = 3.3$ ml

Infusion Pump Rate:

$$\text{Amount of solution} \div \frac{\text{Minutes to administer}}{60 \text{ minutes}} = \text{ml/hr}$$

$$100 \text{ ml} \div \frac{90 \text{ min}}{60 \text{ min}} = 100 \times \frac{60}{90} = 66.6 \text{ or } 67 \text{ ml/hr}$$

Answer: Rate on the infusion pump should be 67 ml/hr to deliver potassium phosphate 10 mM in 90 minutes.

NOTE

When the electrolyte potassium is administered, the maximum infusion rate is 10 mEq/hr.

PRACTICE PROBLEMS: III Intermittent Intravenous Administration

Answers can be found on page 249.

Calculate the fluid rate by using a calibrated cylinder (Buretrol), a secondary set, or an infusion pump, as indicated in each question.

1. Order: cephapirin (Cefadyl) 500 mg, IV, q6h.
   Drug available:

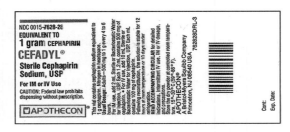

   a. Drug label: add _____ ml of diluent _____; 1 g = _____ ml; 100 mg = 1 ml.

What type of syringe should be used? _____

Set and solution: Buretrol set with a drop factor of 60 gtt/ml; 500 ml of D₅W.

Instructions: Dilute drug in 75 ml of D₅W and infuse over 30 minutes.

b. *Drug Calculation:*

_____

c. *Flow Rate Calculation:*

_____

2. Order: oxacillin 400 mg, IV, q6h.

   Drug available:

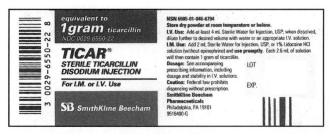

   a. Drug label: add _____ ml of diluent _____; 250 mg = _____ ml; 1 g = _____ ml.

   Set and solution: secondary set with a drop factor of 15 gtt/ml; 500 ml of D₅W.

   Instructions: Dilute drug in 100 ml of D₅W and infuse over 40 minutes.

   b. *Drug Calculation:*

   _____

   c. *Flow Rate Calculation:*

   _____

3. Order: ticarcillin (Ticar) 500 mg, IV, q6h.
   Drug available:

   Set and solution: Buretrol set with a drop factor of 60 gtt/ml; infusion pump; 500 ml of D₅W.

   Instructions: Dilute drug in 75 ml of D₅W and infuse over 40 minutes.

   a. *Drug Calculation:* Add _____ ml to ticarcillin vial (see drug label).

   _____

    b. *Flow Rate Calculation (gtt/min):*
How many drops per minute should the patient receive with use of the Buretrol set?

    _____

    c. *Infusion Pump Rate (ml/hr):*
With an infusion pump, how many ml/hr should be administered?

    _____

4. Order: piperacillin 2.5 g, IV, q6h.
Drug available: piperacillin 4 g vial in powdered form; add 7.8 ml of diluent to yield 10 ml of drug solution (4 g = 10 ml).

   Set and solution: Buretrol set with a drop factor of 60 gtt/ml; infusion pump; 500 ml of D$_5$W.

   Instructions: Dilute drug in 100 ml of D$_5$W and infuse over 30 minutes.

    a. *Drug Calculation:*

    _____

    b. *Flow Rate Calculation (gtt/min):*
How many drops per minute should the patient receive with use of the Buretrol set?

    _____

    c. *Infusion Pump Rate (ml/hr):*
With an infusion pump, how many ml/hr should be administered?

    _____

5. Order: methicillin (Staphcillin) 1 g, IV, q6h.
Drug available: Staphcillin 4 g in powdered form in vial; add 5.7 ml of diluent to yield 8 ml.

   Set and solution: secondary set with a drop factor of 15 gtt/ml; 100-ml bag of D$_5$W; infusion pump.

   Instructions: Dilute drug in 100 ml of D$_5$W and infuse over 40 minutes.

    a. *Drug Calculation:*

    _____

    Explain the procedure for diluting the drug and adding it to the IV bag.

    _____

    b. *Flow Rate Calculation (gtt/min):*
How many drops per minute should the patient receive with use of a secondary set?

    _____

    c. *Infusion Pump Rate (ml/hr):*
With an infusion pump, how many ml/hr should be administered?

    _____

6. Order: ciprofloxacin 250 mg, IV, q12h.

Drug available:

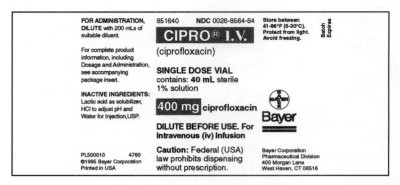

Set and solution: Secondary set with drip factor 15 gtt/ml; 250 ml of D₅W.

Instructions: Add ciprofloxin 250 mg to 250 ml D₅W and infuse over 60 minutes.

a. *Drug Calculation:*

_____

b. *Flow Rate Calculation (gtt/min):*

How many drops per minute should the patient receive?

_____

7. Order: doxycycline (Vibramycin), 100 mg, IV, q12h.

Drug available:

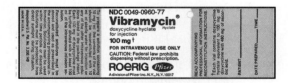

Set and solution: 100 ml of D₅W; secondary set with drop factor 15 gtt/ml; infusion pump.

Instructions: Mix Vibramycin vial with 10 ml of diluent; dilute in 100 ml of D₅W and infuse in 40 minutes.

a. *Flow Rate Calculation (gtt/min):*

_____

b. *Infusion Pump Rate (ml/hr)*

With an infusion pump, how many ml/hr should be administered? _____

8. Order: potassium chloride 20 mEq in 150 ml D₅W infused over 2 hours. Drug available:

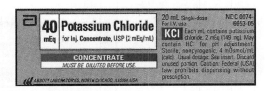

Set and solution: secondary set with drop factor of 15 gtt/ml; 150-ml bottle D₅W; infusion pump.

   a. *Drug Calculation:*

   _____

   b. *Infusion Pump Rate (ml/hr):*
   How many ml/hr should be administered?

   _____

9. Order: magnesium sulfate 5 g in 100 ml D₅W infused over 3 hours. Drug available:

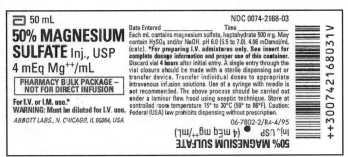

Set and solution: secondary set with drip factor of 15 gtt/ml; 10-ml bag D₅W; infusion pump.

Drug Calculation:

   a. 1 ml = _____ mg (see drug label).

   b. 5 g = _____ ml.

   c. *Infusion Pump Rate (ml/hr):*
   How many ml/hr should be administered?

   _____

10. Order: calcium gluconate 10%, 16 mEq in 100 ml D₅W, infused over 30 minutes.
Drug available:

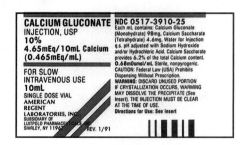

Set and solution: secondary set with a drip factor of 15 gtt/ml; 100-ml bag D₅W; infusion pump.

a. *Drug Calculation:*

_____

b. *Infusion Pump Rate (ml/hr):*
How many ml/hr should be administered?

_____

11. Order: ranitidine (Zantac) 50 mg, IV, q6h.
Set: infusion pump.
Drug available: premixed drug in bag (Zantac 50 mg in 0.45% NaCl [½ NSS]).

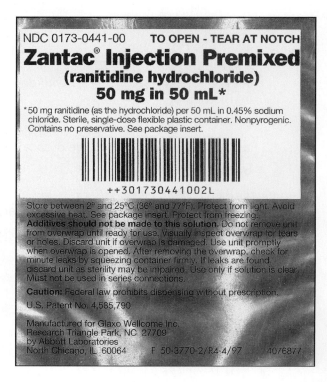

Instructions: Infuse over 15 minutes.

  a. *Infusion Pump Rate:*
  How many ml/hr should be administered?

___

12. Order: cefepime (Maxipime) 750 mg, IV, q12h.
    Set and solution: Infusion pump; 100 ml D$_5$W.
    Drug available:

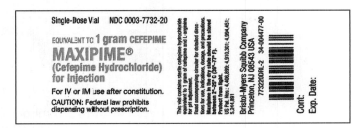

Instructions: Add 8.7 ml of diluent to Maxipime to yield 10 ml of drug solution. Dilute in 100 ml of D$_5$W; infuse over 30 minutes.

  a. *Drug Calculation:*

___

  b. *Infusion Pump Rate (ml/hr):*

___

13. Order: rifampin (Rifadin) 600 mg, IV, daily.
    Set and solution: Infusion pump; 500 ml D$_5$W.
    Drug available: Rifadin, 600 mg sterile powder.

Instructions: Add 10 ml of diluent to the rifampin vial. Dilute rifampin in 500 ml of D$_5$W; infuse over 3 hours.

  a. *Infusion Pump Rate (ml/hr):*

___

14. Order: cefoxitin (Mefoxin) 2 g, IV, q8h.
    Drug available: ADD-Vantage vial.

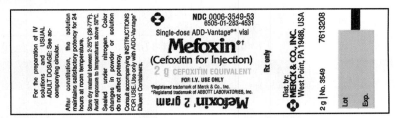

Set and solution: 100 ml of 0.9% NaCl diluent bag for ADD-Vantage; Mefoxin vial for ADD-Vantage.

Instructions: Dilute Mefoxin in 100 ml of NSS (0.9% NaCl) and infuse in 30 minutes.

a. How would you prepare Mefoxin 2 g powdered vial with the diluent bag?
(See page 245 as needed.) _____

b. *Infusion Pump Rate (ml/hr):* _____

15. Order: Hycamtin (toptoecan HCl) 1.5 mg/m²/day, IV, daily for 5 days.
    Adult weight and height: 140 lb, 66 inches.
    Drug available:

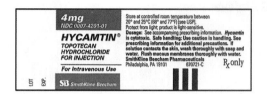

Set and solution: 100 ml of D₅W; infusion pump.

Instructions: Mix Hycamtin with 5.6 ml of diluent, equals 6 ml of Hycamtin;
dilute in 100 ml of D₅W and infuse over 30 minutes.

a. What is the patient's m² (BSA): see page 107.
Drug Calculation: _____
Infusion Pump Rate (ml/hr): _____

16. Order: Velban (vinblantine): initially 3.7 mg/m² as a single dose.
    Adult: Weight 180 lb, height 70 inches.
    Drug available:

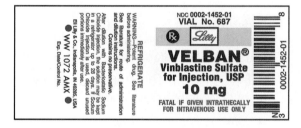

Set and solution: 250 ml of D₅W; infusion pump.

Instructions: Mix vinblastine powdered vial with 10 ml of diluent and inject
solution into 250 ml of D₅W. Infuse over 1 hour.

a. What is the patient's m² (BSA)? _____
Drug Calculation: _____
Infusion Pump Rate (ml/hr): _____

ANSWERS

I Direct IV Injection

1. **a.** 5 ml drug solution
   b. known drug : known minutes ∷ desired drug : desired minutes

      | 5 mg | : | 1 min | ∷ | 50 mg | : | X |

   $$5 X = 50$$
   $$X = 10 \text{ minutes}$$

2. known drug : known minutes :: desired drug : desired minutes
   10 ml : 1 min :: 50 ml : X
$$10\ X = 50$$
$$X = 5\ minutes$$

3. a. 10 ml

 b. known drug : known minutes :: desired drug : desired minutes
   1.5 ml : 1 min :: 10 ml : X
$$1.5\ X = 10$$
$$X = 6.6\ minutes\ or\ 7\ minutes$$

4. a. 5 ml

 b. known drug : known minutes :: desired drug : desired minutes
   10 mg : 1 min :: 50 mg : X
$$10\ X = 50$$
$$X = 5\ minutes$$

5. a. RP: H : V :: D : X
   10 mg : 1 ml :: 6 mg : X
$$10\ X = 6$$
$$X = 0.6\ ml\ morphine$$

or
FE: $\dfrac{H}{V} \times \dfrac{D}{X} = \dfrac{10\ mg}{1\ ml} = \dfrac{6\ mg}{X} =$
$$10\ X = 6$$
$$X = 0.6\ ml$$

 b. known drug : known minutes :: desired drug : desired minutes
   10 mg : 4 min :: 6 mg : X
$$10\ X = 24$$
$$X = 2.4\ minutes$$

6. a. 1 ml

 b. known drug : known minutes :: desired drug : desired minutes
   1 ml : 5 min :: X ml : 1 min
$$5\ X = 1$$
$$X = 0.2\ ml/minutes$$

7. a. DA: ml $= \dfrac{1\ ml \times 2\ \cancel{mg}}{5\ \cancel{mg} \times\ 1} = \dfrac{2}{5} = 0.4$ ml of Haldol

 b. known drug : known minutes :: desired drug : desired minutes
   1 mg : 1 min :: 2 mg : X
$$X = 2\ minutes$$

8. known drug : known minutes :: desired drug : desired minutes

 a. BF: $\dfrac{D}{H} \times V = \dfrac{6\ mg}{4\ mg} \times 1 = 1.5$ ml of Ativan

 b. known drug : known minutes :: desired drug : desired minutes
   2 mg : 1 min :: 6 mg : X
$$2\ X = 6$$
$$X = 3\ minutes$$

9. a. RP: H : V :: D : V
   25 mg : 5 ml :: 20 mg : X ml
$$25\ X = 100$$
$$X = 4\ ml$$

or

$$FE: \frac{H}{V} \times \frac{D}{X} = \frac{25 \text{ mg}}{5 \text{ ml}} \times \frac{20 \text{ mg}}{X \text{ ml}} =$$

(Cross multiply) $\quad\quad\quad$ 25 X = 100

$\quad\quad\quad\quad\quad\quad\quad\quad\quad\quad$ X = 4 ml

or

$$DA: V = \frac{V \times D}{H \times 1}$$

$$ml = \frac{5 \text{ ml} \times \overset{4}{\cancel{20}} \text{ mg}}{\underset{5}{\cancel{25}} \text{ mg} \times 1} = \frac{20}{5} = 4 \text{ ml}$$

b. $\dfrac{\text{Amount of drug}}{\text{Number of minutes}} = \dfrac{4 \text{ ml}}{2 \text{ min}} = 2 \text{ ml/min}$

Answer: Infuse 2 ml of cardizem per minute.

10. **a.** 140 lb ÷ 2.2 = 64 kg

 b. 10 mcg × 64 kg = 640 mcg

 c. Change micrograms (mcg) to milligrams by moving the decimal point three spaces to the *left:*
 $\underset{\smile}{640}$ mcg = 0.640 mg or 0.6 mg.

known drug : known seconds :: desired drug : desired seconds

$\quad$ 1 mg $\quad$: $\quad$ 60 seconds $\quad$ :: $\quad$ 0.6 mg $\quad$: $\quad\quad$ X

$\quad\quad\quad\quad\quad\quad\quad\quad\quad\quad$ X = 36 seconds

Answer: Infuse 0.6 mg of granisetron (Kytril) over 36 seconds.

II Continuous Intravenous Administration

1. **a.** Microdrip set because the patient is to receive 83 ml/hr

 b. Three-step method: (a) $\dfrac{1000}{12} = 83$ ml/hr

 $\quad\quad\quad\quad\quad\quad\quad\quad$ (b) $\dfrac{83}{60} = 1.38$ ml/min

 $\quad\quad\quad\quad\quad\quad\quad\quad$ (c) 1.4 ml/min × 60 gtt/ml = 84 gtt/min

 Using a microdrip set (60 gtt/ml); IV should run at 84 gtt/min.

2. **a.** 1 L = 1000 ml

 b. Each liter should run for 8 hours.

 c. Two-step method: 1000 ÷ 8 = 125 ml/hr

 $$\frac{125 \times \overset{1}{\cancel{15}}}{\underset{4}{\cancel{60}}} = \frac{125}{4} = 31\text{–}32 \text{ gtt/min}$$

 With a 15-gtt/ml drop set, IV should run at 31 to 32 gtt/min.

3. **a.** Microdrip set with drop factor of 60 gtt/ml

 b. One-step method: $\dfrac{250 \times \overset{1}{\cancel{60}}}{24 \times \underset{1}{\cancel{60}}} = 10$ gtt/min

 With a microdrip set, IV should run at 10 gtt/min. KVO usually means 24 hours.

4. **a.** 10 ml of KCl

 b. Use a 10-ml syringe; withdraw 10 ml of KCl and inject into the rubber stopper part of the IV bag.

    c. Microdrip set: 100 gtt/min
      Macrodrip set: drop factor of 20 gtt/ml; 34 gtt/min

5. a. 700 ml of IV fluid is left and 4 hours are left.
   b. Recalculate using 700 ml and 4 hours to run.

     Three-step method: (a) $\dfrac{700}{4} = 175$ ml/hr

                (b) $\dfrac{175}{60} = 2.9$ ml/min

                (c) $2.9 \times 15 = 44$ gtt/min

6. a. 100 gtt/min

     Two-step method: $\dfrac{100 \times \overset{1}{\cancel{60}} \text{ gtt/ml}}{\underset{1}{\cancel{60}} \text{ min}} = 100$ gtt/min

7. a. KCl 40 mEq/20 ml
   b. 20 ml
   c. $\dfrac{1000 \text{ ml}}{125 \text{ ml/hr}} = 8$ hours

8. a. KCl 20 mEq/10 ml
   b. 10 ml
   c. $\dfrac{1000 \text{ ml}}{100 \text{ ml/hr}} = 10$ hours

   d. $\dfrac{100 \text{ ml} \times \overset{1}{\cancel{10}} \text{ gtt/ml}}{\underset{6}{\cancel{60}} \text{ min}} = \dfrac{100}{6} = 16$ to 17 gtt/min

   or

   $\dfrac{1000 \text{ ml} \times \overset{1}{\cancel{10}} \text{ gtt/ml}}{\underset{1}{\cancel{10}} \text{ hr} \times 60 \text{ min}} = \dfrac{1000}{60} = 16$ to 17 gtt/min

III Intermittent Intravenous Administration

1. a. Add 10 ml of sterile or bacteriostatic water (1 g = 10 ml).
   b. *Drug Calculation:* Change 500 mg to grams because the drug label is in grams. Move the decimal point three spaces to the *left:* 500. mg = 0.5 g.

    BF: $\dfrac{D}{H} \times V = \dfrac{0.5}{1} \times 10 \text{ ml} = \dfrac{5}{1} = 5$ ml Cefadyl

    or
    RP: H : V :: D : X
        1 g : 10 ml :: 0.5 g : X ml
           1 X = 10 × 0.5
            X = 5 ml Cefadyl

    or
    FE: $\dfrac{H}{V} \times \dfrac{D}{X} = \dfrac{1 \text{ g}}{10 \text{ ml}} = \dfrac{0.5 \text{ g}}{X \text{ ml}} =$

    (Cross multiply) X = 5 ml of Cefadyl

    or
    DA: ml = $\dfrac{\overset{1}{\cancel{10}} \text{ ml} \times \quad \cancel{1} \text{ g} \quad \times \overset{5}{\cancel{500}} \text{ mg}}{\cancel{1} \text{ g} \times \underset{\underset{1}{100}}{\cancel{1000}} \text{ mg} \times \quad 1} = 5$ ml

c. *Flow Rate Calculation:*

$$\frac{\text{Amount of solution} \times \text{gtt/ml (set)}}{\text{Minutes to administer}} = \frac{75 \text{ ml} \times \overset{2}{\cancel{60}} \text{ gtt/ml}}{\underset{1}{\cancel{30}} \text{ minutes}} = 150 \text{ gtt/min}$$

Regulate flow rate for 150 gtt/min.

2. a. Add 5.7 ml of sterile water.

250 mg = 1.5 ml; 1 g = 6 ml (250 mg is ¼ of a gram; 4 × 1.5 = 6 ml)

b. *Drug Calculation:* Change 400 mg to grams because the drug label is in grams. Move the decimal point three spaces to the *left:* 4̲0̲0̲. mg = 0.4 g.

BF: $\dfrac{0.4}{1} \times 6 \text{ ml} = 2.4 \text{ ml of oxacillin}$

or

RP: 1 g:6 ml :: 0.4 g:X ml

   1 X = 6 × 0.4

    X = 2.4 ml of oxacillin

c. *Flow Rate Calculation:*

$$\frac{100 \text{ ml} \times 15 \text{ gtt/ml (set)}}{40 \text{ minutes}} = 37.5 \text{ or } 38 \text{ gtt/min}$$

Regulate flow rate for 38 gtt/min.

3. a. *Drug Calculation:* ticarcillin 500 mg = 2 ml

b. *Flow Rate Calculation:* amount of solution: 75 ml D₅W + 2 ml of drug solution = 77 ml
For Buretrol set:

$$\frac{77 \text{ ml} \times \overset{3}{\cancel{60}} \text{ gtt/ml (set)}}{\underset{2}{\cancel{40}} \text{ minutes}} = \frac{231}{2} = 115.5 \text{ or } 116 \text{ gtt/min}$$

c. *Infusion Pump Rate:*

$$\text{Amount of solution} \div \frac{\text{Minutes to administer}}{60 \text{ min/hr}} = \text{ml/hr}$$

$$77 \text{ ml} \div \frac{\overset{2}{\cancel{40}} \text{ min to administer}}{\underset{3}{\cancel{60}} \text{ min/hr}} = 77 \times \frac{3}{2} = \frac{231}{2} = 116 \text{ ml/hr}$$

Set pump rate at 116 ml/hr to deliver Ticar 500 mg in 40 minutes.

4. a. *Drug Calculation:*

BF: $\dfrac{D}{H} \times V = \dfrac{2.5 \text{ g}}{\underset{2}{\cancel{4}} \text{ g}} \times \overset{5}{\cancel{10}} \text{ ml} = \dfrac{12.5}{2} = 6.25 \text{ ml}$

or

RP:H : V :: D : X

  4 g:10 ml :: 2.5 g:X ml

     4 X = 25

      X = 6.25 ml

or

FE: $\dfrac{H}{V} \times \dfrac{D}{X} = \dfrac{4\ g}{10\ ml} \times \dfrac{2.5\ g}{X\ ml} =$

(Cross multiply) $\qquad\qquad 4\ X = 25$

$\qquad\qquad\qquad\qquad X = 6.25\ ml$

or

DA: ml $= \dfrac{10\ ml \times 2.5\ \cancel{g}}{4\ \cancel{g} \times 1} = \dfrac{25}{4} = 6.25\ ml$

piperacillin 2.5 g = 6.25 ml

b. *Flow Rate Calculation for Buretrol set:*

$\dfrac{100\ ml \times \overset{2}{\cancel{60}}\ gtt/ml}{\underset{1}{\cancel{30}}\ min/hr} = 200\ gtt/minute$

c. *Infusion Pump Rate:* 100 ml + 6 ml medication = 106 ml

$106\ ml \div \dfrac{\overset{1}{\cancel{30}}\ min\ to\ administer}{\underset{2}{\cancel{60}}\ min/hr} = 106 \times \dfrac{2}{1} = 212\ ml/hr$

Set pump rate at 212 ml/hr to deliver piperacillin 2.5 g in 30 minutes.

5. a. *Drug Calculation:* Staphcillin 4 g = 8 ml. Withdraw 2 ml from vial to yield Staphcillin 1 g.

b. *Flow Rate Calculation for secondary set:*

$\dfrac{\overset{5}{\cancel{100}}\ ml \times 15\ gtt/ml\ (set)}{\underset{2}{\cancel{40}}\ minutes} = \dfrac{75}{2} = 37.5\ or\ 38\ gtt/min$

c. *Infusion Pump Rate:*

$100\ ml \times \dfrac{\overset{2}{\cancel{40}}\ min\ to\ administer}{\underset{3}{\cancel{60}}\ min/hr} = 100 \times \dfrac{3}{2} = \dfrac{300}{2} = 150\ ml/hr$

Set pump rate at 150 ml/hr to deliver Staphcillin 1 g in 40 minutes.

6. a. *Drug Calculation:*

BF: $\dfrac{D}{H} \times V = \dfrac{250\ mg}{\underset{10}{\cancel{400}}\ mg} \times \overset{1}{\cancel{40}}\ ml =$

$\dfrac{250}{10} = 25\ ml$ of ciprofloxacin

FE: $\dfrac{H}{V} \times \dfrac{D}{X} = \dfrac{400}{40} \times \dfrac{250}{X} =$

(Cross multiply) 400 X = 10,000

$\qquad\qquad\qquad X = 25\ ml$ of ciprofloxacin

or

RP:　　H　:　V　::　D　:　X

400 mg : 40 ml :: 250 mg : X ml

400 X = 10,000

X = 25 ml

or

DA: ml $= \dfrac{\overset{1}{\cancel{40}}\ ml \times 250\ \cancel{mg}}{\underset{10}{\cancel{400}}\ \cancel{mg} \times 1} =$

25 ml of ciprofloxacin

b. *Flow Rate Calculation (gtt/min)*

$\dfrac{275\ ml\ (25 + 250) \times 15\ gtt/ml\ (set)}{60\ (1\ hr)} = \dfrac{4125}{60} = 68\ or\ 60\ gtt/min$

7. a. *Flow Rate Calculation (gtt/min)*

$\dfrac{110\ ml\ (10 + 100) \times \overset{3}{\cancel{15}}\ gtt/ml\ (set)}{\underset{8}{\cancel{40}}\ min\ to\ admin} = \dfrac{330}{8} = 41\ gtt/min$

b. *Infusion Pump Rate (ml/hr):*

$$110 \text{ ml} \div \frac{40 \text{ min}}{60 \text{ min}} = 110 \text{ ml} \times \frac{\overset{6}{\cancel{60}}}{\underset{4}{\cancel{40}}} = \frac{660}{4} = 165 \text{ ml/hr}$$

8. a. *Drug calculation:*

BF: $\dfrac{D}{H} \times V = \dfrac{20}{40} \times 20 = \dfrac{400}{40} = 10 \text{ ml KCl}$

or

FE: $\dfrac{H}{V} \times \dfrac{D}{X} = \dfrac{40 \text{ mEq}}{20 \text{ ml}} = \dfrac{20 \text{ mEq}}{X \text{ ml}} =$

(Cross multiply) $40X = 400$

$X = 10 \text{ ml}$

or

RP: $H : V :: D : X$

$40 : 20 :: 20 : X$

$40 X = 400$

$X = 10 \text{ ml KCl}$

or

DA: $\text{ml} = \dfrac{20 \text{ ml} \times \overset{1}{\cancel{20}} \text{ mEq}}{\underset{2}{\cancel{40}} \text{ mEq} \times 1} = \dfrac{20}{2} = 10 \text{ ml}$

Amount of Solution: 150 ml + 10 ml = 160 ml

b. *Infusion Pump Rate:*

$$160 \text{ ml} \div \frac{120 \text{ min to administer}}{60 \text{ min/hr}} = 160 \times \frac{1}{2} = 80 \text{ ml/hr}$$

Set pump rate at 80 ml/hr to deliver KCl 20 mEq in 2 hours.

9. *Drug Calculation:*

a. 1 ml = 500 mg and 2 ml = 1 g.

b. BF: $\dfrac{D}{H} \times V = \dfrac{5}{1} \times 2 = 10 \text{ ml of magnesium sulfate}$

or

RP: $H : V :: D : X$

$1 : 2 :: 5 : X$

$X = 10$

$X = 10 \text{ ml magnesium sulfate}$

or

DA: $\text{ml} = \dfrac{1 \text{ ml} \times \overset{2}{\cancel{1000}} \text{ mg} \times 5 \cancel{g}}{\underset{1}{\cancel{500}} \text{ mg} \times 1 \cancel{g} \times 1} = 10 \text{ ml magnesium sulfate}$

or

FE: $\dfrac{H}{V} \times \dfrac{D}{X} = \dfrac{1 \text{ g}}{2 \text{ ml}} = \dfrac{5 \text{ g}}{X \text{ ml}} =$

(Cross multiply) X = 10 ml of magnesium sulfate

Amount of Solution: 10 ml + 100 ml = 110 ml

c. *Infusion Pump Rate:*

$$110 \text{ ml} \div \frac{\overset{3}{\cancel{180}} \text{ min to administer}}{\underset{1}{\cancel{60}} \text{ min/hr}} = 110 \times \frac{1}{3} = 36.6 \text{ or } 37 \text{ ml/hr}$$

Set pump rate at 37 ml/hr to deliver magnesium sulfate 5 g in 3 hours.

10. a. *Drug Calculation:*

BF: $\dfrac{D}{H} \times V = \dfrac{16 \text{ mEq}}{4.65 \text{ mEq}} \times 10 \text{ ml} = 34.4 \text{ ml}$

or

RP: H   :   V   ::   D   :   X

4.65 mEq : 10 ml :: 16 mEq : X ml

4.65 X = 160

X = 34.4 ml

or

DA: ml = $\dfrac{10\ ml \quad \times\ 16\ m\cancel{Eq}}{4.65\ m\cancel{Eq} \times \quad 1}$ = 34.4 ml

Amount of Solution: 34.4 ml + 100 ml = 134.4 ml

b. *Infusion Pump Rate:*

134.4 ml ÷ $\dfrac{30\ \text{min to administer}}{60\ \text{min/hr}}$ = 134.4 × $\dfrac{2}{1}$ = 268.8 or 269 ml/hr (invert divisor)

11. a. *Amount of Solution:* ÷ $\dfrac{\text{min to administer}}{60\ \text{ml/hr}}$

50 ml ÷ $\dfrac{15\ \text{min}}{60\ \text{min}}$ = 50 ml × $\dfrac{\overset{4}{\cancel{60}}\ \text{min}}{\underset{1}{\cancel{15}}\ \text{min}}$ = 200 ml/hr

Infusion Pump Rate: 200 ml/hr

12. 1 g = 1000 mg (use conversion table as needed) of Maxipime

Drug Calculation:

$\dfrac{D}{H}$ × V = $\dfrac{\overset{3}{\cancel{750}}\ \text{mg}}{\underset{4}{\cancel{1000}}\ \text{mg}}$ × 10 ml = $\dfrac{30}{4}$ = 7.5 ml drug solution

Infusion Pump Rate:

107.5 ml ÷ $\dfrac{30\ \text{min to administer}}{60\ \text{min/hr}}$ = 107.5 ml × $\dfrac{\overset{2}{\cancel{60}}}{\underset{1}{\cancel{30}}}$ = 215 ml/hr pump rate

13. *Amount of Solution:* 10 ml + 500 ml = 510 ml

Infusion Pump Rate: 510 ml ÷ $\dfrac{180\ \text{min}}{60\ \text{min/hr}}$ = 510 ml × $\dfrac{\overset{1}{\cancel{60}}}{\underset{3}{\cancel{180}}}$ = $\dfrac{510}{3}$ = 170 ml/hr

170 ml/hr for 3 hours

14. a. See page 232 for mixing ADD-Vantage drugs. Mix 2 g of cefoxitin (Mefoxin) using ADD-Vantage vial with ADD-Vantage diluent bag.

b. *Infusion Pump Rate (ml/hr)*

100 ml ÷ $\dfrac{30\ \text{minutes to admin}}{60\ \text{min/hr}}$ =

100 ml × $\dfrac{\overset{2}{\cancel{60}}}{\underset{1}{\cancel{30}}}$ = 200 ml/hr

15. a. BSA: 1.74 m², see page 232.

Drug Calculation:

1.5 mg/1.74/day = 2.61 or 2.6 mg per day

BF: $\dfrac{D}{H}$ × V = $\dfrac{2.6\ \text{mg}}{\underset{2}{\cancel{4}}\ \text{mg}}$ × $\overset{3}{\cancel{6}}$ ml = $\dfrac{7.8}{2}$ = 3.9 ml or 4 ml

Infusion Pump Rate (ml/hr):

$$104 \ (100 + 4) \div \frac{30 \text{ min to admin}}{60 \text{ min/hr}} = 104 \times \frac{\overset{2}{\cancel{60}}}{\underset{1}{\cancel{30}}} = 208 \text{ minutes}$$

16. a. 2.05 m² (BSA)
Drug Calculation:
3.7 mg × 2.05 BSA = 7.58 or 7.6 mg
Velban 10 mg diluted in 10 ml
Each mg = 1 ml; 7.6 mg = 7.6 ml

Infusion Pump Rate (ml/hr):

$$257.6 \text{ ml } (7.6 + 250) \div \frac{60}{60} = 257.6 \times \frac{\overset{1}{\cancel{60}}}{\underset{1}{\cancel{60}}} = 257.6 \text{ or } 258 \text{ ml/hr}$$

 Additional practice problems are available on the enclosed CD-ROM in the "Intravenous Calculations" and "Advanced Calculations" sections.

PART IV

CALCULATIONS FOR SPECIALTY AREAS

Pediatrics

CHAPTER 10

OBJECTIVES

- Use the two primary methods of determining pediatric drug dosages.
- State the reason for checking pediatric dosages before administration.
- Describe the dosage inaccuracies that can occur with pediatric drug formulas.
- Identify the steps in determining body surface area from a pediatric nomogram and with the square root method.

OUTLINE

FACTORS INFLUENCING PEDIATRIC DRUG ADMINISTRATION
    Oral
    Intramuscular
    Intravenous
PEDIATRIC DRUG CALCULATIONS
    Dosage per Kilogram Body Weight
    Dosage per Body Surface Area
PEDIATRIC DOSAGE FROM ADULT DOSAGE
    Body Surface Area Formula
    Age Rules

FACTORS INFLUENCING PEDIATRIC DRUG ADMINISTRATION

Drug dosages for children differ greatly from those for adults because of the physiological differences between the two groups. Neonates and infants have immature kidney and liver function, which delays metabolism and elimination of many drugs. Drug absorption in neonates is different as a result of slow gastric emptying. Decreased gastric acid secretion in children younger than 3 years contributes to altered drug absorption. Neonates and infants have a lower concentration of plasma proteins, which can cause toxic effects with drugs that are highly bound to proteins. They have less total body fat and more total body water. Therefore lipid-soluble drugs require smaller doses because less than normal fat is present, and water-soluble drugs can require larger doses because of a greater percentage of body water. As children grow, changes in fat, muscle, body water, and organ maturity can alter the pharmacokinetic effects of drugs. Most drugs are dosed according to weight, and doses are specifically calculated for each child. For example, a dose of cefazolin for a 34-kg, 12-year-old child is larger than a dose for a 7-kg, 8-month-old infant. It is the nurse's responsibility to ensure that a safe drug dosage is given and to closely monitor signs and symptoms of adverse reactions to drugs. The purpose of learning how to calculate pediatric drug doses is to ensure that each child receives the correct dose within the therapeutic range.

Oral

Oral pediatric drug delivery often requires the use of a calibrated measuring device, because most drugs for small children are provided in liquid form. The measuring device can be a small plastic cup, an oral dropper, a measuring spoon, an oral syringe, or a specially designed pediatric medication dispenser such as the Medibottle (Figure 10-1). The Medibottle is a specially designed pediatric medication dispenser that provides optimum drug delivery by allowing small volumes of medication to be swallowed with oral fluids. Some liquid medications come with their own calibrated droppers. The type of measuring device chosen depends on the developmental level of the child. For infants and toddlers, the oral syringe and dropper, Medibottle, provide better drug delivery than is provided by a small cup. A young child who is cooperative is able to use a small cup or measuring spoon. All liquid medications can be drawn up with an oral syringe to ensure accuracy and then are transferred to a small cup or measuring spoon. It may be necessary to refill the cup or spoon with water or juice and to have the child drink that as well, to ensure that all prescribed medication has been administered. Medicine should not be mixed in the infant's or toddler's bottle because the full dose will not be administered if the child doesn't finish the bottle. Any medication with a strong taste should not be mixed in formula because the infant could begin to refuse formula. Avoid giving oral medications to a crying child or infant, who could easily aspirate the medication. Some chewable medications are available for administration to the older child. Because many drugs are enteric-coated or are provided in timed-release form, the child must be told which medications are to be swallowed and not chewed.

Intramuscular

Intramuscular sites are chosen on the basis of the age and muscle development of the child (Table 10-1). All injections should be given in a manner that minimizes physical and psychosocial trauma. The child must be adequately restrained, if necessary, and provided with a momentary distraction. The procedure must be performed quickly, with comfort measures immediately following.

NOTE

The usual needle length and gauge for pediatric clients are ½ to 1 inch long and 22 to 25 gauge. Another method of estimating needle length is to grasp the muscle for injection between the thumb and the forefinger; half the distance would be the needle length.

Intravenous

For children, the maximum amount of intravenous (IV) fluid varies with body weight. Their 24-hour fluid status must be monitored closely to prevent overhydration. The amount of fluid given with IV medication must be considered in the planning of their 24-hour intake (Table 10-2). After the correct dosage

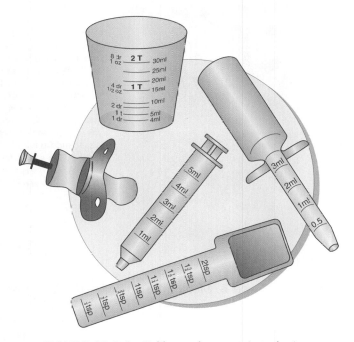

FIGURE 10-1 **A,** Calibrated measuring devices.

Continued

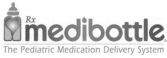

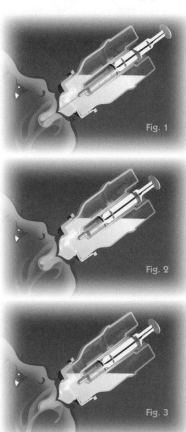

Squirt and Sip Process:

The infant begins to drink the liquid in the medibottle. The parent or caregiver presses the dispenser's plunger to jet a small squirt of medicine or supplements to the tip of the nipple. (Fig. 1) The baby's milk or favorite liquid will then be in position directly behind the medicine in the nipple. (Fig. 2)

With the baby's next sip, this medicine is swallowed and immediately washed down with the milk or favorite liquid. The medicine is undetected by the baby, who tastes only the milk or favorite liquid. (Fig. 3)

Baby swallows several more sips of the milk or favorite liquid before the parent or caregiver presses the plunger again to repeat the Squirt and Sip Process. The entire dose will be administered in 60 seconds, using one ounce of milk or baby's favorite liquid.

FIGURE 10-1, cont'd B, Medibottle. (**B,** from The Medicine Bottle Company, Inc.)

TABLE 10-1

Pediatric Guidelines for Intramuscular Injections According to Muscle Group*

	Amount by Muscle Group (ml)				
	Vastus Lateralis	Rectus Femoris	Ventro-gluteal	Dorsal Gluteal	Deltoid
Neonates	0.5 ml	Not safe	Not safe	Not safe	Not safe
Infants 1-12 months	0.5-1 ml	Not safe	Not safe	Not safe	Not safe
Toddlers 1-2 years	0.5-2 ml	0.5-1 ml	Not safe	Not safe	0.5-1 ml
Preschool to child 3-12 years	2 ml	2 ml	0.5-3 ml	0.5-2 ml	0.5-1 ml
Adolescent 12-18 years	2 ml	2 ml	2-3 ml	2-3 ml	1-1.5 ml

*The safe use of all sites is based on normal muscle development and size of the child. Follow institutional policies and procedures.

TABLE 10-2

Pediatric Guidelines for 24-Hour Intravenous Fluid Therapy

100 ml/kg for first 10 kg body weight
50 ml/kg for the next 10 kg body weight
20 ml/kg after 20 kg body weight

Example: Child's weight 25 kg

100 ml/kg × 10 kg = 1000 ml
50 ml/kg × 10 kg = 500 ml
20 ml/kg × 5 kg = 100 ml
1600 ml for 24 hours, or 66.6 ml/hr, or 67 ml

of drug is obtained, it may need further dilution and to be given over a specified time, as mentioned in Chapter 9. Usually, the drug is diluted with 5 to 60 ml of IV fluid, depending on the drug or dosage, placed in a calibrated cylinder or syringe pump, and infused over 20 to 60 minutes, depending on the type of drug. After the drug has been infused, the cylinder is flushed with 3 to 20 ml of IV fluid to ensure that the child has received all of the medication and to prevent admixture. Refer to Chapter 9 for methods of calculating IV infusion rates.

The safety factors that must be considered when medications are administered to children are similar to those for adults. See Appendix A for more detailed information on safe nursing practice for drug administration.

PEDIATRIC DRUG CALCULATIONS

The two main methods of determining drug dosages for pediatric drug administration are body weight and body surface area (BSA). The first method uses a specific number of milligrams, micrograms, or units for each kilogram of body weight (mg/kg, mcg/kg, unit/kg). Usually, drug data for pediatric dosage (mg/kg) are supplied by manufacturers in a drug information insert. BSA, measured in square meters (m²), is considered a more accurate method than body weight. BSA takes into consideration the relation between basal metabolic rate and surface area, which correlates with blood volume, cardiac output, and organ growth and development. Although BSA has been used primarily to calculate the dosage of antineoplastic agents, BSA is used when there is a narrow margin between therapeutic and toxic doses. Pharmaceutical manufacturers are including BSA parameters (mg/m², mcg/m², units/ m²) in the drug information.

If the manufacturer does not supply data for pediatric dosing, the child's dosage can be determined from the adult dose. The BSA formula is used to calculate the pediatric dose. The BSA formula is considered more accurate than previously used formulas, such as Clark's, Young's, and Fried's rules. Drug calculations performed according to the BSA formula are safer than those done with formulas that rely solely on the child's age or weight. Although the BSA formula has improved the accuracy of drug dosing in infants and children, calculation of drug doses for neonates and preterm infants with this method does not guarantee complete accuracy.

 NOTE

If the manufacturer states in the drug information insert that the medication is not for pediatric use, the alternative formulas should not be used for dosage calculation.

Dosage per Kilogram Body Weight

The following information is needed to calculate the dosage.
a. Physician's order with the name of the drug, the dosage, and the frequency of administration.
b. The child's weight in kilograms:

$$1 \text{ kg} = 2.2 \text{ lb}$$

c. The pediatric dosage as listed by the manufacturer or hospital formulary.
d. Information on how the drug is supplied.

EXAMPLES

PROBLEM 1
a. Order: amoxicillin (Amoxil) 60 mg, po, tid.
   Child's weight: 12½ lb.

b. Change pounds to kilograms.

$$\frac{12.5}{2.2} = 5.7 \text{ kg}$$

c. Pediatric dosage for children who weigh 20 kg: 20-40 mg/kg/day in three equal doses.

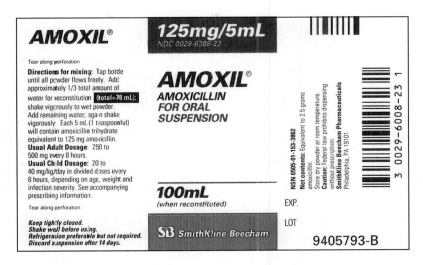

Step 1: Check dosing parameters by multiplying the child's weight by the minimum and maximum daily dose of the drug.

$$20 \text{ mg/kg/day} \times 5.7 \text{ kg} = 114 \text{ mg/day}$$

$$40 \text{ mg/kg/day} \times 5.7 \text{ kg} = 228 \text{ mg/day}$$

Step 2: Multiply the dosage by the frequency to determine the daily dose. The order for amoxicillin 60 mg, po, tid means that three doses will be given per day.

$$60 \text{ mg} \times 3 = 180 \text{ mg}$$

Because the daily dose of amoxicillin 180 mg falls within the recommended range, it is considered a safe dose.

d. Drug preparation:
Use the basic formula (BF), ratio and proportion (RP), or dimensional analysis (DA).
Basic Formula

BF: $\dfrac{D}{H} \times V = \dfrac{60 \text{ mg}}{125 \text{ mg}} \times 5 \text{ ml} = 2.4 \text{ ml}$

or

RP: *Ratio and Proportion*
125 mg:5 ml :: 60 mg:X ml
$\qquad$ 125X = 300
$\qquad\qquad$ X = 2.4 ml

or

Fractional Equation

$\dfrac{H}{V} \times \dfrac{D}{X} = \dfrac{125 \text{ mg}}{5 \text{ ml}} = \dfrac{60 \text{ mg}}{X} =$

(Cross multiply) 125X = 300
$\qquad\qquad\qquad$ X = 2.4 ml

or

DA: ml = $\dfrac{5\ ml\ \times 60\ mg}{125\ mg \times\ 1} = \dfrac{300}{125} = 2.4\ ml$

Answer: amoxicillin 60 mg, po = 2.4 ml

PROBLEM 2

a. Order: ampicillin 350 mg, IV, q6h.
Child's weight and age: 61.5 lb and 9 years old.
Dilution instructions: Mix with 20 ml of D_5/1/4 NSS; infuse over 20 minutes.
Flush with 15 ml.

b. Change pounds to kilograms.

$$\frac{61.5}{2.2} = 27.95\ or\ 28\ kg$$

c. Pediatric dose is 25 to 50 mg/kg/day in divided doses.
Step 1: Multiply weight by minimum and maximum daily dose:

$$25\ mg \times 28\ kg = 700\ mg/day$$

$$50\ mg \times 28\ kg = 1400\ mg/day$$

Step 2: Multiply the dose by the frequency:

$$350\ mg \times 4 = 1400\ mg/day$$

The dose is considered safe because it does not exceed the therapeutic range.

d. Drug available: When diluted, 500 mg = 2 ml. Use your selected formula to calculate the dosage.

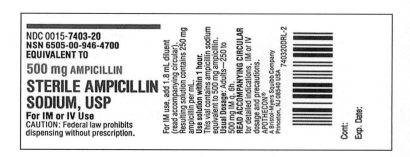

BF: $\dfrac{D}{H} \times V = \dfrac{350\ mg}{500\ mg} \times 2\ ml = 1.4\ ml$

or

RP: 500 mg : 2 ml :: 350 mg : X ml
500X = 700
X = 1.4 ml

or

FE: $\dfrac{H}{V} \times \dfrac{D}{X} = \dfrac{500\ mg}{2\ ml} \times \dfrac{350\ mg}{X} =$
500 X = 700
X = 1.4 ml

or
DA: no conversion factor

$$ml = \frac{2\ ml\ \times \overset{7}{\cancel{350}}\ \cancel{mg}}{\underset{10}{\cancel{500}}\ \cancel{mg} \times\ 1} = \frac{14}{10} = 1.4\ ml$$

Answer: Each dose is 1.4 ml.

e. Amount of fluid to infuse medication:

$$1.4\ ml + 20\ ml\ (dilution) = 21.4\ ml$$

f. Flow rate calculation (60 gtt/ml set):

$$\frac{Amount\ of\ solution \times gtt/ml\ (set)}{Minutes\ to\ administer} = gtt/min$$

$$\frac{21.4\ ml \times \overset{3}{\cancel{60}}\ gtt/ml}{\underset{1}{\cancel{20}}\ minutes} = 64.2\ gtt/min\ or\ 64\ gtt/min$$

g. Infusion pump setting

$$Amount\ of\ solution \div \frac{Minutes\ to\ administer}{60\ min/hr} =$$

$$21.4\ ml \div \frac{20\ minutes}{60\ minutes} =$$

$$21.4 \times \frac{60}{20} = 64.2\ ml/hr\ or\ 64\ ml\ (round\ off)$$

REMEMBER

- The IV flush (3-20 ml) is part of the total IV fluids necessary for medication administration and must be included in patient intake. The flush is started after IV medication infusion is completed, and it is infused at the same rate.
- For a 60 gtt/ml set, the drop per minute rate is the same as the milliliter per minute rate.

Dosage per Body Surface Area

The following information is needed to calculate the dosage:
a. Physician's order with name of drug, dosage, and time frame or frequency.
b. Child's height, weight in kilograms, and age.
c. Information on how the drug is supplied.
d. Pediatric dosage (in m²) as listed by manufacturer or hospital formulary.
e. BSA with square root.
f. BSA nomogram for children (Figure 10-2).

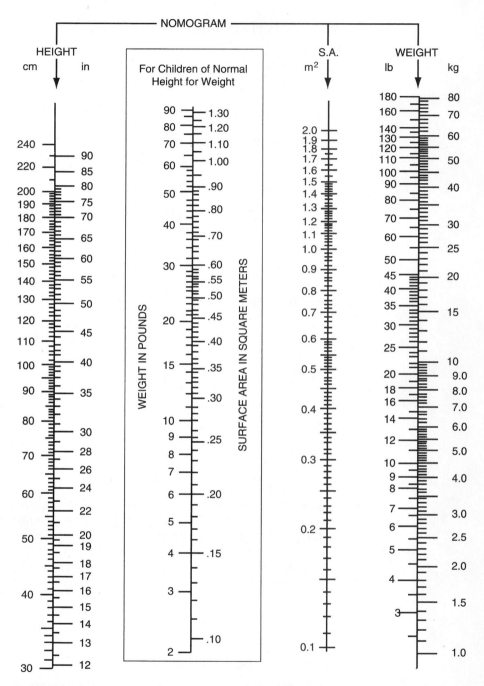

FIGURE 10-2 West Nomogram for Infants and Children. *Directions:* (1) Find height; (2) find weight; (3) draw a straight line connecting the height and weight. Where the line intersects on the S.A. (surface area) column is the body surface area in square meters (m²). (Modified from data by E. Boyd & C. D. West. In Behrman, R. E., Kliegman, R. M., & Jenson, H. B. [2004]. *Nelson textbook of pediatrics.* 17th ed. Philadelphia: W. B. Saunders.)

EXAMPLES

PROBLEM 1
a. Order: methotrexate 50 mg, IV, × 1.
b. Child's height, weight, age: 134 cm, 32.5 kg, 9 yr.
c. Pediatric dose: 25-75 mg/m² wk.
d. Drug preparation: 25 mg/ml.
e. BSA with square root (see BSA metric formula on page 100)

$$\sqrt{\frac{134 \times 32.5}{3600}} = 1.09 \text{ m}^2$$

$$75 \text{ mg/m}^2 \times 1.09 \text{ m}^2 = 81.75 \text{ or } 82 \text{ mg}$$

Compare answer with nomogram.

f. BSA nomogram for children: The child's height (134 cm) and weight (32.5 kg) intersect at 1.11 m² BSA.

Multiply the BSA, 1.11 m², by the minimum and maximum dose. (Substitute BSA for weight.)

$$25 \text{ mg/m}^2 \times 1.11 \text{ m}^2 = 28.0 \text{ mg}$$

$$75 \text{ mg/m}^2 \times 1.11 \text{ m}^2 = 83.0 \text{ mg}$$

This dose is considered safe because it is within the therapeutic range for the child's BSA.

g. Calculate drug dose: For determination of the amount of drug to be administered, either formula can be used:

BF: $\dfrac{D}{H} \times V = \dfrac{50 \text{ mg}}{25 \text{ mg}} \times 1 \text{ ml} = 2 \text{ ml}$

or
FE: $\dfrac{H}{V} \times \dfrac{D}{X} = \dfrac{25 \text{ mg}}{1 \text{ ml}} = \dfrac{50 \text{ mg}}{X \text{ ml}}$
(Cross multiply) 25X = 50
X = 2 ml

or
RP: 25 mg:1 ml :: 50 mg:X ml
25X = 50
X = 2 ml

or
DA: ml $\dfrac{1 \text{ ml} \times \overset{2}{\cancel{50} \text{ mg}}}{\underset{1}{\cancel{25} \text{ mg}} \times 1} = 2 \text{ ml}$

Answer: methotrexate 50 mg = 2 ml

SUMMARY PRACTICE PROBLEMS

In the following dosage problems for oral, IM, and IV administration, determine whether the ordered dose is safe and how much of the drug should be given. Answers are on page 278.

I. Oral

1. Child with rheumatic fever.
Order: penicillin V potassium 250 mg, po, q8h.
Child's weight: 45 lb, age 4 years old.
Pediatric dose: 25-50 mg/kg/day.
Drug available:

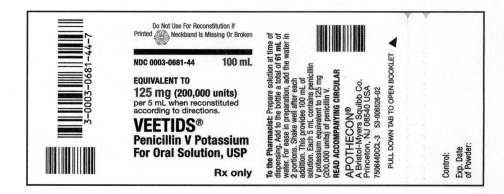

2. Child with seizures.
Order: phenobarbital 25 mg, po, bid.
Child's weight: 7.2 kg, age 9 months.
Pediatric dose: 5-7 mg/kg/day.
Drug available: phenobarbital 20 mg/5 ml.

3. Child with lower respiratory tract infection.
Order: cefprozil (Cefzil) 100 mg, po, q12h.
Child's weight: 17 lb; age: 6 months.
Pediatric dose greater than 6 months: 15 mg/kg/q12h.
Drug available:

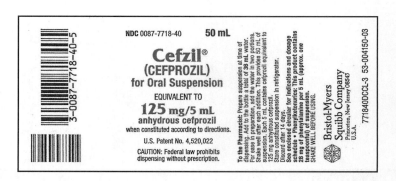

4. Child with pain.
Order: codeine 7.5 mg, po, q4h, prn × 6 doses/day.
Child's height and weight: 43 inches, 50 lb, age 5 years old.
Pediatric dose: 100 mg/m^2/day (see Figure 10-2), or solve by square root.
Drug available: codeine 15 mg tablets.

5. Child with seizures.
   Order: Zarontin 125 mg, po, bid.
   Child's weight: 13 kg, age 36 months.
   Pediatric dose: 15-40 mg/kg/day.
   Drug available:

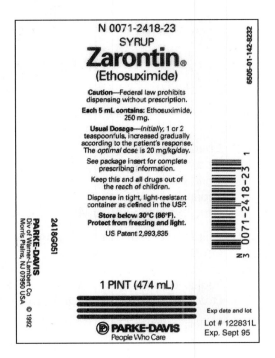

6. Child with seizures.
   Order: Dilantin 40 mg, po, bid.
   Child's weight: 6.7 kg, age 3 months.
   Pediatric dose: 5-7 mg/kg/day.
   Drug available: Dilantin 125 mg/5 ml.

7. Child with a urinary tract infection.
   Order: Gantrisin 1.5 g, po, qid.
   Child's weight: 30.4 kg, age 8 years old.
   Pediatric dose: 120-150 mg/kg/day.
   Drug available: Gantrisin 500 mg tablets.

8. Infant with upper respiratory tract infection.
   Order: Augmentin oral suspension 75 mg, po, q8h.
   Child's weight: 8 kg, age 7 months.
   Pediatric dose: 20-40 mg/kg/day.
   Drug available:

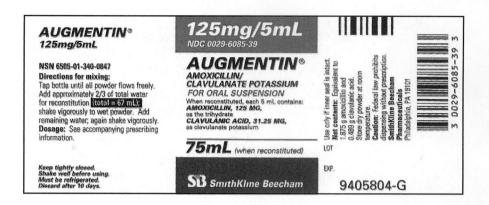

9. Child with poison ivy.
    Order: Benadryl 25 mg, po, q6h.
    Child's weight: 25 kg, age 7 years old.
    Pediatric dose: 5 mg/kg/day.
    Drug available: Benadryl 12.5 mg/5 ml.

10. Child with cystic fibrosis exposed to influenza A.
    Order: Oseltamivir 45 mg, po, bid × 5 days.
    Child's weight and age: 16 kg, 4 years old.
    Pediatric dose: 90 mg/day for 16-23 kg.
    Drug available: Oseltamivir 12 mg/ml.

11. Order: cefaclor (Ceclor) 50 mg, qid.
    Child's weight: 15 lb, age 4 months.
    Pediatric dose: 20-40 mg/kg/day in three to four divided doses.
    Drug available:

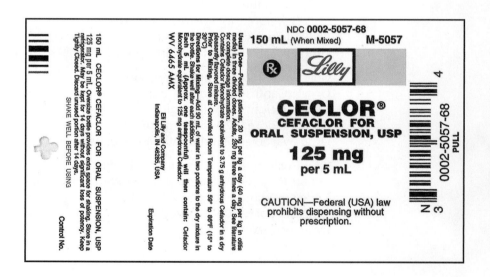

II. Intramuscular

12. Child with pain after surgery.
Order: morphine 4.5 mg/ IM × 1.
Child's weight and age: 45 kg and 14 years old.
Pediatric dose: 0.1 mg/kg.
Drug available: Morphine 10 mg/ml.

13. Child has strep throat (streptococcal pharyngitis).
Order: Bicillin C-R, 1,000,000 units, IM, × 1.
Child's weight: 44 lb.
Pediatric dose: 30-60 lb: 900,000-1,200,000 units daily.
Drug available: Bicillin C-R, 1,200,000 units/2 ml.

14. Child receiving preoperative medication (may solve by nomogram or square root).
Order: hydroxyzine (Vistaril) 25 mg, IM.
Child's height and weight: 47 inches, 45 lb.
Pediatric dose: 30 mg/m^2.
Drug available:

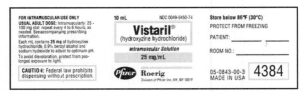

15. Child receiving preoperative medication.
Order: atropine 0.2 mg, IM.
Child's weight: 12 kg, 7 months old.
Pediatric dose: 0.01-0.02 mg/kg/dose, not to exceed 0.4 mg/dose.
Drug available:

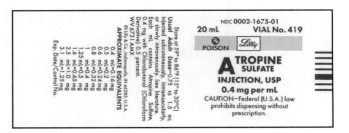

16. Child with cancer.
Order: methotrexate 40 mg, IM, weekly (may solve by nomogram or square root).
Child's height and weight: 56 inches, 100 lb.
Pediatric dose: 7.5-30 mg/m^2/wk.
Drug available: methotrexate 2.5 mg/ml; 25 mg/ml; 100 mg/ml.

17. Order: A newborn is to receive AquaMEPHYTON (vitamin K) 0.5 mg IM immediately after delivery.
Pediatric dose: 0.5-1 mg.

Drug available:

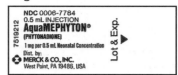 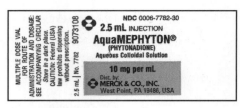

a. Which AquaMEPHYTON container would you select?
b. How many milliliters (ml) should the newborn receive?
c. Is drug dose within the safe range?

III. Intravenous

18. Adolescent with progressive hip pain secondary to rheumatoid arthritis.
Order: morphine sulfate 2.5 mg, IV piggyback, in 10 ml NSS over 5 minutes.
    Flush with 5 ml.
Child's weight: 50 kg, 16 years old.
Pediatric dose: 50-100 mcg/kg/dose for IV.
Drug available:

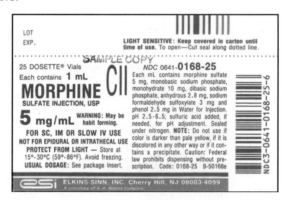

a. How many milliliters should infuse?
b. How many drops/minute should infuse?

19. Treatment to reverse postoperative narcotic depression.
Order: Narcan (naloxone) 1.8 mg IV push.
Child's weight and age: 18 kg and 3 years old.
Pediatric dose: 0.1 mg/kg
Drug available:

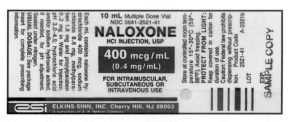

20. Infant with sepsis.
Order: Amikin 40 mg, IV, q12h, in D_5W 5 ml, over 20 minutes. Flush with
    3 ml.
Child's weight: 5.3 kg, 1 year old.

Pediatric dose: 15 mg/kg/day.
Drug available:

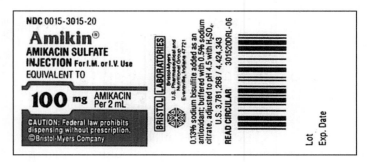

a. How many milliliters should infuse?
b. How many drops/minute should infuse?

21. Treatment for child with cerebral palsy having spasticity after spinal fusion
Order: lorazepam 3 mg IV q6h.
Child's weight and age: 47 kg and 17 years.
Pediatric dose: 0.05-0.1 mg/kg.
Drug available: lorazepam 4 mg/ml.

22. Child with pneumonia.
Order: cefazolin (Ancef) 500 mg, IV, q6h, in D$_5$W 20 ml, over 30 minutes.
Flush with 10 ml.
Child's weight and age: 5.6 kg and 2 months.
Pediatric dose: 25-100 mg/kg/day in four divided doses.
Drug available:

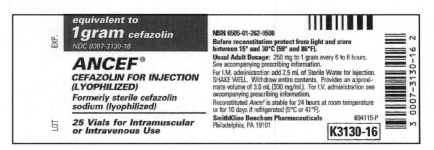

23. Child with sepsis.
Order: gentamicin 10 mg, IV, q8h, in D$_5$W, 4 ml, over 30 minutes. Flush with 3 ml.
Child's height, weight, age: 21 inches, 4 kg, 1 month.
Pediatric dose: greater than 7 days old: 5-7.5 mg/kg/day, three divided doses.
Drug available: gentamicin 10 mg/ml.
a. How many milliliters should infuse?
b. How many drops/minute should infuse?

24. Child with postoperative wound infection.
Order: cefazolin 185 mg, IV, q6h, in D$_5$W 20 ml, over 20 minutes. Flush with 15 ml.
Child's weight: 15 kg.

Pediatric dose: 25-50 mg/kg/day.
Drug available:

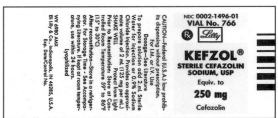

    a. How many milliliters should infuse?
    b. How many drops/minute should infuse?

25. Child with staphylococcus scalded skin syndrome.
Order: clindamycin 50 mg IV q8h.
Dilution instructions: mix in 10 mL NSS over 15 min via syringe pump.
Child's weight and age: 7.5 kg and 5 months old
Pediatric dose: 16-20 mg/kg/day
Drug available: clindamycin 150 mg/ml

26. Child with congestive heart failure.
Order: digoxin 40 mcg, IV, bid, in NSS 2 ml, over 1 minute.
Child's weight and age: 6 lb, 1 month.
Pediatric dose: 2 weeks to 2 years: 25-50 mcg/kg.
Drug available: digoxin 0.1 mg/ml.

27. Child with lymphoma.
Order: Cytoxan 125 mg, IV, in D$_5$½ NSS, 300 ml, over 3 hours, no flush to follow.
Child's weight and height: 16 kg, 75 cm (may solve by nomogram or square root).
Pediatric dose: 60-250 mg/m^2/day.
Drug available:

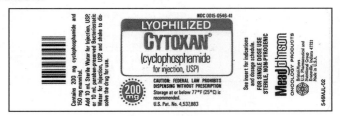

28. Child with severe respiratory tract infection.
Order: kanamycin (Kantrex) 60 mg, IV, q8h.
Child's weight and age: 26 lb, 12 months.
Pediatric dose parameters: 15 mg/kg/day q8-12h, not to exceed 1.5 g per day.
Drug available:

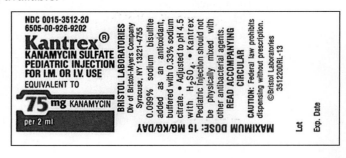

a. How many milliliters of kanamycin will the child receive every 8 hours?

_____

b. How many milliliters of kanamycin will the child receive per day?

_____

c. Is the drug dose within the safe range? _____

29. Child with severe systemic infection.
    Order: tobramycin (Nebcin) 15 mg, IV, q6h.
    Drug available:

NDC 0002-0501-01
2 mL   VIAL No. 782

Ⓡ *Lilly*

NEBCIN®
PEDIATRIC
TOBRAMYCIN
SULFATE
INJECTION
USP

Equiv. to Tobramycin

20 mg
per
2 mL

Multiple Dose
For I.M. or I.V. Use
Must dilute for I.V. use.
YE 1170 AMX
Eli Lilly & Company
Indpls., IN 46285, U.S.A.
Exp. Date/Control No.

Child's weight and age: 10 kg, 18 months.
Pediatric dose parameters: 6-7.5 mg/kg/day in four divided doses.

a. How many milliliters of tobramycin would you give?

_____

b. Is the drug dose within the safe range?

_____

30. Child with acute lymphocytic leukemia.
    Order: daunorubicin HCl 40 mg, IV, daily.
    Pediatric dose parameters: greater than 2 yr: 25-45 mg/m²/day.
    Child's age, weight, and height: 10 years, 72 lb, 60 inches.
    Drug available: daunorubicin 20 mg/4 ml.
    Instructions: Mix in 100 ml D₅W; infuse in 45 minutes via pump.

a. The BSA is _____

b. How many milliliters should be mixed in the D₅W? _____

c. Is the drug dose within the safe range? _____

d. How many milliliters should infuse. _____

31. Child, 7 years old, with pin worms.
    Order: Pyrantel pamoate suspension 250 mg.
    Child's weight: 52 lb.
    Pediatric dose: 11 mg/kg.
    Drug available: Pyrantel pamoate 50 mg/ml.

a. How much does the child weigh in kilograms? _____

b. What dosage should the child receive? _____

c. How many milliliters should the child receive? _____

IV. Neonates

32. Neonate with bradycardia, heart rate less than 60 beats/min.
Order: epinephrine 0.25 mg IV now.
Pediatric dose: 0.1 mg/kg.
Neonate weight: 2.5 kg.
Drug available:

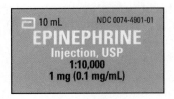

33. Neonate with respiratory depression after delivery, mother received Stadol during labor.
Neonate weight: 8 lb 12 oz.
Order: naxolone 0.04 mg IM now.
Pediatric dose: 0.01 mg/kg.
Drug available: naxolone 0.4 mg/ml.

34. Neonate with bacterial meningitis.
Neonate weight: 2.5 kg.
Order: ampicillin 125 mg IV push over 2 minutes.
Pediatric dose parameters: 50 to 75 mg/kg/dose.
Drug available:

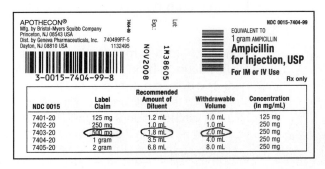

35. Neonate with IV fluids for sepsis.
Neonate weight: 2.5 kg.
Order: $D_{10}W$ 80 ml/kg for 24 hours.

   a. How much $D_{10}W$ should be given in 24 hours?

   b. How many milliliters per hour should be infused?

36. Neonate with sepsis.
Neonate weight: 2.5 kg.
Order: gentamicin 10 mg IV over 24 hours.
Pediatric dosage parameters: 4-5 mg/kg.
Drug available: gentamicin 40 mg/ml.

PEDIATRIC DOSAGE FROM ADULT DOSAGE

Body Surface Area Formula

The following information is needed to calculate the pediatric dosage with the BSA formula:

a. Physician's order with the name of the drug, the dosage, and the time frame or frequency.
b. The child's height and weight.
c. A BSA nomogram for children.
d. The adult drug dosage.
e. The BSA formula:

$$\frac{BSA\ (m^2)}{1.73\ m^2} \times Adult\ dose = Child's\ dose$$

EXAMPLE

PROBLEM 1

a. Erythromycin 80 mg, po, qid.
b. Child's height is 34 inches and weight is 28.5 lb.

Note: *Height and weight do not have to be converted to the metric system.*

c. Height (34 inches) and weight (28.5 lb) intersect the nomogram at 0.57 m². See BSA nomogram, Figure 10-2.
d. The adult drug dosage is 1000 mg/24 hr.
e. BSA formula:

$$\frac{BSA\ (m^2)}{1.73\ m^2} \times Adult\ dose = \frac{0.57\ m^2}{1.73\ m^2} \times 1000\ mg$$
$$= 0.33 \times 1000\ mg$$
$$= 330\ mg/24\ hr$$

Dose frequency:

$$330\ mg \div 4\ doses = 82.5\ \textbf{or}\ 80\ mg\ per\ dose$$

$$80\ mg \times 4\ times\ per\ day = 320\ mg/day$$

Dosage is safe.

Age Rules

Fried's rule and Young's rule are two methods for determining pediatric drug doses based on the child's age. Fried's rule is used primarily for children younger than 1 year of age, whereas Young's rule is used for children between 2 and 12 years of age. In current practice, these rules are infrequently used. Because the maturational development of infants and children is variable, age cannot be an accurate basis for drug dosing.

Fried's Rule:

$$\frac{Age\ in\ months}{150} \times Adult\ dose = Infant\ dose$$

Young's Rule:

$$\frac{\text{Child's age in years}}{\text{Age in years} + 12} \times \text{Adult dose} = \text{Child dose}$$

NOTE

The age rules should not be used if a pediatric dose is provided by the manufacturer.

ANSWERS   Summary Practice Problems

I. Oral

1. Pounds to kilograms: $\dfrac{45 \text{ lb}}{2.2 \text{ lb/kg}} = 20.4 \text{ kg}$

Dosage parameters: 25 mg/kg/day × 20.4 kg = 510 mg/day
50 mg/kg/day × 20.4 kg = 1020 mg/day
Dosage frequency: 250 mg × 3 = 750 mg
Dosage is safe.

BF: $\dfrac{D}{H} \times V = \dfrac{250 \text{ mg}}{125 \text{ mg}} \times 5 \text{ ml} = 10 \text{ ml}$

or
RP: H : V ::   D   : X
125 mg : 5 ml :: 250 mg : X
125 X = 1250
X = 10 ml

or
FE: $\dfrac{H}{V} \times \dfrac{D}{X} = \dfrac{125 \text{ mg}}{5 \text{ ml}} = \dfrac{250 \text{ mg}}{X \text{ ml}}$
(Cross multiply)   125X = 1250
X = 10 ml

2. Dosage parameters: 5 mg/kg/day × 7.2 kg = 36 mg/day
7 mg/kg/day × 7.2 kg = 50.4 mg/day
Dose frequency: 25 mg × 2 = 50 mg
Dosage is safe.

BF: $\dfrac{D}{H} \times V = \dfrac{25 \text{ mg}}{20 \text{ mg}} \times 5 \text{ ml} = 6.25 \text{ ml/dose}$

or
DA: ml $= \dfrac{5 \text{ ml} \times \overset{5}{\cancel{25 \text{ mg}}}}{\underset{4}{\cancel{20 \text{ mg}}} \times 1} = \dfrac{25}{4} = 6.25 \text{ ml}$

3. Dosage parameters: 15 mg/kg, q12h × 8 kg = 120 mg, q12h
Dosage frequency: 100 mg, q12h.
Dosage is safe.

BF: $\dfrac{D}{H} \times V = \dfrac{100 \text{ mg}}{125 \text{ mg}} \times 5 \text{ ml} = 4 \text{ ml/dose}$

or
FE: $\dfrac{H}{V} \times \dfrac{D}{X} = \dfrac{125 \text{ mg}}{5 \text{ ml}} = \dfrac{100 \text{ mg}}{X}$
125X = 500
X = 4 ml

4. Height and weight intersect at 0.84 m² with nomogram.
   Dosage parameters: 100 mg/0.84 m²/day = 84 mg/day
   Dose frequency: 84 mg/day ÷ 6 = 14 mg/dose
   Dosage is safe.
   BSA with the Square Root: BSA Pounds and Inches Formula, see page 277.

$$\sqrt{\frac{43 \times 50}{3131}} = \sqrt{0.686} = 0.828 \text{ or } 0.83 \text{ m}^2$$

   Dosage parameters: 100 mg/0.83 m² = 83 mg/day (compare with nomogram)
   Dosage frequency: 83 mg/day/6 = 13.8 or 14 mg per dose
   Dosage is safe.

   BF: $\dfrac{D}{H} \times V = \dfrac{7.5 \text{ mg}}{15 \text{ mg}} \times 1 = 0.50$ or ½ tablet

   or

   RP: H : V ::   D   : X
         15 mg : 1 ml :: 7.5 mg : X
                  15 X = 7.5
                     X = ½ tablet

5. Dosage parameters: 15 mg/kg/day × 13 kg = 195 mg/day
                      40 mg/day × 13 kg = 520 mg/day
   Dose frequency: 125 mg × 2 = 250 mg/day
   Dosage is safe.

   BF: $\dfrac{D}{H} \times V = \dfrac{125 \text{ mg}}{250 \text{ mg}} \times 5 \text{ ml} = 2.5 \text{ ml}$

6. Dosage parameters: 5 mg/kg/day × 6.7 kg = 33.5 mg/day
                      7 mg/kg/day × 6.7 kg = 46.9 mg/day
   Dose frequency: 40 mg × 2 = 80 mg/day
   Dosage exceeds the therapeutic range. Dosage is *not safe.*

7. Dosage parameters: 120 mg/kg/day × 30.4 kg = 3648 mg or 3.6 g
                      150 mg/kg/day × 30.4 kg = 4560 mg or 4.5 g
   Dose frequency: 1 g × 4 = 4 g or 4000 mg
   Dose is safe.

   BF: $\dfrac{D}{H} = \dfrac{1000 \text{ mg}}{500 \text{ mg}} = 2$ tablets/dose

   or

   DA: tab = $\dfrac{1 \text{ tab} \times \overset{2}{\cancel{1000}} \text{ mg} \times \cancel{1.0} \text{ g}}{\underset{1}{\cancel{500}} \text{ mg} \times \cancel{X} \text{ g} \times 1} = 2$ tablets

8. Dosage parameters: 20 mg/kg/day × 8 kg = 160 mg/day
                      40 mg/kg/day × 8 kg = 320 mg/day
   Dose frequency: 75 mg × 3 = 225 mg
   Dosage is safe.

BF: $\dfrac{D}{H} \times V = \dfrac{75 \text{ mg}}{125 \text{ mg}} \times 5 \text{ ml} = 3 \text{ ml}$

or

RP: $\quad$ H $\quad$: V $\quad$ :: $\quad$ D $\quad$:X

$\qquad$ 125 mg:5 ml::75 mg:X

$\qquad\qquad$ 125X = 375

$\qquad\qquad\qquad$ X = 3 ml

or

FE: $\dfrac{H}{V} \times \dfrac{D}{X} = \dfrac{125 \text{ mg}}{5 \text{ ml}} \times \dfrac{75 \text{ mg}}{X} =$

$\qquad\qquad$ 125X = 375

$\qquad\qquad\qquad$ X = 3 ml

9. Dosage parameters: 5 mg/kg/day $\times$ 25 kg = 125 mg/day
   Dose frequency: 25 mg $\times$ 4 = 100 mg/day
   Dosage is safe.

   BF: $\dfrac{D}{H} \times V = \dfrac{25 \text{ mg}}{12.5 \text{ mg}} \times 5 \text{ ml} = 10 \text{ ml}$

   or

   DA: ml $= \dfrac{5 \text{ ml} \times \overset{2}{\cancel{25}} \text{ mg}}{\underset{1}{\cancel{12.5}} \text{ mg} \times 1} = 10 \text{ ml}$

   or

   FE: $\dfrac{H}{V} \times \dfrac{D}{X} = \dfrac{12.5 \text{ mg}}{5 \text{ ml}} \times \dfrac{25 \text{ mg}}{X \text{ ml}} =$

   $\qquad\qquad$ 125X = 125

   $\qquad\qquad\qquad$ X = 10 ml

10. Dosing parameters: 90 mg/day
    Dosing frequency: 45 mg $\times$ 2 = 90 mg
    Dose is safe.

    BF: $\dfrac{D}{H} \times V = \dfrac{45 \text{ mg}}{12 \text{ mg}} \times 1 \text{ ml} = 3.75 \text{ ml}$

    or

    DA: ml $= \dfrac{1 \text{ ml} \times 45 \text{ mg}}{12 \text{ mg} \times 1} = 3.75 \text{ ml}$

11. 15 lb $\div$ 2.2 = 6.8 kg
    Dosage parameters: 20 mg $\times$ 6.8 kg = 136 mg/day
    40 mg $\times$ 6.8 kg = 272 mg/day
    Dose frequency: 50 mg $\times$ 4 = 200 mg/day
    Dosage is safe.

    BF: $\dfrac{D}{H} \times V = \dfrac{50}{125} \times 5 = \dfrac{250}{125} = 2 \text{ ml}$

    or

    RP: $\quad$ H $\quad$: V $\quad$ :: $\quad$ D $\quad$: X

    $\qquad$ 125 mg:5 ml :: 50 mg:X ml

    $\qquad\qquad$ 125X = 250

    $\qquad\qquad\qquad$ X = 2 ml

    or

    DA: ml $= \dfrac{5 \text{ ml} \times \overset{2}{\cancel{50}} \text{ mg}}{\underset{5}{\cancel{125}} \text{ mg} \times 1} = \dfrac{10}{5} = 2 \text{ ml}$

    or

    FE: $\dfrac{H}{V} \times \dfrac{D}{X} = \dfrac{12.5 \text{ mg}}{5 \text{ ml}} \times \dfrac{50 \text{ mg}}{X} =$

    $\qquad\qquad$ 125X = 250

    $\qquad\qquad\qquad$ X = 2 ml

II. Intramuscular

12. Dosing parameters: 0.1 mg/kg $\times$ 45 kg = 4.5 mg.
    Dosing frequency: one time.
    Dosage is safe.

BF: $\dfrac{D}{H} \times V = \dfrac{4.5 \text{ mg}}{10 \text{ mg}} \times 1 = 0.45$ ml

or

DA: ml $= \dfrac{1 \text{ ml} \times 4.5 \text{ mg}}{10 \text{ mg}} = \dfrac{4.5}{10} = 0.45$ ml

13. Dosage parameters: Child's weight is 44 lb, which falls in the 30 to 60 lb pediatric dose range. Dose frequency: The one-time dose of 1,000,000 units falls within the pediatric dose range. Dosage is safe.

BF: $\dfrac{D}{H} \times V = \dfrac{1,000,000 \text{ Units}}{1,200,000 \text{ Units}} \times 2 = 1.6$ ml

14. Height and weight intersect at 0.82 m² with the nomogram.
    BSA with Square Root (Pounds and Inches Formula)

$$\sqrt{\dfrac{47 \text{ inches} \times 45 \text{ pounds}}{3131}} = \sqrt{0.675} = 0.82 \text{ m}^2 \text{ (same as the nomogram)}$$

Dosage parameters: 30 mg/m² × 0.82 m² = 24.6 mg or 25 mg
Dose frequency: 25 mg IM/dose
Dosage is safe.

BF: $\dfrac{D}{H} \times V = \dfrac{25 \text{ mg}}{25 \text{ mg}} \times 1 = 1.0$ ml

or

DA: ml $= \dfrac{1 \text{ ml} \times \overset{1}{\cancel{25 \text{ mg}}}}{\underset{1}{\cancel{25 \text{ mg}}} \times 1} = 1$ ml

15. Dosing parameters: 0.01 mg/kg/dose × 12 kg = 0.12 mg/dose
    0.02 mg/kg/dose × 12 kg = 0.24 mg/dose

Dosage is safe.

BF: $\dfrac{D}{H} \times V = \dfrac{0.2}{0.4} \times 1 = 0.5$ ml

16. Height and weight intersect at 1.38 m² with the nomogram.
    Dosing parameters for nomogram: 7.5 mg × 1.38 m² = 10.35 mg/wk
    30 mg × 1.38 m² = 41.4 mg/wk

BSA with Square Root (Pounds and Inches Formula)

$$\sqrt{\dfrac{56 \text{ inches} \times 100 \text{ pounds}}{3131}} = \sqrt{1.788} = 1.34 \text{ m}^2$$

Dosing parameter for BSA formula: 7.5 mg × 1.34 m² = 10.05 mg/wk
30 mg × 1.34 m² = 40.2 mg/wk

Dose frequency: 40 mg/wk IM
Dosage is safe.

BF: $\dfrac{D}{H} \times V = \dfrac{40 \text{ mg}}{100 \text{ mg}} \times 1 \text{ ml} = 0.4$ ml

or
$$\text{DA: ml} = \frac{1 \text{ ml} \times 40 \text{ mg}}{100 \text{ mg } 1} = \frac{40 \text{ mg}}{100 \text{ mg}} = 0.4 \text{ ml}$$

17. **a.** Preferred selection is AquaMEPHYTON 1 mg = 0.5 ml

    b. *AquaMEPHYTON 1 mg = 0.5 ml:*

        $$\text{BF: } \frac{D}{H} \times V = \frac{0.5 \text{ mg}}{1.0 \text{ mg}} \times 0.5 \text{ ml} = \frac{0.25}{1.0} = 0.25 \text{ ml}$$

    or

    RP: H : V ::   D :X

          1 mg:0.5 ml :: 0.5 mg:X

                  X = 0.25 mg

    AquaMEPHYTON 10 mg = 1 ml:

    $$\text{BF: } \frac{D}{H} \times V = \frac{0.5 \text{ mg}}{10 \text{ mg}} \times 1.0 \text{ ml} = \frac{0.5}{10} = 0.05 \text{ ml}$$
    or
$$\text{FE: } \frac{H}{V} \times \frac{D}{X} = \frac{10 \text{ mg}}{1 \text{ ml}} \times \frac{0.5 \text{ mg}}{X \text{ ml}} =$$
$$10 X = 0.5$$
$$X = 0.05 \text{ ml}$$

    For AquaMEPHYTON 1 mg = 0.5 ml, give 0.25 ml (use a tuberculin syringe).

    For AquaMEPHYTON 10 mg = 1 ml, give 0.05 ml (use a tuberculin syringe; however, it would be difficult to give this small amount.)

    c. Drug dose is within the safe range.

III. Intravenous

18. Dosage parameters: 50 mcg/kg/dose × 50 kg = 2500 mcg/dose or 2.5 mg/dose

                      100 mcg/kg/dose × 50 kg = 5000 mcg/dose or 5 mg/dose

    Dosage is safe.

    $$\text{BF: } \frac{D}{H} \times V = \frac{2.5}{5} \times 1 = 0.5 \text{ ml}$$

    or
$$\text{DA: ml} = \frac{1 \text{ ml} \times 2.5 \text{ mg}}{5 \text{ mg} \times 1} = \frac{1}{2} \text{ or } 0.5 \text{ ml}$$

    Amount of fluid to be infused: 0.5 ml + 10 ml = 10.5 ml

    $$\frac{10.5 \text{ ml} \times 60 \text{ gtt/ml}}{5 \text{ minutes}} = 125 \text{ gtt/min}$$

    Total fluid for medication infusion plus flush: 10.5 ml + 5 ml = 15.5 ml.

19. Dosing parameter: 0.1 mg/kg × 18 kg = 1.8 mg.

    Dosage is safe.

    $$\text{BF: } \frac{D}{H} \times V = \frac{1.8 \text{ mg}}{0.4 \text{ mg}} \times 1 \text{ ml} = 4.5 \text{ ml}$$

20. Dosage parameters: 15 mg/kg/day × 5.3 = 79.5 mg/day.

    Dose frequency: 40 mg IV × 2 = 80 mg.

    79.5 mg is rounded off to 80 mg. The dosage is safe.

    $$\text{BF: } \frac{D}{H} \times V = \frac{40 \text{ mg}}{100 \text{ mg}} \times 2 = 0.8 \text{ ml}$$

or

RP: H   :   V   ::   D   : X

100 mg : 2 ml :: 40 mg : X

100X = 80

X = 0.8 ml

or

FE: $\dfrac{H}{V} \times \dfrac{D}{X} = \dfrac{100\ mg}{2\ ml} \times \dfrac{40\ mg}{X} =$

100 X = 80

X = 0.8 ml

Amount of fluid to be infused: 0.8 ml + 5 ml = 5.8 ml

$$\dfrac{5.8\ ml \times \overset{3}{\cancel{60}}\ gtt/ml}{\underset{1}{\cancel{20}}\ minutes} = 17.4\ gtt/min\ or\ 17\ gtt/min$$

Total fluid for medication infusion plus flush: 5.8 ml + 3 ml = 8.8 ml.

21. Dosing parameters: 0.05 mg/kg × 47 kg = 2.35 mg

0.1 mg/kg × 47 kg = 4.7 mg

Dose is safe.

BF: $\dfrac{D}{H} \times V = \dfrac{3\ mg}{4\ mg} \times 1\ ml = 0.75\ ml$

or

RP: H   :   V   ::   D   : X

4 mg : 1 ml :: 3 mg : X

4X = 3

X = 0.75 ml

or

FE: $\dfrac{H}{V} \times \dfrac{D}{X} = \dfrac{4\ mg}{1\ ml} \times \dfrac{3\ mg}{X} =$

4 X = 3

X = 0.75 ml

22. Dosage parameters: 25-100 mg/kg/day in four divided doses.

25 mg × 5.6 kg = 140 mg/day

100 mg × 5.6 kg = 560 mg/day

560 mg ÷ 4 = 140 mg/dose

Dose frequency: 500 mg × 4 = 2000 mg/day

Dose exceeds therapeutic range of 560 mg/day. Dosage is *not safe.*

23. Dosage parameters: 5 mg/kg/day × 4 kg = 20 mg/day

7.5 mg/kg/day × 4 kg = 30 mg/day

Dose frequency: 10 mg × 3 times/day = 30 mg

Dosage is safe.

BF: $\dfrac{D}{H} \times V = \dfrac{10\ mg}{10\ mg} \times 1\ ml = 1\ ml$

or

RP: H : V :: D : X

10 mg : 1 ml :: 10 mg : X ml

10 X = 10

X = 1 ml

or

DA: ml $= \dfrac{1\ ml \times \overset{1}{\cancel{10}}\ mg}{\underset{1}{\cancel{10}}\ mg \times\ 1} = 1\ ml$

or

FE: $\dfrac{H}{V} \times \dfrac{D}{X} = \dfrac{10\ mg}{1\ ml} \times \dfrac{10\ mg}{X\ ml} =$

10 X = 10

X = 1 ml

Amount of fluid to be infused: 1 ml + 4 ml = 5 ml

$$\dfrac{5\ ml \times \overset{2}{\cancel{60}}\ gtt/ml}{\underset{1}{\cancel{30}}\ minutes} = 10\ gtt/min$$

Total fluid for medication infusion plus flush: 5 ml + 3 ml = 8 ml

24. Dosage parameters: 25 mg/kg/day $\times$ 15 kg = 375 mg/day
$\qquad\qquad\qquad\qquad$ 50 mg/kg/day $\times$ 15 kg = 750 mg/day

Dose frequency: 185 mg $\times$ 4 = 740 mg/day

Dosage is safe. 250 mg = 2 mg or 125 mg = 1 ml

BF: $\dfrac{D}{H} \times V = \dfrac{185 \text{ mg}}{125 \text{ mg}} \times 1 \text{ ml} = 1.48$ or 1.5 ml

or

RP: $\qquad$ H $\quad$: V $\quad$ :: $\quad$ D $\quad$: X
$\qquad\qquad$ 125 mg : 1 ml :: 185 mg : X
$\qquad\qquad\qquad$ 125X = 185
$\qquad\qquad\qquad\qquad$ X = 1.5 ml

Amount of fluid to be infused: 1.5 ml + 20 ml = 21.5 ml

$$\frac{21.5 \text{ ml} \times \overset{3}{\cancel{60}} \text{ gtt/ml}}{\underset{1}{\cancel{20}} \text{ minutes}} = 64.5 \text{ gtt/min}$$

Total fluid for medication infusion plus flush: 21.5 ml + 15 ml = 36.5 ml

25. Dosing parameter: 16 mg/kg/day $\times$ 7.5 kg = 120 mg/day
$\qquad\qquad\qquad\qquad$ 20 mg/kg/day $\times$ 7.5 kg = 150 mg/day

Dosing frequency: 50 mg $\times$ 3 = 150 mg

Dosage is safe.

BF: $\dfrac{D}{H} \times V = \dfrac{50 \text{ mg}}{150 \text{ mg}} \times 1 \text{ ml} = 0.33$ ml or 0.3 ml

or

RP: H $\quad$: V $\quad$ :: $\quad$ D $\quad$: X
$\qquad$ 150 mg : 1 ml :: 50 mg : X ml
$\qquad\qquad$ 150 X = 50
$\qquad\qquad\qquad$ X = $\dfrac{50}{150}$ = 0.3 ml

or

DA: ml = $\dfrac{1 \text{ ml} \times \overset{1}{\cancel{50 \text{ mg}}}}{\underset{3}{\cancel{150 \text{ mg}}} \times 1} = 0.33$ ml or 0.3 ml

or

FE: $\dfrac{H}{V} \times \dfrac{D}{X} = \dfrac{150 \text{ mg}}{1 \text{ ml}} \times \dfrac{50 \text{ mg}}{X \text{ ml}} =$
$\qquad\qquad\qquad$ 150 X = 50
$\qquad\qquad\qquad\qquad$ X = $\dfrac{50}{150}$ = 0.3 ml

26. Dosage parameters: 25 mcg/kg/day $\times$ 2.72 kg = 68 mcg
$\qquad\qquad\qquad\qquad$ 50 mcg/kg/day $\times$ 2.72 kg = 136 mcg

Dose frequency: 40 mcg $\times$ 2 = 80 mcg

0.1 mg = 100 mcg (μg)

Dosage is safe.

BF: $\dfrac{D}{H} \times V = \dfrac{40 \text{ mcg}}{100 \text{ mcg}} \times 1 = 0.4$ ml

27. Height and weight intersect at 0.6 m² according to the nomogram.
Dosing parameters for nomogram: 60 mg/m²/day × 0.6 m² = 36 mg/day.
$\qquad\qquad\qquad\qquad\qquad$ 250 mg/m²/day × 0.6 m² = 150 mg/day.

BSA with the Square Root (Metric Formula)

$$\frac{\sqrt{16 \text{ kg} \times 75 \text{ cm}}}{3600} = \sqrt{0.333} = 0.58 \text{ m}^2$$

Dosage parameters for BSA formula: 60 mg/m²/day × 0.58 m² = 34.8 mg/day
$\qquad\qquad\qquad\qquad\qquad\qquad$ 250 mg/m²/day × 0.58 m² = 145 mg/day

Dosage is safe.

BF: $\dfrac{D}{H} \times V = \dfrac{125 \text{ mg}}{200 \text{ mg}} \times 10 \text{ ml} = 6.25 \text{ ml}$

or

DA: ml $= \dfrac{10 \text{ ml} \times \overset{5}{\cancel{125} \text{ mg}}}{\underset{8}{\cancel{200} \text{ mg}} \times 1} = \dfrac{50}{8} = 6.25 \text{ ml}$

28. a. BF: $\dfrac{60}{75} \times 2 \text{ ml} = \dfrac{120}{75} = 1.6 \text{ m of kanamycin}$

    or
RP: 75 mg : 2 ml :: 60 mg : X
$\qquad$ 75X = 120
$\qquad\qquad$ X = 1.6 mg of kanamycin

    or
FE: $\dfrac{H}{V} \times \dfrac{D}{X} = \dfrac{75 \text{ mg}}{2 \text{ ml}} \times \dfrac{60 \text{ mg}}{X} =$
$\qquad\qquad$ 75 X = 120
$\qquad\qquad\qquad$ X = 1.6 ml

b. 4.8 ml/day
c. Dosage parameters: 15 mg × 12 kg = 180 mg/day
$\qquad\qquad\qquad\qquad\qquad$ 60 mg × 3 (q8h) = 180 mg/day
Drug dose per day is within the safe range.

29. a. BF: $\dfrac{15}{\underset{10}{\cancel{20}}} \times \overset{1}{\cancel{2}} \text{ ml} = \dfrac{15}{10} = 1.5 \text{ ml of Nebcin}$

    or
RP: 20 mg : 2 ml :: 15 mg : X
$\qquad\qquad$ 20X = 30
$\qquad\qquad\qquad$ X = 1.5 ml of Nebcin

b. Pediatric dosage parameters: 6 mg/10 kg/day = 60 mg/day
$\qquad\qquad\qquad\qquad\qquad$ 7.5 mg/10 kg/day = 75 mg/day
$\qquad\qquad\qquad\qquad\qquad$ 15 mg × 4 (q6h) = 60 mg/day
Drug dose per day is within the safe range.

30. a. The BSA is 1.16.
b. 8 ml of daunorubicin HCl mixed in 100 ml D₅W.
c. Dosage parameters: 25 mg × 1.16 m² = 29 mg/day
$\qquad\qquad\qquad\qquad\qquad$ 45 mg × 1.16 m² = 52.2 mg/day or 52 mg/day
Child is to receive 40 mg of daunorubicin HCl per day.
Drug dose is within the safe range.

$$108 \text{ ml} \div \frac{45 \text{ min}}{60 \text{ min}} = 108 \times \frac{\overset{4}{\cancel{60}}}{\underset{3}{\cancel{45}}} = 144 \text{ ml}$$

Pump setting: 144 ml/hr

31. a. Child weighs 23.6 kg
b. 23.6 kg × 11 mg/kg = 259.6 or 260 mg
c. 260 mg/50 mg/ml = 5.2 ml

IV. Neonates

32. 0.1 mg/kg × 2.5 kg = 0.25 mg

BF: $\dfrac{0.25 \text{ mg}}{0.1 \text{ mg}} \times 1 \text{ ml} = 2.5 \text{ ml}$

or
DA: ml = $\dfrac{1 \text{ ml} \times 0.25 \text{ mg}}{0.1 \text{ mg} \times 1} = \dfrac{0.25}{0.1} = 2.5 \text{ ml}$

or
FE: $\dfrac{H}{V} \times \dfrac{D}{X} = \dfrac{0.1 \text{ mg}}{1 \text{ ml}} \times \dfrac{0.25 \text{ mg}}{X} =$

$0.1 \text{ X} = 0.25$
$\text{X} = 2.5 \text{ ml}$

33. $\dfrac{8.75}{2.2} = 3.97 \text{ kg or 4 kg}$

0.01 mg/kg × 4 kg = 0.04 mg dose
Drug dose is safe.

BF: $\dfrac{D}{H} \times V = \dfrac{0.04 \text{ mg}}{0.4 \text{ ml}} \times 1 \text{ ml} = 0.1 \text{ ml}$

or
RP: H   :   V   ::   D   :   X
    0.4 mg : 1 ml :: 0.04 mg : X ml
          0.4X = 0.04
             X = 0.1 ml

34. Dosage parameters:
50 mg/kg × 2.5 kg = 125 mg
75 mg/kg × 2.5 kg = 187.5 mg
Drug dose is within safe range

BF: $\dfrac{125 \text{ mg}}{500 \text{ mg}} \times 2 \text{ ml} = 0.5 \text{ ml}$

or
DA: ml = $\dfrac{2 \text{ ml} \times \overset{1}{125} \text{ mg}}{\underset{4}{500} \text{ mg} \times 1} = \dfrac{2}{4} = 0.5 \text{ ml}$

or
FE: $\dfrac{H}{V} \times \dfrac{D}{X} = \dfrac{500 \text{ mg}}{2 \text{ ml}} \times \dfrac{125 \text{ mg}}{X} =$

$500 \text{ X} = 250$
$\text{X} = 0.5 \text{ ml}$

35. a. 80 ml/kg × 2.5 kg = 200 ml $D_{10}W$ in 24 hours

b. $\dfrac{200 \text{ ml}}{24 \text{ hr}} = 8.3 \text{ ml/hr}$

36. Dosage parameters: 4 mg/kg × 2.5 kg = 10 mg
                        5 mg/kg × 2.5 kg = 12.5 mg

Drug dose is safe.

BF: $\dfrac{D}{H} \times V = \dfrac{10 \text{ mg}}{40 \text{ mg}} \times 1 \text{ ml} = 0.25 \text{ ml}$

or
   RP: H   :   V   ::   D   :   X
       40 mg : 1 ml :: 10 mg : X ml
            40X = 10
              X = 0.25 ml

Additional practice problems are available on the enclosed CD-ROM in the "Pediatric Calculations" section.

Critical Care

OBJECTIVES

- Calculate the prescribed concentration of a drug in solution.
- Identify the units of measure designated for the amount of drug in solution.
- Describe the four determinants of infusion rates.
- Calculate the concentration of drug per unit time for a specific body weight.
- Recognize the variables needed for the basic fractional formula.
- Describe how the titration factor is used when infusion rates are changed.
- Recognize the methods of determining the total amount of drug infused over time.

OUTLINE

Medication administration has become increasingly individualized for critically ill patients. Nurses are responsible for safe and accurate delivery of these drugs. Administration of potent drugs in milligrams, micrograms, or units per body weight or unit time requires extreme accuracy in calculations. Physicians determine the amount of drug to be mixed in the intravenous (IV) solution and designate infusion rates or the dosage per kilogram of body weight per unit time. Some institutions have their own guidelines for preparation of medication in the critical care areas. Research studies have shown a high incidence of error in drug calculations among nurses and physicians. Many institutions have initiated policies of drug infusion standardization, especially for the concentration of solution, to limit infusion errors.

Nationally, efforts are under way to standardize continuous infusions of vasoactive drugs in conjunction with programmable infusion pump technology called "smart" pumps. These pumps have drug menus entered into their software with safe dosing limits attached. The unit will alarm if limits are reached, and it actually prevents infusions beyond the safe dose range. The "smart" pump technology contains a "drug library" with a database of thousands of medications that allows physicians to tailor medication doses and rates. Infusion pump technology eventually will have a customized program for each drug it delivers.

Because some institutions have their own guidelines for preparations and medication in the critical care areas, the medication often comes in premixed bags or bottles from the pharmacy ready for infusion. Still, in some facilities, these drugs are prepared by the nurse. The nurse must know what data are needed for each drug and apply those parameters to whatever IV equipment is available. Wide use of volumetric IV infusion pumps has improved the safety of individualized drug administration. The accuracy of the infusion rate with the pump has almost eliminated the need for drop counting, but nurses are still responsible for all other infusion rates. Each drug has its own dosing parameters. Some drugs are dosed in the concentration per hour or minute and others are administered in micrograms, milligrams, or units per kilogram of body weight. The nurse must be familiar with the specific dosing parameters to ensure the accuracy of infusion rates.

Only four components are necessary for the correct calculation of drugs used in critical care. These are as follows:

1. Concentration of the solution
2. Concentration per hour or per minute
3. Volume per hour or per minute
4. Dosage per kilogram body weight per minute

Many other formulas and methods may be used to calculate these four components, but these are basic for administering all drugs for continuous infusion.

CALCULATING AMOUNT OF DRUG OR CONCENTRATION OF A SOLUTION

The first step in administering a medication is to determine the concentration of the solution, which is the amount of drug in each milliliter of solution. This is written as units per milliliter, milligrams per milliliter, or micrograms per milliliter and must be calculated for each problem. For all problems, remember to convert to like units before solving.

Calculating Units per Milliliter

EXAMPLES

PROBLEM: Infuse heparin 5000 units in D_5W 250 ml at 30 ml/hr. What will be the concentration of heparin in each milliliter of D_5W?

Method: units/ml

Set up a ratio and proportion. Solve for X.	5000 units : 250 ml :: X units : ml

$$250 X = 5000$$
$$X = 20 \text{ units}$$

Answer: The D_5W with heparin will have a concentration of 20 units/ml of solution.

Calculating Milligrams per Milliliter

EXAMPLES

PROBLEM: Infuse lidocaine 2 g in 500 ml D_5W at 2 mg/min. What will be the concentration of lidocaine in each milliliter of D_5W?

Method: mg/ml

Convert grams to milligrams. Set up a ratio and proportion and solve for X.	2 g = 2000 mg 2000 mg : 500 ml :: X mg : ml

$$500 X = 2000$$
$$X = 4 \text{ mg}$$

Answer: The D_5W with lidocaine has a concentration of 4 mg/ml of solution.

Calculating Micrograms per Milliliter

EXAMPLES

PROBLEM: Infuse dobutamine 250 mg in 500 ml D_5W at 650 mcg/min. What is the concentration of dobutamine in each milliliter of D_5W?

Method: mcg/ml

Convert milligrams to micrograms. Set up a ratio and proportion and solve for X.	250 mg = 250,000 mcg 250,000 mcg : 500 ml :: X mcg : ml

$$500 X = 250,000$$
$$X = 500 \text{ mcg/ml}$$

Answer: The D_5W with dobutamine will have a concentration of 500 mcg/ml of solution.

PRACTICE PROBLEMS: I Calculating Concentration of a Solution

Answers can be found on page 307.

1. Order: heparin 10,000 units in 250 ml D$_5$W at 30 ml/hr.

_____

2. Order: aminophylline 250 mg in 500 ml D$_5$W at 50 ml/hr.

_____

3. Order: regular insulin 100 units in 500 ml NSS at 30 ml/hr.

_____

4. Order: lidocaine 1 g in 1000 ml D$_5$W at 30 ml/hr.

_____

5. Order: norepinephrine 4 mg in 500 ml D$_5$W at 15 ml/hr.

_____

6. Order: dopamine 500 mg in 250 ml D$_5$W at 10 ml/hr.

_____

7. Order: dobutamine 400 mg in 250 ml D$_5$W at 20 ml/hr.

_____

8. Order: Isuprel 2 mg in 250 ml D$_5$W at 10 ml/hr.

_____

9. Order: streptokinase 750,000 units in 50 ml D$_5$W over 30 minutes.

_____

10. Order: nitroprusside 50 mg in 500 ml D$_5$W at 50 mcg/min.

_____

11. Order: aminophylline 1 g in 250 ml D$_5$W at 20 ml/hr.

_____

12. Order: Pronestyl 2 g in 250 ml D$_5$W at 16 ml/hr.

_____

13. Order: heparin 25,000 units in 250 ml D$_5$W at 5 ml/hr.

_____

14. Order: aminophylline 1 g in 500 ml D$_5$W at 40 cc/hr.

_____

15. Order: nitroglycerin 50 mg in 250 ml D$_5$W at 50 mcg/min.

_____

16. Order: alteplase 100 mg in NSS 100 ml over 2 hours.

_____

17. Order: theophylline 800 mg in D$_5$W 500 ml at 0.5 mg/kg.

_____

18. Order: milrinone 20 mg in D$_5$W 100 ml at 0.50 mcg/kg/min.

_____

19. Order: streptokinase 1.5 million units in D$_5$W 100 ml over 60 minutes.

_____

20. Order: amiodarone 150 mg in D$_5$W 100 ml over 10 minutes.

_____

CALCULATING INFUSION RATE FOR CONCENTRATION AND VOLUME PER UNIT TIME

The second step for administering medication is to calculate the _infusion rate_ of drug per _unit time._ Infusion rates can mean two things: the rate of volume (ml) given or the rate of concentration (units, mg, mcg) administered. _Unit time_ means per hour or per minute. For drugs administered by continuous infusion, the four most important determinants are the concentration per hour and minute and the volume per hour and minute. Infusion rates of potent drugs are usually part of the physician's order and may be stated in concentration or volume per unit time.

Many hospitals have policies requiring that all potent drugs be delivered via volumetric infusion pump. New technology has produced pumps that are programmable and calculate the drug dosage. The information entered in the pump's control panel is (1) the name of the drug, (2) the amount of the drug, (3) the amount of the solution, and (4) the patient's weight in kilograms. The nurse enters the ordered dose and the correct dosage parameters, i.e., mg/min, units/hr, mcg/min. The pump automatically delivers the appropriate dosage.

Not all facilities have infusion pumps with advanced technology; therefore, the nurse must be able to calculate the infusion rates. For infusion pumps that deliver ml/hr, the volume per hour of the drug must be known. _Remember:_ If an infusion device is unavailable, a microdrip IV administration set is the appropriate set to use because the drops per minute rate (gtt/min) corresponds to the volume per hour rate (ml/hr).

Complete infusion rates for volume and concentration are given in the examples and practice problems. In clinical practice, not all the data are needed for each drug. For heparin, the concentration per minute is not as vital as the concentration per hour, whereas for vasoactive drugs such as dobutamine, the concentration per minute is essential information and the concentration per hour is not. The same methods of calculation are used for both drugs, and the same information can be obtained. The nurse must have knowledge of pharmacology and clinical practice to determine the most useful data.

Concentration and Volume per Hour and Minute With a Drug in Units

EXAMPLES

PROBLEM: Infuse heparin 5000 units in D_5W 250 ml at 30 ml/hr. Concentration of solution is 20 units/ml. (Also note that volume/hour is given.) How many milliliters will be infused per minute?

Find volume per minute:

Method: ml/min

Set up a ratio and proportion. Use volume/hour, 30 ml/hr, or 30 ml/60 min as the known variable.	30 ml:60 min :: X ml: min 60 X = 30 X = 0.5 ml

Answer: The infusion rate for volume per minute is 0.5 ml/min and the hourly rate is 30 ml/hr.

What is the concentration per minute and hour?
Find concentration per minute:

Method: units/min

Multiply the concentration of solution by the volume per minute.	20 units/ml × 0.5 ml/min = 10 units/min

Find concentration per hour:

Method: units/hr

Multiply the volume per minute by 60 min/hr.	10 units/min × 60 min/hr = 600 units/hr

Answer: The concentration per minute of heparin is 10 units/min and the concentration per hour is 600 units/hr.

Concentration and Volume per Hour and Minute With a Drug in Milligrams

EXAMPLES

PROBLEM: Infuse lidocaine 2 g in D_5W 500 ml at 2 mg/min. Concentration of solution is 4 mg/ml. (Also note that concentration/minute is given.) How many milligrams will be infused per hour?

Find concentration per hour:

Method: mg/hr

| Find the concentration/minute. Multiply concentration/ minute × 60 min/hr. | lidocaine 2 mg/min
2 mg/min × 60 min = 120 mg/hr |

Answer: The amount of lidocaine infused per hour is 120 mg/hr.

How many milliliters of lidocaine will be infused in 1 hour?
Find volume per hour:

Method: ml/hr

| Calculate concentration of solution. Divide the concentration/hour by the concentration of solution. | lidocaine 4 mg/ml
$\dfrac{120 \text{ mg/hr}}{4 \text{ mg/ml}} = 30 \text{ ml/hr}$ |

Answer: The infusion rate in milliliters for lidocaine 2 mg/min is 30 ml/hr.

How many milliliters of lidocaine will be infused in 1 minute?

| Divide the concentration/minute by the concentration of the solution. | $\dfrac{2 \text{ mg/min}}{4 \text{ mg/ml}} = 0.5 \text{ ml/min}$ |

Answer: The infusion rate for lidocaine 2 mg/min is 0.5 ml/min.

Concentration and Volume per Hour and Minute With a Drug in Micrograms

EXAMPLES

PROBLEM: Infuse dobutamine 250 mg in D_5W 500 ml at 650 mcg/min. Concentration of solution is 500 mcg/ml. (Also note that concentration/ minute is given in the order.) How many micrograms will be infused in 1 hour?

Find concentration per hour:

Method: mcg/hr

| Find the concentration/minute. Multiply concentration/minute by 60 min/hr. | dobutamine 650 mcg/min
650 mcg/min × 60 min/hr = 39,000 mcg/hr |

Answer: The concentration of dobutamine infused per hour is 39,000 mcg/hr.

How many milliliters of dobutamine will be infused in 1 hour?
Find volume per hour:

Method: ml/hr

| Calculate concentration of solution. Divide the concentration/hour by the concentration of solution. | dobutamine 500 mcg/ml $$\frac{39{,}000 \text{ mcg/hr}}{500 \text{ mcg/ml}} = 78 \text{ ml/hr}$$ |

Answer: The infusion rate for dobutamine 650 mcg/min is 78 ml/hr.

How many milliliters of dobutamine should be infused in 1 minute? Find volume per minute:

Method: ml/min

| Divide concentration/minute by concentration of solution. | $$\frac{650 \text{ mcg/min}}{500 \text{ mcg/ml}} = 1.3 \text{ ml/min}$$ |

Answer: The infusion rate for dobutamine is 1.3 ml/min.

PRACTICE PROBLEMS: II Calculating Infusion Rate

Answers can be found on page 309.

Use the examples to find the following information:

- Concentration of the solution
- Infusion rates per unit time:
  a. Volume per minute
  b. Volume per hour
  c. Concentration per minute
  d. Concentration per hour

1. Order: heparin 1000 units in D_5W 500 ml at 50 ml/hr.

2. Order: nitroprusside 100 mg in D_5W 500 ml at 60 ml/hr.

3. Order: nitroprusside 25 mg in D_5W 250 ml at 50 mcg/min.

4. Order: dopamine 800 mg in D_5W 500 ml at 400 mcg/min.

5. Order: norepinephrine 2 mg in D_5W 250 ml at 45 ml/hr.

6. Order: dobutamine 1000 mg in D_5W 500 ml at 12 ml/hr.

7. Order: dobutamine 250 mg in D$_5$W 250 ml at 10 ml/hr.

_____

8. Order: lidocaine 2 g in D$_5$W 500 ml at 4 mg/min.

_____

9. Order: dopamine 400 mg in D$_5$W 250 ml at 60 ml/hr.

_____

10. Order: isoproterenol 4 mg in D$_5$W 500 ml at 65 ml/hr.

_____

11. Order: morphine sulfate 50 mg in 150 ml NSS at 3 mg/hr.

_____

12. Order: regular Humulin insulin 50 units in 250 ml NSS at 4 units/hr.

_____

13. Order: aminophylline 2 g in 250 ml D$_5$W at 20 ml/hr.

_____

14. Order: nitroglycerin 50 mg in 250 ml D$_5$W at 24 ml/hr.

_____

15. Order: heparin 25,000 units in 500 ml D$_5$W at 10 ml/hr.

_____

16. Order: amiodarone 900 mg in D$_5$W 500 ml at 33.3 ml/hr.

_____

17. Order: procainamide 1 g in D$_5$W 250 ml at 4 mg/min.

_____

18. Order: diltiazem 100 mg in 100 ml NSS at 10 mg/hr.

_____

19. Order: streptokinase 750,000 units in 250 ml NSS at 100,000 units/hr.

_____

20. Order: bretylium 1 g in 250 ml D$_5$W at 1 mg/min.

_____

CALCULATING INFUSION RATES OF A DRUG FOR SPECIFIC BODY WEIGHT PER UNIT TIME

The last method is calculating infusion rates for the amount of drug per unit time for a specific body weight. The weight parameter is an accurate means of dosing for a therapeutic effect. The metric system is used for all drug dosing, so pounds must be changed to kilograms. The physician orders the *desired dose per kilogram of body weight* and the *concentration of the solution.* From this information, infusion rates can be calculated for administering an individualized dose. Accurate daily weights are essential for the correct dosage.

The previous methods for calculating *concentration of solution* and *infusion rates* for concentration and volume are used, with one addition. The *concentration per minute* is obtained by multiplying the *body weight* by the *desired dose per kilogram per minute,* which must be done before the other infusion rates can be calculated. For many vasoactive drugs given as examples in this chapter, the most useful information clinically is the concentration per minute for the specific body weight, volume per minute, and volume per hour, because these parameters determine the infusion pump settings.

New volumetric infusion pumps now can deliver fractional portions of a milliliter from tenths to hundredths in addition to calculating dosages for infusion rates. If the infusion pumps available do not have this feature and the volume per hour is a fractional amount, it must be rounded off to a whole number (1.8 ml/hr = 2 ml/hr). When calculating concentration per minute and hour and volume per minute, carry out the problem to three decimal places, if necessary, before rounding off. The volume per hour, if fractional, can then be rounded off, making the volume per hour as accurate as possible. There are two exceptions to rounding off fractional infusion rates:

1. If the patient's condition is labile, the difference between 1 or 2 ml could be important.
2. Because physicians order the medication, they must be consulted if rounding off would significantly change the drug dosage.

Micrograms per Kilogram Body Weight

EXAMPLES

PROBLEM: Infuse dobutamine 250 mg in 500 ml D₅W at 10 mcg/kg/min. Patient weighs 143 lb. Concentration of solution is 500 mcg/ml. How many micrograms of dobutamine would be infused per minute? Per hour?

Convert pounds to kilograms:

| Divide pounds by 2.2. | $\dfrac{143\ \text{lb}}{2.2\ \text{lb/kg}} = 65\ \text{kg}$ |

Find concentration per minute:

Method: mcg/min

| Multiply patient's weight by the desired dose of mcg/kg/min. | $65\ \text{kg} \times 10\ \text{mcg/kg/min} = 650\ \text{mcg/min}$ |

Find concentration per hour:

Method: mcg/hr

| Multiply concentration/min by 60 min/hr. | 650 mcg/min × 60 min/hr = 39,000 mcg/hr |

Answer: The concentration of dobutamine infused per minute and per hour is 650 mcg/min and 39,000 mcg/hr for the patient's body weight.

How many milliliters of dobutamine will be infused per minute? Per hour? Find volume per minute:

Method: ml/min

| Divide the concentration/minute by the concentration of the solution. | $\dfrac{650 \text{ mcg/min}}{500 \text{ mcg/ml}} = 1.3 \text{ ml/min}$ |

Find volume per hour:

Method: ml/hr

| Multiply volume/minute by 60 min/hr. | 1.3 ml/min × 60 min/hr = 78 ml/hr |

Answer: The volume of dobutamine infused per minute is 1.3 ml/min, and the infusion rate is 78 ml/hr.

BASIC FRACTIONAL FORMULA

A fractional equation can create a basic formula that can be used as another quick method to determine any one of the following quantities: concentration of solution, volume per hour, and desired concentration per minute (× kilogram of body weight, if required). The equation has one constant, the drop rate of the IV set, 60 gtt/ml. The unknown quantity can be represented by X. (See Chapter 3 for fractional equations.) The basic formula is not accurate to the nearest hundredth, as are the other methods in this section:

$$\frac{\text{Concentration of solution (units, mg, mcg/ml)}}{\text{Drop rate of set (60 gtt/ml)}} =$$

$$\frac{\text{Desired concentration/min} \times \text{kg body weight}}{\text{Volume/hr (ml/hr or gtt/min)}}$$

Using Basic Formula to Find Volume per Hour or Drops per Minute

EXAMPLES

PROBLEM: Infuse heparin 5000 units in 250 ml D$_5$W at 0.15 units/kg/min.

Patient weighs 70 kg. The concentration of solution is 20 units/ml.

Desired concentration/minute: 0.15 units/kg/min $\times$ 70 kg = 10.5 units/min

$$\frac{20 \text{ units/ml}}{60 \text{ gtt/ml}} = \frac{10.5 \text{ units/min}}{X \text{ (ml/hr or gtt/min)}}$$
$$20 X = 630$$
$$X = 31 \text{ ml/hr or } 31 \text{ gtt/min}$$

Using Basic Formula to Find Desired Concentration per Minute

EXAMPLES

PROBLEM: Infuse lidocaine 2 g in 500 ml D_5W at 30 ml/hr. The concentration of the solution is 4 mg/ml.

$$\frac{4 \text{ mg/ml}}{60 \text{ gtt/ml}} = \frac{X}{30 \text{ ml/hr}}$$
$$60 X = 120$$
$$X = 2 \text{ mg/min}$$

Using Basic Formula to Find Concentration of Solution

EXAMPLES

PROBLEM: Infuse dobutamine 250 mg in D_5W 500 ml at 10 mcg/kg/min with rate of 78 ml/hr. Patient weights 65 kg.

$$\text{Desired concentration per minute} = 10 \text{ mcg/kg/min} \times 65 \text{ kg}$$
$$= 650 \text{ mcg/min}$$
$$\frac{X}{60 \text{ gtt/ml}} = \frac{650 \text{ mcg/min}}{78 \text{ ml/hr}}$$
$$78 X = 39{,}000$$
$$X = 500 \text{ mcg/ml}$$

PRACTICE PROBLEMS: III Calculating Infusion Rate for Specific Body Weight

Answers can be found on page 317.

Determine the infusion rates for specific body weight by calculating the following:

• Concentration of the solution

• Weight in kilograms

• Infusion rates:

  a. Concentration per minute

  b. Concentration per hour (not always measured)

  c. Volume per minute

  d. Volume per hour

You can use the basic fractional formula and compare answers.

1. Infuse dobutamine 500 mg in 250 ml D$_5$W at 5 mcg/kg/min. Patient weighs 182 lb.

2. Infuse amrinone 250 mg in 250 ml NSS at 5 mcg/kg/min. Patient weighs 165 lb.

3. Infuse dopamine 400 mg in 250 ml D$_5$W at 10 mcg/kg/min. Patient weighs 140 lb.

4. Infuse nitroprusside 100 mg in 500 ml D$_5$W at 3 mcg/kg/min. Patient weighs 55 kg.

5. Infuse dobutamine 1000 mg in 500 ml D$_5$W at 15 mcg/kg/min. Patient weighs 110 lb.

6. Infuse propofol (Diprivan) 500 mg/50 ml infusion bottle at 10 mcg/kg/min. Patient weighs 187 lb.

7. Infuse alfentanil (Alfenta) 10,000 mcg in D$_5$W 250 ml at 0.5 mcg/kg/min. Patient weighs 175 lb.

8. Infuse milrinone (Primacor) 20 mg in D$_5$W 100 ml at 0.375 mcg/kg/min. Patient weighs 160 lb.

9. Infuse theophylline 400 mg in D$_5$W 500 ml at 0.55 mg/kg/hr. Patient weighs 70 kg. Hourly rate only.

10. Infuse esmolol 2.5 g in NSS 250 ml at 150 mcg/kg/min. Patient weighs 148 lb.

TITRATION OF INFUSION RATE

Titration of drugs administered by infusion is based on (1) *concentration of solution,* (2) *infusion rates,* (3) *specific concentration per kilogram of body weight,* and (4) *titration factor.* The *titration factor* is the concentration of drug per drop in units (units/gtt), milligrams (mg/gtt), or micrograms (mcg/gtt). For the programmable volumetric infusion pump, the titration factor is the increment of increase or decrease in units, micrograms, or milligrams. If the only IV equip-

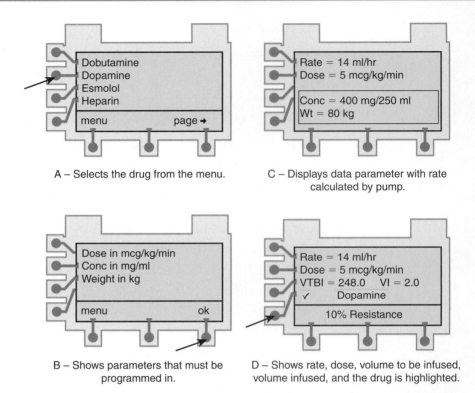

A – Selects the drug from the menu.

C – Displays data parameter with rate calculated by pump.

B – Shows parameters that must be programmed in.

D – Shows rate, dose, volume to be infused, volume infused, and the drug is highlighted.

FIGURE 11-1 Examples of display screen of a dose rate calculator on an advanced infusion pump. (Modified from Volumetric Infusion Manual, 1999, Alaris Medical Systems, San Diego, CA.)

ment available has the ml/hr feature, the titration factor of concentration per drop can be used. Advanced volumetric infusion pumps can infuse medication volume in increments of 0.1 ml/hr. Other pump features include a drug-specific dose calculator that allows the nurse to select a drug name, input the dosage, the concentration of the drug, and the weight of the patient (Figure 11-1). These infusion pumps make drug delivery and titration safer and easier. Any dose changes can be easily reprogrammed by the drug-specific dose calculator. The safety features of the advanced infusion pumps decrease medication errors. Many drug manufacturers are recommending infusion pumps for the delivery of all vasoactive medications used in critical care.

Calculating the titration factor is necessary when the technology of the advanced infusion pumps is unavailable. The titration factor can be added to or subtracted from the baseline infusion rate to determine the exact concentration of an infusion. Because the titration method of drug administration is primarily used when a patient's condition is labile, calculating the titration factor gives the nurse the means of determining the exact amount of drug to be infused.

Charts for drug infusion, developed by drug manufacturers, can be used to adjust infusion rates for drug titrations. Often, the amount of drug being infused falls between calibrations on the charts. When this occurs, the titration factor can be used to determine the exact concentration of drug being administered. The titration factor can also be used to verify the correct selection from the chart.

EXAMPLES

PROBLEM: Infuse Isuprel 2 mg in 250 ml D$_5$W. Titrate 1-3 mcg/min to maintain heart rate greater than 50 beats/min and less than 130 beats/min and blood pressure greater than 90 mm Hg systolic.

a. Find concentration of solution:

Convert mg to mcg. Set up ratio and proportion.	2 mg = 2000 mcg 2000 mcg:250 ml :: X mcg:ml 250 X = 2000 X = 8 mcg 8 mcg/ml

b. Infusion rate by volume per unit time:
Desired infusion rate by concentration is stated in the problem.
Note that the upper dosage and lower dosage must be determined.

Find volume rate per minute: ml/min:

Divide concentration/ minute by concentration of solution.	*Lower* $\dfrac{1\ \text{mcg/min}}{8\ \text{mcg/ml}}$ = 0.125 ml/min	*Upper* $\dfrac{3\ \text{mcg/min}}{8\ \text{mcg/ml}}$ = 0.375 ml/min

Find volume rate per hour: ml/hr (equivalent to gtt/min):

Multiply volume rate/minute by 60 min.	*Lower* 0.125 ml/min × 60 min/hr = 7.5 ml/hr

Upper
0.375 ml/hr × 60 min/hr
= 22.5 ml/hr

Dosage range is 7.5 ml/hr at 1 mcg/min, the lowest dose ordered, to 22.5 ml/hr at 3 mcg/min, the highest dose ordered.

Determine Titration Factor Using Infusion Pump

When the amount of fluid being titrated is 1 ml or greater (0.1 ml/hr lowest increment of infusion), the concentration of the solution multiplied by the volume per hour will give the total concentration to be given in 1 hour. The total volume in 1 hour divided by 60 min/hr will yield the concentration per minute.

EXAMPLE

Increase Isuprel from 7.5 ml/hr to 9 ml/hr.

Multiply concentration of solution by volume/hr. Then divide by 60 min/hr.	$9 \text{ ml/hr} \times 8 \text{ mcg/ml} = 72 \text{ mcg/hr}$ $$\frac{72 \text{ mcg/hr}}{60 \text{ min/hr}} = 1.2 \text{ mcg/min}$$

When increments of less than 1 ml are being titrated, multiply the concentration by the lowest increment of infusion.

Multiply concentration of solution by 0.1 ml/hr to get the concentration/hr.	$8 \text{ mcg/ml} \times 0.1 \text{ ml/hr} = 0.8 \text{ mcg/hr}$

Find rate in mcg/min by dividing concentration/hr by 60 min/hr.	$$\frac{0.8 \text{ mcg/hr}}{60 \text{ min/hr}} = 0.013 \text{ mcg/min}$$

Titration factor is 0.8 mcg/hr or 0.013 mcg/min for the solution of Isuprel 2 mg in 250 ml D_5W with 0.1 ml/hr as the lowest increment of infusion. If the baseline rate is 7.5 ml/hr and 1 mcg/min, increasing the rate by 0.1 ml/hr to 7.6 ml/hr will increase the per minute dose to 1.013 mcg/minute. Since Isuprel is ordered in mcg/min, using the titration factor in mcg/min would give a very accurate dose if increases or decreases are needed.

Increasing or Decreasing Infusion Rates Using Infusion Pump

When increasing infusion rate (0.1 ml/hr lowest increment of infusion) from baseline, multiply the titration factor by the number of increases and add to beginning rate.

EXAMPLE

Baseline Data

Order	Isuprel 2 mg in 250 ml
Concentration of solution	8 mcg/ml
Beginning rate	1 mcg/min
Volume per hour	7.5 ml/hr
Lowest increment of infusion	0.1 ml/hr (lowest pump setting)
Titration factors	0.8 mcg/hr or 0.013 mcg/min

Since the order is given in mcg/min, the titration factor of mcg/min should be used. To increase infusion rate from 7.5 ml/hr to 7.7 ml/hr, a 0.2 ml increase on the infusion pump, multiply titration factor by 2. Multiply 2×0.013 mcg/min = 0.028 mcg/min, then add to baseline of 1 mcg/min and now the concentration per minute is 1.028 mcg/min. Incremental increases can be easily calculated by multiplying the titration factor by the number of increases, then adding to baseline.

EXAMPLE

Hourly Rate (ml/hr)	Titration Factor	Concentration/ min (ADD)
7.5 ml/hr	0.013 mcg/min	1 mcg/min
7.6 ml/hr	0.013 mcg/min × 1 = 0.013	1.013 mcg/min
7.7 ml/hr	0.013 mcg/min × 2 = 0.026	1.026 mcg/min
7.8 ml/hr	0.013 mcg/min × 3 = 0.039	1.039 mcg/min

To titrate downward, multiply titration factor by the number of decreases and subtract each decrease from current infusion rate.

EXAMPLE

Hourly Rate (ml/hr)	Titration Factor	Concentration/min (SUBTRACT)
10 ml/hr	0.013 mcg/min	1.325 mcg/min
9.8 ml/hr	0.013 mcg/min × 2 = 0.026	1.299 mcg/min
9.4 ml/hr	0.013 mcg/min × 6 = 0.078	1.247 mcg/min

Determine Titration Factor Using a Microdrip IV Set

A microdrip IV set has a drop factor of 60 gtts/ml, so the number of drops per minute is the same as the hourly rate. In a situation where infusion pumps are not available, a microdrip IV set may be the only option to deliver small amounts of IV medication. Using the Isuprel data, the ml/hr rate will be 7.5 gtt counted per minute from the drip chamber. The titration factor is the amount of Isuprel in each drop.

Determine the titration factor:

Find rate in gtt/min. Divide concentration/minute by gtt/min.	7.5 gtt/min $\dfrac{1 \text{ mcg/min}}{7.5 \text{ gtt/min}} = 0.133$ mcg/gtt

The *titration factor* is 0.133 mcg/gtt in a solution of Isuprel 2 mg in 250 ml D_5W. In other words, changing drops per minute results in a corresponding change in milliliters per hour. If the baseline infusion rates are **1 mcg/min** for concentration and **7.5 ml/hr** for volume, increasing the infusion rate by **1 gtt/min** changes the concentration/minute by **0.133 mcg** and increases the hourly volume by **1 ml** to give a rate of **8.5 ml/hr.**

Increasing or Decreasing Infusion Rates Using a Microdrip IV Set

To increase the infusion rate by 5 gtt/min from a baseline rate of 1 mcg/min, set up a ratio and proportion or multiply the titration factor (mcg/gtt) by 5 to obtain the increment of increase.

EXAMPLES

Set up a ratio and proportion with rate in gtt/min as the known variable.	$7.5 \text{ gtt} : 1 \text{ mcg} :: 5 \text{ gtt} : X \text{ mcg}$ $7.5 X = 5$ $X = 0.666 \text{ mcg}$ $5 \text{ gtt}/0.66 \text{ mcg}$

or

Multiply titration factor in mcg/gtt by 5.	$0.133 \text{ mcg/gtt} \times 5 \text{ gtt} = 0.665 \text{ mcg}$

Adding 5 gtt/min increases the volume infusion rate by 5 ml/hr, from 7.5 to 12.5 ml/hr. The concentration of drug delivered is increased by 0.665 mcg/min to 1.665 mcg/min. For example,

$$\begin{array}{ll} 1.000 \text{ mcg/min} & \text{baseline rate} \\ + \underline{0.665} \text{ mcg/min} & \text{increment of rate increased} \\ 1.665 \text{ mcg/min} & \text{adjusted infusion rate} \end{array}$$

Suppose the infusion rate was 3 mcg/min and a decrease was needed. To decrease the infusion rate by 10 gtt, set up another ratio and proportion or multiply the titration factor (mcg/gtt) by 10.

EXAMPLES

Set up a ratio and proportion with rate in gtt/mcg as the known variable.	$7.5 \text{ gtt} : 1 \text{ mcg} :: 10 \text{ gtt} : X \text{ mcg}$ $7.5 X = 10$ $X = 1.33 \text{ mcg}$ $1.33 \text{ mcg}/10 \text{ gtt}$

or

Multiply titration factor in mcg/gtt by 10.	$0.133 \text{ mcg/gtt} \times 10 \text{ gtt} = 1.33 \text{ mcg}$

Subtracting 10 gtt/min decreases the infusion rate by 10 ml/hr, from 22.5 to 12.5 ml/hr. The amount of drug delivered is decreased by 1.33 mcg/min to 1.67 mcg/min. For example,

$$\begin{array}{ll} 3.00 \text{ mcg/min} & \text{baseline infusion rate} \\ - \underline{1.33} \text{ mcg/min} & \text{increment of rate decreased} \\ 1.67 \text{ mcg/min} & \text{adjusted infusion rate} \end{array}$$

PRACTICE PROBLEMS: IV Titration of Infusion Rate

Answers can be found on page 321.

1. What are the units of measure for the following terms?

   a. Concentration of solution per minute for specific body weight

   _____

b. Concentration of solution

_____

c. Volume per hour

_____

d. Concentration per minute

_____

e. Volume per minute

_____

f. Concentration per minute

_____

g. Titration factor

_____

2. Order: nitroprusside 50 mg in 250 ml D_5W. Titrate 0.5 to 1.5 mcg/kg/min to maintain mean systolic blood pressure at 100 mm Hg. Patient weighs 70 kg.

Find the following:

a. Concentration of solution

_____

b. Concentraton per minute

_____

c. Volume per minute and hour

_____

d. Titration factor for infusion pump; for microdrop set

_____

e. Increase infusion rate of 10.5 ml/hr by 0.5 ml to 11 ml/hr with infusion pump. What is the concentration per minute?

_____

f. Increase infusion rate from 11 ml/hr to 20 ml/hr. What is the concentration per minute?

_____

g. Increase the infusion rate of 11 gtt/min by 5 gtt. What is the concentration per minute? What is the volume per hour?

_____

h. Increase the infusion rate of 16 gtt/ml by 13 gtt. What is the concentration per minute? What is the volume per hour?

_____

3. Order: dopamine 400 mg in 250 ml D$_5$W. Titrate beginning at 4 mcg/kg/min to maintain a mean systolic blood pressure of 100 to 120 mm Hg. Patient weighs 75 kg.

Find the following:

a. Concentration of solution

_____

b. Concentration per minute

_____

c. Volume per minute and hour

_____

d. Titration factor for infusion pump; for microdrip set

_____

e. With the infusion pump, increase infusion rate from 11.4 ml/hr to 12 ml/hr. What is the concentration per minute?

_____

f. With the infusion pump, increase the infusion rate to 12.5 ml/hr. What is the concentration per minute?

_____

g. Using a microdrip set, increase the infusion rate of 13 gtt/min by 7 gtt. What is the concentration per minute? What is the volume per hour?

_____

h. Using a microdrop set, decrease the infusion rate of 20 ml/hr (20 gtt/min) by 5 gtt. What is the concentration per minute? What is the volume per hour?

_____

TOTAL AMOUNT OF DRUG INFUSED OVER TIME

Determining the total amount of drug infused over time is useful when changes in drug therapy occur. If adverse effects, toxic levels, therapeutic failure, or discontinuance of a drug occurs, knowing the amount that was administered can be important for charting and for determining future therapies.

For this calculation, the concentration of the drug in solution must be known, as must the time that drug therapy began to the nearest minute. Again, with 60-gtt sets, the hourly rate is the same as the drip rate per minute.

EXAMPLES

PROBLEM: Heparin 10,000 units in 250 ml D$_5$W at 30 ml/hr has been infusing for 3 hours. The drug is discontinued.

How much heparin did the patient receive?

Find concentration of solution:

Set up a ratio and proportion. Solve for X.	10,000 units : 250 ml :: X units : ml 250 X = 10,000 X = 40 units 40 units/ml

Find concentration per hour:

Multiply concentration of solution by volume/hour.	40 units/ml × 30 ml/hr = 1200 units/hr

Calculate total amount of drug infused:

Multiply concentration/hour by length of administration.	1200 units/hr × 3 hr = 3600 units/hr

Answer: The total amount of heparin infused over 3 hours was 3600 units.

PRACTICE PROBLEMS: V Total Amount of Drug Infused Over Time

Answers can be found on page 323.

Solve for the amount of drug infused over time.

1. In 1 hour, a patient received two boluses of lidocaine 100 mg and an IV infusion of 4 mg/ml at 40 ml/hr for 30 minutes. How many milligrams have been infused?

    Note: Do not exceed 300 mg/hr of lidocaine.

2. Heparin 20,000 units in 500 ml D$_5$W at 50 ml/hr has been infused for 5½ hours. The drug is discontinued. How much heparin has been given?

ANSWERS

I Calculating Concentration of a Solution

1. 10,000 units : 250 ml :: X units : ml
    250 X = 10,000
    X = 40 units
The concentration of solution is 40 units/ml.

2. 250 mg : 500 ml ∷ X mg : ml
$$500\ X = 250$$
$$X = 0.5\ mg$$
The concentration of solution is 0.5 mg/ml.

3. 100 units : 500 ml ∷ X units : ml
$$500\ X = 100$$
$$X = 0.2\ units$$
The concentration of solution is 0.2 units/ml.

4.   1 g = 1000 mg
1000 mg : 1000 ml ∷ X mg : ml
$$1000\ X = 1000$$
$$X = 1\ mg$$
The concentration of solution is 1 mg/ml.

5.   4 mg = 4000 mcg
4000 mcg : 500 ml ∷ X mcg : ml
$$500\ X = 4000$$
$$X = 8\ mcg$$
The concentration of solution is 8 mcg/ml.

6. 500 mg : 250 ml ∷ X mcg : ml
$$250\ X = 500$$
$$X = 2\ mg$$
The concentration of solution is 2 mg/ml.

7. 400 mg : 250 ml ∷ X mg : ml
$$250\ X = 400$$
$$X = 1.6\ mg$$
The concentration of solution is 1.6 mg/ml.

8.   2 mg = 2000 mcg
2000 mcg : 250 ml ∷ X mcg : ml
$$250\ X = 2000$$
$$X = 8\ mcg$$
The concentration of solution is 8 mcg/ml.

9. 750,000 units : 50 ml ∷ X units : ml
$$50\ X = 750,000$$
$$X = 15,000\ units$$
The concentration of solution is 15,000 units/ml.

10.   50 mg = 50,000 mcg
50,000 mcg : 500 ml ∷ X mcg : ml
$$500\ X = 50,000$$
$$X = 100\ mcg$$
The concentration of solution is 100 mcg/ml.

11.   1 g = 1000 mg
1000 mg : 250 ml ∷ X mg : ml
$$250\ X = 1000$$
$$X = 4\ mg$$
The concentration of solution is 4 mg/ml.

12.   2 g = 2000 mg
   2000 mg:250 ml :: X mg:ml
             250 X = 2000
                  X = 8 mg
The concentration of solution is 8 mg/ml.

13. 25,000 units:250 ml :: X mg:ml
                250 X = 25,000
                     X = 100 units
The concentration of solution is 100 units/ml.

14.   1 g = 1000 mg
   1000 mg:500 ml :: X mg:ml
             500 X = 1000
                  X = 2 mg
The concentration of solution is 2 mg/ml.

15.   50 mg = 50,000 mcg
   50,000 mcg:250 ml :: X mcg:ml
                250 X = 50,000 mcg
                     X = 200 mcg
The concentration of solution is 200 mcg/ml.

16. 100 mg:100 ml :: X mg:ml
             100 X = 100
                  X = 1 mg/ml
The concentration of solution is 1 mg/ml.

17. 800 mg:500 ml :: X mg:ml
             500 X = 800
                  X = 1.6 mg/ml
The concentration of solution is 1.6 mg/ml.

18. 20 mg:100 ml :: X mg:ml
             100 X = 20
                  X = 0.2 mg/ml
The concentration of solution is 0.2 mg/ml.

19. 1,500,000 units:100 ml :: X mg:ml
                100 X = 1,500,000
                     X = 15,000 units/ml
The concentration of solution is 15,000 units/ml.

20. 150 mg:100 ml :: X mg:ml
             100 X = 150
                  X = 1.5 mg/ml
The concentration of solution is 1.5 mg/ml.

II Calculating Infusion Rate

1. *Concentration of solution:*
   1000 units:500 ml = X units:ml
             500 X = 1000
                  X = 2 units
The concentration of solution is 2 units/ml.

Infusion rates:

a. Volume/min:

    50 ml:60 min :: X ml:min

          60 X = 50

              X = 0.833 ml or 0.83 ml or 0.8 ml

                  0.8 ml/min

b. Volume/hr:

    50 ml/hr

c. Concentration/min:

    2 units/ml × 0.8 ml/min = 1.60 units/min

d. Concentration/hr:

    1.60 units/min × 60 min/hr = 96 units/hr

2. *Concentration of solution.*

    100 mg:500 ml :: X mg:ml

          500 X = 100

             X = 0.2 mg

The concentration of solution is 0.2 mg/ml.

Infusion rates:

a. Volume/min:

    60 ml:60 min :: X ml:min

          60 X = 60

             X = 1 ml

                1 ml/min

b. Volume/hr:

    60 ml/hr

c. Concentration/min:

    0.2 mg/ml × 1 ml/min = 0.2 mg/min

d. Concentration/hr:

    0.2 mg/min × 60 min/hr = 12 mg/hr

3. *Concentration of solution:*

          25 mg = 25,000 mcg

    25,000 mcg:250 ml :: X mcg:ml

          250 X = 25,000

             X = 100 mcg

The concentration of solution is 100 mcg/ml.

Infusion rates:

a. Volume/min:

$$\frac{50 \text{ mcg/min}}{100 \text{ mcg/ml}} = 0.5 \text{ ml/min}$$

b. Volume/hr:

    0.5 ml/min × 60 min/hr = 30 ml/hr

c. Concentration/min:

    50 mcg/min

d. Concentration/hr:

    50 mcg/min × 60 min/hr = 3000 mcg/hr

4. *Concentration of solution:*

$$800 \text{ mg} = 800,000 \text{ mcg}$$
$$800,000 \text{ mcg}:500 \text{ ml} :: X \text{ mcg}:\text{ml}$$
$$500 \text{ X} = 800,000$$
$$X = 1600 \text{ mcg}$$

The concentration of solution is 1600 mcg/ml.

Infusion rates:

a. Volume/min:
$$\frac{400 \text{ mcg/min}}{1600 \text{ mcg/ml}} = 0.25 \text{ ml/min}$$

b. Volume/hr:
0.25 ml/min × 60 min/hr = 15 ml/hr

c. Concentration/min:
400 mcg/min

d. Concentration/hr:
400 mcg/min × 60 min/hr = 24,000 mcg/hr

5. *Concentration of solution:*

$$2 \text{ mg} = 2000 \text{ mcg}$$
$$2000 \text{ mcg}:250 \text{ ml} :: X \text{ mcg}:\text{ml}$$
$$250 \text{ X} = 2000$$
$$X = 8 \text{ mcg}$$

The concentration of solution is 8 mcg/ml.

Infusion rates:

a. Volume/min:
$$45 \text{ ml}:60 \text{ min} :: X \text{ ml}:\text{min}$$
$$60 \text{ X} = 45$$
$$X = 0.75 \text{ ml/min}$$

b. Volume/hr:
45 ml/hr

c. Concentration/min:
8 mcg/ml × 0.75 ml/min = 6 mcg/min

d. Concentration/hr:
6 mcg/min × 60 min/hr = 360 mcg/hr

6. *Concentration of solution:*

$$1000 \text{ mg} = 1,000,000 \text{ mcg}$$
$$1,000,000 \text{ mcg}:500 \text{ ml} :: X \text{ mcg}:\text{ml}$$
$$500 \text{ X} = 1,000,000$$
$$X = 2000 \text{ mcg}$$

The concentration of solution is 2000 mcg/ml.

Infusion rates:

a. Volume/min:
$$12 \text{ ml}:60 \text{ min} :: X \text{ ml}:\text{min}$$
$$60 \text{ X} = 12$$
$$X = 0.2 \text{ ml}$$
$$0.2 \text{ ml/min}$$

   b. Volume/hr:
   12 ml/hr
   c. Concentration/min:
   2000 mcg/ml $\times$ 0.2 ml/min = 400 mcg/min
   d. Concentration/hr:
   400 mcg/min $\times$ 60 min/hr = 24,000 mcg/hr
7. *Concentration of solution:*

$$250 \text{ mg} = 250,000 \text{ mcg}$$
$$250,000 \text{ mcg} : 250 \text{ ml} :: X \text{ mcg} : \text{ml}$$
$$250 X = 250,000$$
$$X = 1000 \text{ mcg}$$

The concentration of solution is 1000 mcg/ml.
Infusion rates:
   a. Volume/min:

$$10 \text{ ml} : 60 \text{ min} :: X \text{ ml} : 1 \text{ min}$$
$$60 X = 10 \text{ ml}$$
$$X = 0.1666 \text{ ml or } 0.17 \text{ ml}$$
$$0.17 \text{ ml/min}$$

   b. Volume/hr:
   10 ml/hr
   c. Concentration/min:
   1000 mcg/ml $\times$ 0.17 ml/min = 170 mcg/min
   d. Concentration/hr:
   170 mcg/min $\times$ 60 min/hr = 10,200 mcg/hr
8. *Concentration of solution:*

$$2 \text{ g} = 2000 \text{ mg}$$
$$2000 \text{ mg} : 500 \text{ ml} :: X \text{ mg} : \text{ml}$$
$$500 X = 2000$$
$$X = 4 \text{ mg}$$

The concentration of solution is 4 mg/ml.
Infusion rates:
   a. Volume/min:

$$\frac{4 \text{ mg/ml}}{4 \text{ mg/min}} = 1 \text{ ml/min}$$

   b. Volume/hr:
   1 ml/min $\times$ 60 min/hr = 60 ml/hr
   c. Concentration/min:
   4 mg/min
   d. Concentration/hr:
   4 mg/min $\times$ 60 min/hr = 240 mg/hr
9. *Concentration of solution:*

$$400 \text{ mg} : 250 \text{ ml} :: X \text{ mg} : \text{ml}$$
$$250 X = 400$$
$$X = 1.6 \text{ mg}$$

The concentration of solution is 1.6 mg/ml.

Infusion rates:
a. Volume/min:

60 ml:60 min :: X ml:min

60 X = 60

X = 1 ml

1 ml/min

b. Volume/hr:

60 ml/hr

c. Concentration/min:

1.6 mg/ml × 1 ml/min = 1.6 mg/min

d. Concentration/hr:

1.6 mg/min × 60 min/hr = 96 mg/hr

10. *Concentration of solution:*

4 mg = 4000 mcg

4000 mcg:500 ml :: X mcg:ml

500 X = 4000

X = 8 mcg

The concentration of solution is 8 mcg/ml.

Infusion rates:
a. Volume/min:

65 ml:60 min :: X ml:min

60 X = 65

X = 1.083 ml or

1.08 ml/min

b. Volume/hr:

65 ml/hr

c. Concentration/min:

8 mcg/ml × 1.08 ml/min = 8.64 mcg/min

d. Concentration/hr:

8.64 mcg/min × 60 min/hr = 518.4 mcg/hr or 518 mcg/hr

11. *Concentration of solution:*

50 mg:150 ml :: X mg:ml

150 X = 50

X = 0.33 mg

The concentration of solution is 0.33 mg/ml.

Infusion rates:
a. Concentration/min:

3 mg:60 min :: X mg:min

60 X = 3

X = 0.05 mg/min

b. Concentration/hr:

3 mg/hr

c. Volume/min:

$$\frac{0.05 \text{ mg/min}}{0.33 \text{ mg/ml}} = 0.15 \text{ ml/min}$$

    d. Volume/hr:

$$\frac{3 \text{ mg/hr}}{0.33 \text{ mg/ml}} = 9.09 \text{ or } 9 \text{ ml/hr}$$

12. *Concentration of solution:*

    50 units : 250 ml ∷ X mg : ml

             250 X = 50

                X = 0.2 units

The concentration of solution is 0.2 units/ml.

Infusion rates:

    a. Concentration/min:

        4 units : 60 min ∷ X units : min

             60 X = 4

                X = 0.066 units/min

    b. Concentration/hr:

        4 units/hr

    c. Volume/min:

$$\frac{0.7 \text{ units/min}}{0.2 \text{ units/ml}} = 0.33 \text{ ml/min}$$

    d. Volume/hr:

$$\frac{4 \text{ units/hr}}{0.2 \text{ units/ml}} = 20 \text{ ml/hr}$$

13. *Concentration of solution:*

            2 g = 2000 mg

    2000 mg : 250 ml ∷ X mg : ml

             250 X = 2000

                X = 8 mg

The concentration of solution is 8 mg/ml.

Infusion rates:

    a. Volume/hr = 20 ml/hr

    b. Volume/min:

        20 ml : 60 min ∷ X ml : min

             60 X = 20

                X = 0.3 ml/min

    c. Concentration/min:

        8 mg/ml × 0.3 ml/min = 2.4 mg/min

    d. Concentration/hr:

        2.4 mg/min × 60 min/hr = 144 mg/hr

14. *Concentration of solution:*

            50 mg = 50,000 mcg

    50,000 mcg : 250 ml ∷ X mg : ml

             250 X = 50,000

                X = 200 mcg

The concentration of solution is 200 mcg/ml.

Infusion rates:

a. Volume/hr = 24 ml/hr

b. Volume/min:

24 ml/hr:60 min/hr :: X ml:min

60 X = 24

X = 0.4 ml/min

c. Concentration/min:

200 mcg/ml × 0.4 ml/min = 80 mcg/min

d. Concentration/hr:

80 mcg/min × 60 min = 4800 mcg/hr

15. *Concentration of solution:*

25,000 units:500 ml :: X units:ml

500 X = 25,000

X = 50 units

The concentration of solution is 50 units/ml.

Infusion rates:

a. Volume/hr:

10 ml/hr

b. Volume/min:

10 ml:60 min/hr :: X ml:min

60 X = 10

X = 0.166 ml/min

c. Concentration/hr:

50 units/ml × 10 ml/hr = 500 units/hr

d. Concentration/min:

50 units/ml × 0.166 ml/min = 8.3 units/min

16. *Concentration of solution:*

900 mg:500 ml :: X mg:ml

500 X = 900

X = 1.8 mg/ml

The concentration of solution is 1.8 mg/ml.

Infusion rates:

a. Volume/hr:

33.3 ml/hr

b. Volume/min:

33.3 ml:60 min :: X ml:min

60 X = 33.3

X = 0.55 ml/min

c. Concentration/hr:

1.8 mg/ml × 33.3 min/hr = 59.4 mg/hr

d. Concentration/min:

1.8 mg/ml × 0.55 ml/min = 0.99 mg/ml or 1.0 mg/ml

17. *Concentration of solution:*

$$1 \text{ g} = 1000 \text{ mg}$$
$$1000 \text{ mg} : 250 \text{ ml} :: X \text{ mg} : \text{ml}$$
$$250 \text{ X} = 1000$$
$$X = 4 \text{ mg/ml}$$

The concentration of solution is 4 mg/ml.

Infusion rates:

a. Volume/min:
$$\frac{4 \text{ mg/min}}{4 \text{ mg/ml}} = 1 \text{ ml/min}$$

b. Volume/hr:
1 ml/min $\times$ 60 min/hr = 60 ml/hr

c. Concentration/hr:
4 mg/min $\times$ 60 min/hr = 240 mg/hr

d. Concentration/min:
4 mg/min

18. *Concentration of solution:*

$$100 \text{ mg} : 100 \text{ ml} :: X \text{ mg} : \text{ml}$$
$$100 \text{ X} = 100$$
$$X = 1 \text{ mg/ml}$$

The concentration of solution is 1 mg/ml.

Infusion rates:

a. Volume/hr:
$$\frac{10 \text{ mg/hr}}{1 \text{ mg/ml}} = 10 \text{ ml/hr}$$

b. Volume/min:
$$\frac{10 \text{ ml/hr}}{60 \text{ min/hr}} = 0.166 \text{ ml/min}$$

c. Concentration/hr:
10 mg/hr

d. Concentration/min:
1 mg/ml $\times$ 0.166 ml/min = 0.166 mg/min or 0.17 mg/min

19. *Concentration of solution:*

$$750,000 \text{ units} : 250 \text{ ml} :: X \text{ units} : \text{ml}$$
$$250 \text{ X} = 750,000$$
$$X = 3000 \text{ units/ml}$$

The concentration of solution is 3000 units/ml.

Infusion rates:

a. Volume/hr:
$$\frac{100,000 \text{ units/hr}}{3000 \text{ units/ml}} = 33.3 \text{ ml/hr}$$

b. Volume/min:
$$\frac{33.3 \text{ ml/hr}}{60 \text{ min/hr}} = 0.55 \text{ ml/min}$$

c. Concentration/hr:
100,000 units/hr

d. Concentration/min:

$$\frac{100,000 \text{ units/hr}}{60 \text{ min/hr}} = 1666.6 \text{ units/min or 1667 units/min}$$

20. *Concentration of solution:*

$$1 \text{ g} = 1000 \text{ mg}$$
$$1000 \text{ mg}:250 \text{ ml} :: X \text{ mg}:\text{ml}$$
$$250 \text{ X} = 1000$$
$$X = 4 \text{ mg/ml}$$

The concentration of solution is 4 mg/ml.

Infusion rates:

a. Volume/min:

$$\frac{1 \text{ mg/min}}{4 \text{ mg/ml}} = 0.25 \text{ ml/min}$$

b. Volume/hr:

0.25 ml/min × 60 min/hr = 15 ml/hr

c. Concentration/hr:

4 mg/ml × 15 ml/hr = 60 mg/hr

d. Concentration/min:

1 mg/min

III Calculating Infusion Rate for Specific Body Weight

1. *Concentration of solution:*

lb to kg

$$500 \text{ mg} = 500,000 \text{ mcg} \qquad \frac{182}{2.2} = 82.7 \text{ kg}$$
$$500,000:250 \text{ ml} :: X \text{ mcg}:\text{ml}$$
$$250 \text{ X} = 500,000$$
$$X = 2000 \text{ mcg}$$

The concentration of solution is 2000 mcg/ml.

Infusion rates:

a. Concentration/min:

Body weight × Desired dose/kg/min

82.7 kg × 5 mcg/kg/min

= 413.5 mcg/min

b. Concentration/hr:

413.5 mcg/min × 60 min/hr = 24,810 mcg/hr

c. Volume/min:

$$\frac{413.5 \text{ mcg/min}}{2000 \text{ mcg/ml}} = 0.206 \text{ ml/min or 0.2 ml/min}$$

d. Volume/hr:

0.2 ml/min × 60 min/hr = 12 ml/hr

2. *Concentration of solution:*

lb to kg

$$250 \text{ mg} = 250,000 \text{ mcg} \qquad \frac{165}{2.2} = 75 \text{ kg}$$
$$250,000 \text{ mcg}:250 \text{ ml} :: X \text{ mcg}:\text{ml}$$
$$250 \text{ X} = 250,000$$
$$X = 1000 \text{ mcg}$$

The concentration of solution is 1000 mcg/ml.

Infusion rates:

a. Concentration/min:

Body weight $\times$ Desired dose/kg/min

75 kg $\times$ 5 mcg/kg/min = 375 mcg/min

b. Concentration/hr:

375 mcg/min $\times$ 60 min/hr = 22,500 mcg/hr

c. Volume/min:

$$\frac{375 \text{ mcg/min}}{1000 \text{ mcg/ml}} = 0.375 \text{ ml/min}$$

d. Volume/hr:

0.375 ml/min $\times$ 60 min/hr = 22.5 ml/hr

3. *Concentration of solution:*

lb to kg

400 mg = 400,000 mcg

400,000 mg : 250 ml ∷ X mg : ml

$$\frac{140}{2.2} = 63.6 \text{ kg}$$

250 X = 400,000

X = 1600 mcg

The concentration of solution is 1600 mcg/ml.

Infusion rates:

a. Concentration/min:

Body weight $\times$ Desired dose/kg/min

63.6 kg $\times$ 10 mcg/kg/min

= 636 mcg/min

b. Concentration/hr:

636 mcg/min $\times$ 60 min/hr = 38,160 mcg/hr

c. Volume/min:

$$\frac{636 \text{ mcg/min}}{1600 \text{ mcg/ml}} = 0.39 \text{ ml/min}$$

d. Volume/hr:

0.39 ml/min $\times$ 60 min/hr = 23.4 ml/hr

4. *Concentration of solution:*

Patient weight

100 mg = 100,000 mcg   55 kg

100,000 mcg : 500 ml ∷ X mg : ml

500 X = 100,000

X = 200 mcg

The concentration of solution is 200 mcg/ml.

Infusion rates:

a. Concentration/min:

3 mcg/kg/min $\times$ 55 kg = 165 mcg/min

b. Concentration/hr:

165 mcg/min $\times$ 60 min/hr = 9900 mcg/hr

c. Volume/min:

$$\frac{165 \text{ mcg/min}}{200 \text{ mcg/ml}} = 0.825 \text{ ml/min}$$

d. Volume/hr:

0.825 ml/min $\times$ 60 min/hr = 49.5 ml/hr

5. *Concentration of solution:*

lb to kg

1000 mg = 1,000,000 mcg $\quad \dfrac{110}{2.2} = 50 \text{ kg}$

1,000,000 mcg : 500 ml :: X mcg : ml

500 X = 1,000,000

X = 2000 mcg

The concentration of solution is 2000 mcg/ml.

Infusion rates:

a. Concentration/min:

Body weight × Desired dose/kg/min

50 kg × 15 mcg/kg/min

= 750 mcg/min

b. Concentration/hr:

750 mcg/min × 60 min/hr = 45,000 mcg/hr

c. Volume/min:

$\dfrac{750 \text{ mcg/min}}{2000 \text{ mcg/ml}} = 0.375 \text{ ml/min}$

d. Volume/hr:

0.375 ml/min × 60 min/hr = 22.5 ml/hr

6. *Concentration of solution:*

lb to kg

500 mg : 50 ml :: X mg : ml $\quad \dfrac{187}{2.2} = 85 \text{ kg}$

50 X = 500

X = 10 mg/ml

The concentration of solution is 10 mg/ml or 10,000 mcg/ml.

Infusion rates:

a. Concentration/min:

Body weight × Desired dose/kg/min

85 kg × 10 mcg/kg/min

= 850 mcg/min

b. Concentration/hr:

850 mcg/min × 60 min/hr = 51,000 mcg/hr or 51 mg/hr

c. Volume/min:

$\dfrac{850 \text{ mcg/min}}{10,000 \text{ mcg/ml}} = 0.085 \text{ ml/min}$

d. Volume/hr:

0.085 ml/min × 60 min/hr = 5.1 ml/hr

7. *Concentration of solution:*

lb to kg

10,000 mcg : 250 ml :: X mcg : ml $\quad \dfrac{175}{2.2} = 79.5 \text{ kg}$

250 X = 10,000

X = 40 mcg/ml

Infusion rates:

a. Concentration/min:

Body weight × Desired dose/kg/min

79.5 kg × 0.5 mcg/kg/min

= 39.75 mcg/min

  b. Concentration/hr:
  39.75 mcg/min × 60 min/hr = 2385 mcg/hr or 2.4 mg/hr
  c. Volume/min:
  $$\frac{39.75 \text{ mcg/min}}{40 \text{ mcg/ml}} = 0.99 \text{ ml/min or 1 ml/min}$$
  d. Volume/hr:
  0.99 ml/min × 60 min/hr = 59.6 ml/hr

8. *Concentration of solution:*

lb to kg

20 mg:100 ml :: X mg:ml $\dfrac{160}{2.2} = 72.7$ kg
    100 X = 20
      X = 0.2 mg/ml
        or 200 mcg/ml

Infusion rates:
  a. Concentration/min:
  Body weight × Desired dose/kg/min
      72.7 kg × 0.375 mcg/kg/min
        = 27.2 mcg/min
  b. Concentration/hr:
  27.2 mcg/min × 60 min/hr = 1632 mcg/hr or 1.6 mg/hr
  c. Volume/min:
  $$\frac{27.2 \text{ mcg/min}}{200 \text{ mcg/ml}} = 0.136 \text{ ml/min}$$
  d. Volume/hr:
  0.136 ml/min × 60 min/hr = 8.16 ml/hr or 8.2 ml/hr

9. *Concentration of solution:*

Patient weight

400 mg:500 ml :: X mg:ml   70 kg
      500 X = 400
        X = 0.8 mg/ml

Infusion rates:
  a. Concentration/hr:
  Body weight × Desired dose/kg/min
      70 kg × 0.55 mg/kg/min
        = 38.5 mg/hr
  b. Volume/hr:
  $$\frac{38.5 \text{ mg/hr}}{0.8 \text{ mg/ml}} = 48.125 \text{ ml/hr or 48 ml/hr}$$

10. *Concentration of solution:*

lb to kg

2500 mg:250 ml :: X mg:ml $\dfrac{148}{2.2} = 67.2$ or 67.3 kg
    250 X = 2500
      X = 10 mg/ml

Infusion rates:
a. Concentration/min:
   Body weight × Desired dose/kg/min
   $$67.3 \times 150 \text{ mcg/kg/min}$$
   $$= 10{,}080 \text{ mcg/min or } 10 \text{ mg/min}$$
b. Concentration/hr:
   10 mg/min × 60 min/hr = 600 mg/hr
c. Volume/min:
   $$\frac{10 \text{ mg/min}}{10 \text{ mg/ml}} = 1 \text{ ml/min}$$
d. Volume/hr:
   1 ml/min × 60 min/hr = 60 ml/hr

IV Titration of Infusion Rate

1. a. (units, mg, mcg)/kg/min
   b. (units, mg, mcg)/ml
   c. ml/hr
   d. (units, mg, mcg)/min
   e. ml/min
   f. (units, mg, mcg)/min
   g. (units, mg, mcg)/min with infusion pump
      (units, mg, mcg)/gtt with microdrip IV set
2. a. Concentration of solution:
   $$50 \text{ mg} = 50{,}000 \text{ mcg}$$
   $$50{,}000 \text{ mcg} : 250 \text{ ml} :: X \text{ mcg} : 1 \text{ ml}$$
   $$250 X = 50{,}000$$
   $$X = 200 \text{ mcg}$$
   The concentration of solution is 200 mcg/ml.
   b. Concentration/min:
   Lower: 0.5 mcg/kg/min × 70 kg = 35 mcg/min
   Upper: 1.5 mcg/kg/min × 70 kg = 105 mcg/min
   c. Volume/min and volume/hr:
   Lower
   $$\frac{35 \text{ mcg/min}}{200 \text{ mcg/ml}} = 0.175 \text{ ml/min} \times 60 \text{ min/hr} = 10.5 \text{ or } 11 \text{ ml/hr}$$
   Upper
   $$\frac{105 \text{ mcg/min}}{200 \text{ mcg/ml}} = 0.525 \text{ ml/min} \times 60 \text{ min/hr} = 31.5 \text{ or } 32 \text{ ml/hr}$$
   d. Titration factor for infusion pump
   200 mcg/ml × 0.1 ml/hr = 20 mcg/hr $$\frac{20 \text{ mcg/hr}}{60 \text{ min/hr}} = 0.333 \text{ or } 0.3 \text{ mcg/min}$$

   Titration factor for microdrip
   11 ml/hr = 11 gtt/min $$\frac{35 \text{ mcg}}{11 \text{ gtt/min}} = 3.18 \text{ or } 3 \text{ mcg/gtt}$$

  e. Base rate 10.5 ml/hr or 35 mcg/min.

$5 \times 0.33/min = 1.65$ mcg/min or 1.7 mcg/min

Add to base rate 35 mcg/min

$$\frac{+1.7 \text{ mcg/min}}{36.7 \text{ mcg/min}}$$

  f. 200 mcg/hr $\times$ 20 ml/hr = 4000 mcg/hr

$$\frac{4000 \text{ mcg/hr}}{60 \text{ min/hr}} = 66.6 \text{ mcg/min}$$

  g. Concentration/min and volume/hr using a microdrip set

5 gtt $\times$ 3 mcg/gtt = 15 mcg

15 mcg + 35 mcg/min = 50 mcg/min

5 gtt + 11 gtt/min = 16 gtt/min or 16 ml/hr

  h. Concentration/min and volume/hr using a microdrip set

13 gtt $\times$ 3 mcg/gtt = 39 mcg

39 mcg + 50 mcg = 89 mcg/min

13 gtt + 16 gtt = 29 gtt/ml or 29 ml/hr

3. **a.** Concentration of solution:

400 mg = 400,000 mcg

400,000 mcg:250 ml :: X mcg:1 ml

250 X = 400,000 mcg

X = 1600 mcg

The concentration of solution is 1600 mcg/ml.

  b. Concentration/min:

4 mcg/kg/min $\times$ 75 kg = 300 mcg/min

  c. Volume/min and volume/hr:

$$\frac{300 \text{ mcg/min}}{1600 \text{ mcg/ml}} = 0.1875 \text{ ml/min} \times 60 \text{ min/hr} = 11.25 \text{ or } 11 \text{ ml/hr}$$

Titration factor for infusion pump

1600 mcg/ml $\times$ 0.1 ml/hr = 160 mcg/hr

$$\frac{160 \text{ mcg/hr}}{60 \text{ min/hr}} = 2.66 \text{ or } 2.7 \text{ mcg/min}$$

  d. Titration factor for microdrip

11 ml/hr = 11 gtt/min

$$\frac{300 \text{ mcg/min}}{11 \text{ gtt/min}} = 27.2 \text{ or } 27 \text{ mcg/gtt}$$

  e. Base rate 11 ml/hr or 300 mcg/min

6 $\times$ 2.7 mcg/min = 16.2 mcg/min

$$\begin{array}{r} 300 \text{ mcg/min} \\ \underline{16.25} \text{ mcg/min} \\ 316.2 \text{ mcg/min} \end{array}$$

  f. 12.5 ml/hr $\times$ 1600 mcg/ml = 333 mcg/min

  g. Concentration/min and volume/hr using a microdrip set

20 gtt/min $\times$ 27 mcg/gtt = 540 mcg/min

7 gtt + 13 gtt/min = 20 gtt/min or 20 ml/hr

  h. Concentration/min and volume/hr using a microdrip set

15 gtt/min $\times$ 27 mcg/gtt = 405 mcg/min

20 gtt/min − 5 gtt = 15 gtt/min or 15 ml/hr

V Total Amount of Drug Infused Over Time

1. Lidocaine bolus:

   100 mg
   +100 mg
   200 mg

   Lidocaine IV infusion:

   a. Concentration of solution: given as 4 mg/ml in problem.

   b. Concentration/hr:

   4 mg/ml × 40 ml/hr = 160 mg/hr

   c. Concentration over ½ hour:

   $$160 \text{ mg/hr} \times \frac{30 \text{ min}}{60 \text{ min/hr}} = 80 \text{ mg over 30 min}$$

   d. Amount of IV drug infused:

Lidocaine per two boluses:	200 mg
Lidocaine per IV infusion:	+80 mg
	280 mg total amount infused over 1 hr

   Note: The infusion rate is close to exceeding the maximum therapeutic range, which is 200 to 300 mg/hr.

2. Concentration of solution:

   20,000 units : 500 ml ∷ X units : 1 ml

   $$500 \text{ X} = 20,000$$
   $$\text{X} = 40 \text{ units}$$

   a. The concentration of solution is 40 units/ml.

   b. Concentration/hr:

   40 units/ml × 50 ml/hr = 2000 units/hr

   c. Amount of IV drug infused over 5½ hours:

   $$2000 \text{ units} \times \frac{30 \text{ min}}{60 \text{ min/hr}} = 1000 \text{ units over } \tfrac{1}{2} \text{ hr}$$

   200 units × 5 hr = 10,000 units/5 hr

   10,000 units
   +1,000 units
   11,000 units over 5½ hr

 Additional practice problems are available on the enclosed CD-ROM in the "Advanced Calculations" section.

CHAPTER 12

Pediatric Critical Care

OBJECTIVES

- Recognize factors that contribute to errors in drug and fluid administration.
- Identify the steps in calculating dilution parameters.
- Determine the accuracy of the dilution parameters in a drug order.

OUTLINE

FACTORS INFLUENCING INTRAVENOUS ADMINISTRATION

CALCULATING ACCURACY OF DILUTION PARAMETERS

In delivery of emergency drugs with complex dilution calculations, it is important for the nurse to evaluate the accuracy of the physician's order and to ensure that a child does not receive excessive fluids. Many institutions are attempting to standardize the concentration of the solution for various pediatric intravenous (IV) dosages to decrease the occurrence of miscalculations. National efforts are under way to standardize intravenous emergency drugs for infusion to eliminate medication errors.

As noted in Chapter 11, the concepts of concentration of the solution, infusion rates for concentration and volume, and concentration of a drug for specific body weight per unit time that are employed in adult critical care are also used to prepare pediatric doses.

FACTORS INFLUENCING INTRAVENOUS ADMINISTRATION

Excess fluid can be given when the fluid volume of the emergency drug is not considered in the 24-hour fluid intake. Long IV tubing can be another source of fluid excess and can cause errors in drug delivery. When the priming or filling volume of the IV tubing is not considered, the child may receive extra fluid, especially if medication is added to the primary IV set via a secondary IV set. IV medication may not reach the child if the IV infusion rate is low, such as 1 ml/hr, or if the IV tubing has not been primed or filled with the medication before infusion. Most pediatric departments are developing protocols for safe and consistent IV drug delivery.

CALCULATING ACCURACY OF DILUTION PARAMETERS

The nurse may find it necessary to calculate the dilution parameters of a drug order that specifies the concentration per kilogram per minute and the volume per hour infusion rate. The physician should determine all drug dose parameters, including concentration per kilogram per minute, volume per hour, and dilution parameters. The nurse should check the accuracy of the dilution parameters to ensure that the correct drug dosage is given. These methods are also used to prepare the pediatric dose. In many pediatric critical care areas, IV fluids for drug administration are limited to prevent fluid overload. If the physician changes the drug dosage, rather than increasing the volume (ml), the concentration of the solution will be changed. It is important that all health care providers follow the policies and procedures of their institution regarding medication administration.

EXAMPLE

PROBLEM 1: A 5-year-old child, weight 14 kg, is in septic shock.
Order: Dopamine 5 mcg/kg/min at 1.3 ml/hr.
Dilute as follows: 160 mg dopamine in 46 ml D_5W to make a total volume of 50 ml.
Dosage: 2-20 mcg/kg/min.
Drug available: Dopamine 40 mg/ml.

The following steps are needed to determine whether dilution orders will result in the correct concentration of solution to deliver 5 mcg/kg/min at 1.3 ml/hr.

Step 1: Find infusion rates for concentration per unit time.

  1. Determine concentration per minute.

  Child's weight × concentration/kg/min =
  14 kg × 5 mcg/kg/min = 70 mcg/min

  2. Determine the concentration per hour.

  70 mcg/min × 60 min/hr = 4200 mcg/hr = 4.2 mg/hr

Step 2: Find concentration of solution.
  Divide the concentration per hour by volume per hour.

$$\frac{4200 \text{ mcg/hr}}{1.3 \text{ ml/hr}} = 3230 \text{ mcg/ml or } 3.2 \text{ mg/ml}$$

Step 3: Find infusion rate per hour. Divide concentration per hour by concentration of solution to determine whether infusion rate is correct.

$$\frac{4.2 \text{ mg/hr}}{3.2 \text{ mg/ml}} = 1.3 \text{ ml/hr}$$

Step 4: Find the accuracy of the dilution order.
  Determine how much dopamine must be added to D_5W to make a total volume of 50 ml.
  Set up a ratio and proportion.
  3.2 mg : 1 ml = X : 50 ml
  X = 160 mg

Dilution order is correct.

Preparation of Drug Dosage

$$\frac{D}{H} \times V = \frac{160}{40} \times 1 = 4 \text{ ml} \quad \textbf{or} \quad H : V :: D : V$$
$$40 \text{ mg} : 1 \text{ ml} :: 160 \text{ mg} : X \text{ ml}$$
$$40 X = 160$$
$$X = 4 \text{ ml}$$

Answer: Add 4 ml of dopamine 40 mg/ml to 46 ml D_5W for a total volume of 50 ml.

NOTE: The total volume in the syringe is 50 ml and is the sum of drug volume (4 ml) plus diluent volume (46 ml). To verify, divide 160 mg dopamine by 50 ml total volume in syringe:

$$\frac{160 \text{ mg}}{50 \text{ ml}} = 3.2 \text{ mg/ml}$$

If 4 ml dopamine 40 mg/ml were added to 50 ml of D_5W, the volume in the syringe would be 54 ml (4 ml dopamine plus 50 ml D_5W). The resulting concentration of that solution would be 2.96 mg/ml (160 mg/54 ml).

PROBLEM 2: A 3-week-old premature infant, weight 1.6 kg, is in shock.

Order: Dobutamine 2.5 mcg/kg/min at 0.4 ml/hr.

Dilute as follows: 30 mg dobutamine in 47.6 ml D_5W to make a total volume of 50 ml.

Dosage: 2.5-40 mcg/kg/min.

Drug available: Dobutamine 250 mg/20 ml.

Determine accuracy of dilution order to deliver 2.5 mcg/kg/min at 0.4 ml/hr.

Step 1: Find infusion rates for concentration per unit time.
> **1.** Determine the concentration per minute.

$$\text{Child's weight} \times \text{concentration/kg/min} =$$
$$1.6 \text{ kg} \quad \times \quad 2.5 \text{ mcg/kg/min} \quad = 4 \text{ mcg/min}$$

> **2.** Determine the concentration per hour.

$$4 \text{ mcg/min} \times 60 \text{ min/hr} = 240 \text{ mcg/hr} = 0.24 \text{ mg/hr}$$

Step 2: Find the concentration of solution.
> Divide the concentration per hour by volume per hour.

$$\frac{240 \text{ mcg/hr}}{0.4 \text{ ml/hr}} = 600 \text{ mcg/ml or } 0.6 \text{ mg/ml}$$

Step 3: Find infusion rate per hour. Divide concentration per hour by concentration of the solution to determine whether infusion rate is correct.

$$\frac{0.24 \text{ mg/hr}}{0.6 \text{ mg/ml}} = 0.4 \text{ ml/hr}$$

Step 4: Find the accuracy of the dilution order.
> Determine how much dobutamine must be added to D_5W to make a total volume of 50 ml.
> Set up a ratio and proportion.

$$0.6 \text{ mg:1 ml } = X:50 \text{ ml}$$
$$X = 30 \text{ mg}$$

Dilution order is correct.

Preparation of Drug Dosage

$$\frac{D}{H} \times V = \frac{30}{250} \times 20 = 2.4 \text{ ml}$$

or

$$\begin{array}{ccccccc} H & : & V & :: & D & : & V \\ 250 \text{ mg} & : & 20 \text{ ml} & :: & 30 \text{ mg} & : & X \text{ ml} \end{array}$$
$$250X = 600$$
$$X = 2.4 \text{ ml}$$

Answer: Add 2.4 ml of dobutamine 250 mg/20 ml to 47.6 ml D_5W for a total volume of 50 ml.

PROBLEM 3: For the same infant, the physician increases the dose of dobutamine. Again, fluids must be limited, and another concentration must be prepared.

Order: Dobutamine 15 mcg/kg/min at 1.8 ml/hr.

Dilute as follows: 40 mg dobutamine in 46.8 ml D_5W to make a total volume of 50 ml.

Dosage: 2.5-40 mcg/kg/min.

Drug available: dobutamine 250 mg/20 ml.

Determine accuracy of rate order to deliver 15 mcg/kg/min at 1.8 ml/hr.

Step 1: Find infusion rates for concentration per unit time.

    1. Determine the concentration per minute.

$$\begin{array}{c} \text{Child's weight} \times \text{concentration/kg/min} = \\ 1.6 \text{ kg} \quad \times \quad 15 \text{ mcg/kg/min} \quad = 24 \text{ mcg/min} \end{array}$$

    2. Determine the concentration per hour.

$$24 \text{ mcg/min} \times 60 \text{ min/hr} = 1440 \text{ mcg/hr} = 1.44 \text{ mg/hr}$$

Step 2: Find concentration of solution.

    Divide the concentration per hour by volume per hour.

$$\frac{1440 \text{ mcg/hr}}{1.8 \text{ ml/hr}} = 800 \text{ mcg/ml or } 0.8 \text{ mg/ml}$$

Step 3: Find infusion rate per hour. Divide concentration per hour by concentration of the solution to determine whether infusion rate is correct.

$$\frac{1.44 \text{ mg/hr}}{1.8 \text{ mg/ml}} = 0.8 \text{ ml/hr}$$

Answer: The rate order is *correct* and is 0.8 ml/hr.

Step 4: Find the accuracy of the dilution order.

    Determine how much dopamine must be added to D_5W to make a total volume of 50 ml.

    Set up a ratio and proportion.

$$\begin{array}{c} 0.8 \text{ mg:1 ml} = \text{X:50 ml} \\ \text{X} = 40 \text{ mg} \end{array}$$

Dilution order is correct.

Preparation of Drug Dosage

$$\frac{D}{H} \times V = \frac{40}{250} \times 20 = 3.2 \text{ ml}$$

or

$$\begin{array}{ccccc} H & : & V & :: & D & : & V \\ 250 \text{ mg} & : & 20 \text{ ml} & :: & 40 \text{ mg} & : & \text{X ml} \\ & & & 250\text{X} & = & 800 \\ & & & \text{X} & = & 3.2 \text{ ml} \end{array}$$

Answer: Add 3.2 ml of dobutamine 250 mg/20 ml to 46.8 ml D_5W for a total volume of 50 ml.

SUMMARY PRACTICE PROBLEMS

Determine whether dilution orders will yield the correct concentration of solution.

1. A 5-year-old child with acute status asthmaticus.
   Child weighs 21 kg.
   Order: Terbutaline 0.1 mcg/kg/min. Dilute 25 mg terbutaline in 25 ml D_5W to make a total volume of 50 ml. Infuse at 0.25 ml/hr.
   Pediatric dose: 0.02-0.25 mcg/kg/min.
   Drug available: Terbutaline 1 mg/ml.

2. A 9-year-old child who is intubated postoperatively.
   Child weighs 30 kg.
   Order: Fentanyl 0.03 mcg/kg/min. Dilute 2.5 mg fentanyl in 25 ml 0.9% saline to make a total volume of 50 ml. Infuse at 1 ml/hr.
   Pediatric dose: 0.01-0.05 mcg/kg/min.
   Drug available: Fentanyl 2.5 mg/50 ml.

3. A 1-year-old child with septic shock.
   Child weighs 9 kg.
   Order: Dopamine 5 mcg/kg/min. Dilute 40 mg dopamine in 49.5 ml D_5W to make a total volume of 50 ml. Infuse at 3.4 ml/hr.
   Pediatric dose: 2-20 mcg/kg/min.
   Drug available: Dopamine 400 mg/5 ml.

4. A 3-year-old child with hypertension related to a tumor.
   Child weighs 16 kg.
   Order: Sodium nitroprusside 2 mcg/kg/min. Dilute 50 mg nitroprusside in 45 ml D_5W to make a total volume of 50 ml. Infuse at 3 ml/hr.
   Pediatric dose: 200-500 mcg/kg/hr.
   Drug available: Sodium nitroprusside 50 mg/5 ml.

5. A 10-year-old child with diabetic ketoacidosis.
   Child weighs 32 kg.
   Order: Regular Humulin insulin 0.1 units/kg/hr. Dilute: Regular Humulin insulin 50 units in 49.5 ml 0.9% saline, total volume 50 ml at 6.4 ml/hr.
   Pediatric dose: 0.1 units/kg/hr.
   Drug available: 100 units/ml.

6. A 2-day-old child with patent ductus arteriosus.
   Child weighs 3.4 kg.
   Order: Alprostadil 0.1 mcg/kg/min.
   Dilute 0.1 mg of alprostadil in 50 ml D_5W to run at 2 ml/hr.
   Pediatric dosage: 0.05-0.1 mcg/kg/min.
   Drug available: Alprostadil 500 mcg/ml.

7. A 7-year-old child with pulmonary embolism.
   Child weighs 20 kg.
   Order: Heparin 25 units/kg/hr using a premixed bag with a standard concentration of 200 units/ml. Run at 2.5 ml/hr.
   Pediatric dosage: 15-25 units/kg/hr.
   Drug available: 50,000 units/250 ml.

ANSWERS Summary Practice Problems

1. *Step 1:* Infusion rates for concentration/unit time.
   Concentration per minute.
   $$21 \text{ kg} \times 0.1 \text{ mcg/kg/min} = 2.1 \text{ mcg/min}$$
   Concentration per hour.
   $$2.1 \text{ mcg/min} \times 60 \text{ min/hr} = 126 \text{ mcg/hr} = 0.126 \text{ mg/hr}$$
   Step 2: Concentration of solution.
   $$\frac{126 \text{ mcg/hr}}{0.25 \text{ ml/hr}} = 504 \text{ mcg/ml} = 0.5 \text{ mg/ml}$$
   Step 3: Infusion rate calculation, volume/hr.
   $$\frac{0.126 \text{ mg/hr}}{0.5 \text{ mg/ml}} = 0.25 \text{ ml/hr}$$
   Step 4: Accuracy of dilution order.

   $$\text{BF:} \frac{D}{H} \times V = \frac{25}{1} \times 1 = \frac{25}{1} = 25 \text{ ml}$$

   or
   RP: 0.5 mg : 1 ml :: X mg/50 ml
   X = 25 mg
   Order is correct.

2. *Step 1:* Infusion rates for concentration/unit time.
   Concentration per minute.
   $$30 \text{ kg} \times 0.03 \text{ mcg/kg/min} = 0.9 \text{ mcg/min}$$
   Concentration per hour.
   $$0.9 \text{ mcg/min} \times 60 \text{ min/hr} = 54 \text{ mcg/hr} = 0.054 \text{ mg/hr}$$
   Step 2: Concentration of solution.
   $$\frac{54 \text{ mcg/hr}}{1 \text{ ml/hr}} = 54 \text{ mcg/ml} = 0.05 \text{ mg/ml}$$
   Concentration does not match ordered concentration of 0.025 mg/ml, so order is *incorrect.*
   Step 3: Infusion rate calculation, volume/hr.
   $$\frac{0.054 \text{ mg/hr}}{0.025 \text{ mg/ml}} = 2.16 \text{ ml/hr}$$
   Rate does not match ordered rate of 1 ml/hr, so order is *incorrect.*
   Step 4: Accuracy of dilution order.

   $$\text{BF:} \frac{D}{H} \times V = \frac{2.5}{2.5} \times 50 = \frac{125}{2.5} = 50 \text{ ml}$$

   50 ml of drug is required, so dilution is *incorrect.*
   or
   RP: 0.05 mg : 1 ml :: X mg/50 ml
   X = 2.5 mg
   Fentanyl is supplied as 2.5 mg in 50 ml = 0.05 mg/ml. To obtain the ordered dilution 0.025 mg/ml, 1.25 mg of fentanyl would need to be placed in a total volume of 50 ml (1.25 divided by 50 = 0.025 mg/ml), and the infusion run at 2.16 ml/hr.

3. *Step 1:* Infusion rate for concentration/unit time.

Concentration per minute.

$$9 \text{ kg} \times 5 \text{ mcg/kg/min} = 45 \text{ mcg/min}$$

Concentration per hour.

$$45 \text{ mcg/min} \times 60 \text{ min/hr} = 2700 \text{ mcg/hr} = 2.7 \text{ mg/hr}$$

Step 2: Concentration of solution.

$$\frac{2700 \text{ mcg/hr}}{3.4 \text{ ml/hr}} = 794 \text{ mcg/ml or } 0.8 \text{ mg/ml } (0.794 \text{ mg/ml before round})$$

Step 3: Infusion rate calculation, volume/hr.

$$\frac{2.7 \text{ mg/hr}}{0.8 \text{ mg/ml}} = 3.4 \text{ ml/hr } (3.375 \text{ ml/hr before rounding})$$

Step 4: Accuracy of dilution order.

$$\text{BF: } \frac{D}{H} \times V = \frac{40}{400} \times 5 = \frac{200}{400} = 0.5 \text{ ml}$$

or

RP: 400 mg : 5 ml :: 40 mg : X ml

400 X :: 200 ml

X :: 0.5 ml

4. *Step 1:* Infusion rates for concentration/unit time.

a. Concentration per minute.

$$16 \text{ kg} \times 2 \text{ mcg/kg/min} = 32 \text{ mcg/min}$$

b. Concentration per hour.

$$32 \text{ mcg/min} \times 60 \text{ min/hr} = 1920 \text{ mcg/hr} = 1.92 \text{ mg/hr}$$

Step 2: Concentration of solution.

$$\frac{1920 \text{ mcg/hr}}{3 \text{ ml/hr}} = 640 \text{ mcg/ml} = 0.64 \text{ mg/ml}$$

Calculated concentration of solution does not agree with concentration ordered. Order is *incorrect.*

Step 3: Infusion rate calculation, volume/hr.

$$\frac{1.92 \text{ mg/hr}}{1 \text{ mg/ml}} = 1.9 \text{ ml/hr}$$

This is the correct infusion rate.

Step 4: Accuracy of dilution order.

$$\text{BF: } \frac{D}{H} \times V = \frac{50}{50} \times 5 = \frac{250}{50} = 5 \text{ ml}$$

or

RP: 50 mg : 5 ml :: 50 mg : X ml

50 X = 250 ml

X = 5 ml

5. *Step 1:* Infusion rates for concentration/unit time.

Concentration per hour.

$$32 \text{ kg} \times 0.1 \text{ units/kg/hr} = 3.2 \text{ units/hr}$$

Step 2: Concentration of solution.

$$\frac{3.2 \text{ units/hr}}{6.4 \text{ ml/hr}} = 0.5 \text{ units/ml}$$

Step 3: Infusion rate calculation, volume/hr.

$$\frac{3.2 \text{ units/hr}}{0.5 \text{ units/ml}} = 6.4 \text{ ml/hr}$$

Step 4: Accuracy of dilution order.

RP: 50 units : 1 ml :: X units/50 ml

X = 25 units

Dilution order as written is *incorrect.* 25 units is placed in 50 ml to obtain a concentration of 0.5 units/ml. 50 units in 50 ml would result in a concentration of 1 unit/ml.

6. *Step 1:* Infusion rates for concentration/unit time.

    a. Concentration per minute.

$$3.4 \text{ kg} \times 0.1 \text{ mcg/kg/min} = 0.34 \text{ mcg/min}$$

    b. Concentration per hour.

$$0.34 \text{ mcg/kg/min} \times 60 \text{ min} = 20.4 \text{ mcg/hr} = 0.02 \text{ mg/hr}$$

Step 2: Concentration of solution.

$$\frac{20.4 \text{ mcg/hr}}{2 \text{ ml/hr}} = 10.2 \text{ mcg/ml} = 0.01 \text{ mg/ml}$$

Step 3: Infusion rate calculation, volume/hr.

$$\frac{0.02 \text{ mg/hr}}{0.01 \text{ mg/ml}} = 2 \text{ ml/hr}$$

Step 4: Accuracy of dilution order.

RP: 0.1 mg : 50 ml :: X mg : 1 ml

50X = 0.1

X = 0.002 mg/ml

Dilution order is incorrect. 0.002 mg/1 ml = 2 mcg/ml. Ordered concentration is 10 mcg/ml. 0.5 mg in 50 ml would be required for a concentration of 10 mcg/ml.

7. *Step 1:* Infusion rates for concentration.

    Concentration per hour.

$$20 \text{ kg} \times 25 \text{ units/kg/hr} = 500 \text{ units/hr}$$

Step 2: Concentration of solution.

$$\frac{500 \text{ units/hr}}{2.5 \text{ ml/hr}} = 200 \text{ units/ml}$$

Step 3: Infusion rate calculation, volume/hr.

$$\frac{500 \text{ units/hr}}{200 \text{ units/ml}} = 2.5 \text{ ml/hr}$$

Step 4: Accuracy of dilution order.

RP: 50000 units : 250 ml :: X units : 1 ml

250 X = 50000

X = 200 units/ml

Order is correct.

Labor and Delivery

OBJECTIVES

- State the complication related to intravenous fluid administration in the high-risk mother.
- Recognize the different types of fluid administration used in cases of high-risk labor.
- Determine the infusion rates of a drug in solution when the drug is prescribed by concentration or volume.

OUTLINE

Drug calculations for labor and delivery are the same as those used in critical care. Determinations of the concentration of the solution, infusion rates, and titration factors are the primary calculation skills used. Accurate calculations are essential, as is the monitoring of intravenous (IV) fluid intake for medications and anesthetic procedures. Impaired renal filtration in patients with preeclampsia and the antidiuretic effect of tocolytic drugs make the monitoring of fluid intake vital. Accurate measurement of IV fluid intake along with pulmonary assessment can decrease the risk of fluid overload and the sequelae of acute pulmonary edema in women at high risk for complications.

Physicians' orders and hospital protocols give specific guidelines for administering IV drugs. Carefully labeling all IV fluids, IV medications, and IV lines is essential in preventing drug errors. The nurse is responsible for managing the IV drug therapy, monitoring the patient's fluid balance, and assessing the patient's response to drug therapy.

FACTORS INFLUENCING INTRAVENOUS FLUID AND DRUG MANAGEMENT

The most important concept in labor and delivery is that the drugs given to the mother also affect the unborn baby. Therefore the responses of both the mother and the unborn baby must be closely monitored. Vital signs and laboratory results, such as platelets, liver function studies, renal function, magnesium levels, reflexes, and contraction patterns, are the main indicators of the mother's status. For the fetus, fetal heart pattern is the primary guide.

TITRATION OF MEDICATIONS WITH MAINTENANCE INTRAVENOUS FLUIDS

Women in labor receive IV fluids to prevent dehydration when oral intake is contraindicated. IV drugs are given to stimulate labor, treat preeclampsia, or inhibit preterm labor. Normally, 500 to 1000 ml of IV fluids may be given to initially hydrate the mother, especially in preterm labor or before administration of regional anesthesia. Any IV medications that are given by titration are a part of the hourly IV rate. The patient has a primary IV line and a secondary IV line for medications. All IV medications should be delivered by a volumetric pump, which ensures that the specified volume and correct dosage are delivered.

Titration of drugs is frequently done for women with preeclampsia and women experiencing preterm labor. The most common use of titration is for the induction or augmentation of labor. In the following example, an oxytocic drug is given, and the primary IV rate is adjusted with the secondary IV drug line to achieve a therapeutic effect and maintain adequate maternal hydration. Note that the drug is ordered to be given by concentration and that the infusion rates for volume per minute and hour must be determined.

Administration by Concentration

EXAMPLES

1. Give IV fluids at 100 ml/hr with LRS.
2. Mix 10 units of oxytocin in 1000 NSS. Start at 1 milliunits/min, increase by 1 or 2 milliunits/min, every 15-30 min, until uterine contractions are 2 to 3 minutes apart. Do not exceed 40 milliunits/min.

Note: *1 Unit = 1000 milliunits*

Available: Secondary set:
        oxytocin 10 units/ml
        1000 ml NSS
        IV set drop factor 20 gtt/ml
        infusion pump
      Primary set:
        1000 ml Lactated Ringer's (LR)
        IV set drop factor 20 gtt/ml
        infusion pump

For the *secondary* IV set, the following calculations must be made:
1. Concentration of solution.
2. Infusion rates: volume per minute and volume per hour.
3. Titration factor in concentration per minute (milliunits/min).

For the *primary* IV set, the following calculations must be made:
1. Pump is used; set the rate at ml/hr.
2. Balance primary IV flow with secondary IV rate to achieve 100 ml/hr.

Secondary IV (see Chapter 7 for formulas)
1. Concentration of solution:
$$10 \text{ units}:1000 \text{ ml} :: X:1 \text{ ml}$$
$$1000 \ X = 10$$
$$X = 0.01 \text{ units or 10 milliunits}$$
The concentration of solution is 10 milliunits/ml.

2. Infusion rates for volume:

$$\frac{\text{Concentration/minute}}{\text{Concentration of solution}} = \text{Volume/min} \times 60 \text{ min} = \text{Volume/hr}$$

Volume per minute   **Volume per hour**

$$\frac{1 \text{ milliunit/min}}{10 \text{ milliunits/ml}} = 0.1 \text{ ml/min} \times 60 \text{ min} = 6 \text{ ml/hr}$$

$$\frac{2 \text{ milliunits/min}}{10 \text{ milliunits/ml}} = 0.2 \text{ ml/min} \times 60 \text{ min} = 12 \text{ ml/hr}$$

$$\frac{5 \text{ milliunits/min}}{10 \text{ milliunits/ml}} = 0.5 \text{ ml/min} \times 60 \text{ min} = 30 \text{ ml/hr}$$

3. Titration factor (see Chapter 11): to increase the concentration by increments of 1 milliunit/min, the hourly rate on the pump must be increased by 6 ml/hr. The titration factor for this problem is 6 ml/hr. To increase the concentration to a higher rate, multiply the rate of increase times 6 ml/hr. (Example: to increase infusion to 5 milliunits/min, multiply 5 by 6 ml = 30 ml/hr.)

For the secondary IV line, the concentration of the solution is 10 milliunits/ml of oxytocin, with the infusion rate of 6 ml/hr to be increased in increments of 1 to 2 milliunits every 15 to 30 minutes until contractions are 2 to 3 minutes apart.

Primary IV

The secondary IV rate will start at 6 ml/hr; therefore the primary rate will be 94 ml/hr. (A balance is needed to achieve 100 ml/hr.)

For every increase in rate from the secondary line, a corresponding decrease must be made with the primary IV line. If the rate of the secondary line exceeds the ordered hourly rate, the primary IV line may be shut off completely. The concentration of the solution may be changed by the physician if the mother is receiving too much fluid.

Administration by Volume

In the previous example, the oxytocin was ordered to be infused by concentration (milliunits/min), which is the recommended method for patient safety. Sometimes in clinical practice, the infusion rate may be ordered by volume (ml/hr).

EXAMPLES

Mix 30 units of oxytocin in 500 ml NSS. Start at 1 ml/hr and increase by 1 to 2 ml every 15-30 min until uterine contractions are 2 to 3 minutes apart. Notify physician before exceeding 40 milliunits/min.

To determine the concentration per hour of infusion, multiply concentration of the solution by volume/hr = concentration/hr:

$$60 \text{ milliunits/ml} \times 1 \text{ ml/hr} = 60 \text{ milliunits/hr}$$

To determine the concentration of the infusion per minute, divide:

$$\frac{\text{Concentration/hr}}{60 \text{ min/hr}} = \text{Concentration/min}$$

$$\frac{60 \text{ milliunits/hr}}{60 \text{ min/hr}} = 1 \text{ milliunit/min}$$

Therefore an oxytocin solution with a concentration of 60 milliunits/ml infused at 1 ml/hr will administer 1 milliunit of the drug per minute.

INTRAVENOUS LOADING DOSE

Some situations require IV medications to be infused over a short period to obtain a serum level for a therapeutic effect. This type of IV drug administration is called a *loading dose.*

In the following example, a patient with preeclampsia receives a loading dose of magnesium sulfate, followed by a maintenance dose of magnesium sulfate via the secondary IV line. A primary IV line is also maintained after the loading dose is given. At the end of this example, the total IV intake is determined for an 8-hour period.

EXAMPLES

1. Mix magnesium sulfate 40 g in 1000 ml of sterile NSS.
2. Infuse 4 g over 20 minutes, then maintain at 2 g/hr.
3. Start LRS at 75 ml/hr after magnesium sulfate loading dose.

Available: Secondary set:
magnesium sulfate 50% (5 g in 10-ml ampules)
1000 ml IV fluid.
IV set 20 gtts/ml
infusion pump
Primary set:
1000 ml LRS
IV set drop factor 20 gtt/ml
infusion pump

For the *secondary* IV line, the following calculations must be made:

1. Dose of magnesium sulfate in IV.
2. Concentration of solution.
3. Volume of loading dose and flow rate for infusion pump (see Chapter 9).
4. Infusion rate: volume per hour of magnesium sulfate infusion.

For the *primary* IV line, the following calculation must be made:

1. Drop rate per minute.

For the total IV intake, the following solutions must be added:

1. Volume of loading dose.
2. Volume of secondary IV for 8 hours.
3. Volume of primary IV for 8 hours.

Secondary IV

1. $\dfrac{D}{H} \times V = \dfrac{40 \text{ g}}{5 \text{ g}} \times 10 \text{ ml} = 80 \text{ ml of magnesium sulfate or 8 ampules}$

2. Concentration of solution:

$$40 \text{ g} = 40,000 \text{ mg}$$
$$40,000 \text{ mg} : 1000 \text{ ml} :: X : 1 \text{ ml}$$
$$1000 X = 40,000$$
$$X = 40 \text{ mg}$$

The concentration of solution is 40 mg/ml.

3. Volume of loading dose:

$$4 \text{ g} = 4000 \text{ mg}$$
$$40 \text{ mg} : 1 \text{ ml} :: 4000 \text{ mg} : X \text{ ml}$$
$$40 X = 4000$$
$$X = 100 \text{ ml}$$

Flow rate for the pump:

$$100 \text{ ml} \div \frac{20 \text{ min}}{60 \text{ min/hr}} = 100 \times \frac{\overset{3}{\cancel{60}}}{\underset{1}{\cancel{20}}} = 300 \text{ ml/hr}$$

The rate on the infusion pump for the 4-g infusion of magnesium sulfate over 20 minutes is 300 ml/hr. When the infusion rate is this high, it must be monitored closely, and the patient must be observed for response to drug therapy.

4. Infusion rate: volume per hour:

$$2 \text{ g} = 2000 \text{ mg}$$

$$\frac{\text{Concentration/hr}}{\text{Concentration of solution}} = \text{Volume/hr} \qquad \frac{2000 \text{ mg/hr}}{40 \text{ mg/ml}} = 50 \text{ ml/hr}$$

The rate on the pump for the 2 g/hr infusion is 50 ml/hr.

Primary IV
After the loading dose of magnesium sulfate, the primary IV will run at 75 ml/hr.

Total IV Intake Over 8 Hours

Volume of loading dose		100 ml
Volume of secondary IV	50 ml × 8 =	400 ml
Volume of primary IV	75 ml × 8 =	+ 600 ml
		1100 ml

Because fluid overload is a potential problem for patients with preeclampsia, all IV fluids must be calculated accurately and the use of infusion pumps is essential.

INTRAVENOUS FLUID BOLUS

An IV fluid *bolus* is a large volume, 500 to 1000 ml, of IV fluid infused over a short time (1 hour or less). A bolus may be given before administration of regional anesthesia or to a patient experiencing preterm labor.

In the next example, calculate the flow rate of an IV bolus from the primary IV followed by an infusion of a tocolytic drug given by titration. At the end of this example, calculate the patient's fluid intake for 8 hours.

EXAMPLES

1. Start 1000 LRS at 300 ml/10 min, then reduce to 125 ml/hr.
2. Mix terbutaline 7.5 mg in 500 ml of NSS; start at 2.5 mcg/min; increase 2.5 mcg/min every 20 min until contractions subside.

Available: Primary set:
           1000 ml LRS
           IV set drop factor 20 gtt/ml
           infusion pump
      Secondary set:
           terbutaline 1 mg/ml
           500 ml NSS
           IV set 20 gtt/ml
           infusion pump

For the *secondary* IV line, the following calculations must be made:

1. The dose of terbutaline in IV.
2. Concentration of solution.
3. Infusion rates: volume per minute and hour.
4. Titration factor for 2.5 mcg/ml.

For the *primary* IV line, determine the following:

1. Set pump to infuse 300 ml over 10 minutes and then 100 ml/hr.
2. Balance the primary IV with the secondary IV to achieve a rate of 100 ml/hr. Total the IV fluids for 8 hours.

Secondary IV

1. $\dfrac{D}{H} \times V = \dfrac{7.5 \text{ mg}}{1 \text{ mg}} \times 1 \text{ ml} = 7.5 \text{ ml of terbutaline}$

2. Concentration of solution:

$$7.5 \text{ mg} = 7500 \text{ mcg}$$
$$7500 \text{ mcg} : 500 \text{ ml} :: X \text{ mcg} : 1 \text{ ml}$$
$$500 \text{ X} = 7500$$
$$X = 15 \text{ mcg}$$

The concentration of solution is 15 mcg/ml.

3. Infusion rates: volume per minute and volume per hour.

$$\dfrac{2.5 \text{ mcg/min}}{15 \text{ mcg/ml}} = 0.16 \text{ ml/min} \times 60 \text{ min/hr} = 9.9 \text{ ml/hr or } 10 \text{ ml/hr}$$

4. Titration factor: to increase the concentration by increments of 2.5 mcg/min, the volume of the increment of change must be calculated per minute and per hour:

$$\frac{\text{Concentration/minute}}{\text{Concentration of solution}} = \text{ml/min} \qquad \frac{2.5 \text{ mcg/min}}{15 \text{ mcg/ml}} = 0.166 \text{ ml/min}$$

$$\text{Volume/min} \times 60 \text{ min/hr} = \text{Volume/hr}$$
$$0.166 \text{ ml/min} \times 60 \text{ min/hr} = 9.96 \text{ ml/hr or } 10 \text{ ml}$$

The titration factor is 0.166 ml/min or 10 ml/hr. Increasing or decreasing the infusion rate by 2.5 mcg/min will correspond to an increase or decrease in volume by 0.166 ml/min or 10 ml/hr.

Primary IV

1. Set infusion pump at 300 ml over 10 minutes, then reduce rate to 90 ml/hr.

Total IV Intake Over 8 Hours

Volume of loading dose		300 ml
Volume of primary set	115 ml × 8 =	920 ml
Volume of secondary set	80 ml × 8 =	+ 80 ml
		1300 ml

Assume that an average of 80 ml/hr of terbutaline was given.

SUMMARY PRACTICE PROBLEMS

1. Preeclamptic labor.

   a. Mix magnesium sulfate 20 g in 500 ml NSS

   b. Infuse 4 g over 30 minutes, then maintain at 2 g/hr.

   c. Start LRS 1000 ml at 75 ml/hr after loading dose of magnesium sulfate.

   Available: Secondary set:
   magnesium sulfate 50% (5 g in 10 ml)
   1000 ml NSS
   IV set 20 gtt/ml
   infusion pump
   Primary set:
   1000 ml LRS
   IV set 20 gtt/ml

Determine the following:

   a. Secondary IV:
   (1) Magnesium sulfate dosage.
   (2) Concentration of solution.
   (3) Volume of loading dose and infusion rate for pump.
   (4) Infusion rate per hour of magnesium sulfate.

   b. Primary IV: 75 ml/hr.

   c. Total fluid intake for 8 hours.

2. Oxytocin/Pitocin for augmentation of labor

   a. Give LR 500 ml over 30 minutes, then infuse at 75 ml/hr.

   b. Mix 15 units of oxytocin/Pitocin in 250 ml NSS.

   Start infusion at 2 milliunits/hr, increase by 1 to 2 milliunits until labor pattern is established and contractions are 2 to 3 minutes apart. Notify physician before exceeding 40 milliunits per minute.

   Available: Secondary set
           Oxytocin 10 units/ml
           250 ml NSS
           IV set 20 gtt/ml
         Infusion pump
           Primary set
           1000 LR
           IV set 20 gtt/ml

For secondary IV line, the following calculations must be made:

1. Dose of oxytocin for IV

2. Concentration of solution

3. Infusion rate: Volume per minute and hour

4. Titration factor in milliunits per minute

   For primary IV line, the following calculation must be made:

1. Infusion rate for 500 ml over 30 minutes

ANSWERS Summary Practice Problems

1. a. Secondary IV:

(1) Magnesium sulfate dosage:

$$\frac{D}{H} \times V = \frac{20\ g}{5\ g} \times 10\ ml = 40\ ml \text{ or 4 ampules of magnesium sulfate}$$

(2) Concentration of solution:

$$20\ g = 20,000\ mg$$
$$20,000\ mg:500\ ml :: X\ mg:1\ ml$$
$$500\ X = 20,000$$
$$X = 40\ mg$$

The concentration of solution is 40 mg/ml.

(3) Volume of loading dose:

$$4\ g = 4000\ mg$$
$$40\ mg:1\ ml :: 4000\ mg:X\ ml$$
$$40\ X = 4000$$
$$X = 100\ ml$$

Infusion rate for 30 minutes:

$$100\ ml \div \frac{30\ min}{60\ min/hr} = 100 \times \frac{\overset{2}{\cancel{60}}}{\underset{1}{\cancel{30}}} = 200\ ml/hr$$

(4) Infusion rate: volume per hour:

$$2 \text{ g} = 2000 \text{ mg}$$

$$\frac{2000 \text{ mg/hr}}{40 \text{ mg/ml}} = 50 \text{ ml/hr}$$

b. Primary IV:
After the loading dose: Set IV rate 75 ml/hr.

c. Total IV intake over 8 hours:

Volume of loading dose		100 ml
Volume of secondary IV	50 ml × 8 =	400 ml
Volume of primary IV	75 ml × 8 =	+600 ml
		1100 ml

2. Augmentation of Labor

   a. Secondary IV:

   1. Oxytocin dosage: $\dfrac{D}{H} \times V = \dfrac{15 \text{ units}}{10 \text{ units}} \times 1 \text{ ml} = 1.5 \text{ ml}$

   Add 1.5 ml of oxytocin to 250 ml of NSS.

   2. Concentration of solution

   15 units = 15,000 milliunits

   15,000 milliunits: 250 ml = X milliunits : 1 ml

   $$250X = 15,000$$
   $$X = 60 \text{ milliunits/ml}$$

   3. Infusion rate: $\dfrac{\text{Concentration/minute}}{\text{Concentration of solution}} = \dfrac{2 \text{ milliunits/min}}{60 \text{ milliunits/ml}}$

   $$= 0.033 \text{ ml/min}$$

   4. Titration factor: $\dfrac{2 \text{ milliunits/min}}{60 \text{ milliunits/ml}} = 0.033 \text{ ml/min} \times 60 \text{ min/hr} = 1.9 \text{ ml/hr or 2 ml/hr}$

   $$\dfrac{3 \text{ milliunits/min}}{60 \text{ milliunits/ml}} = 0.05 \text{ ml/min} \times 60 \text{ min/hr} = 3 \text{ ml/hr}$$

   $$\dfrac{4 \text{ milliunits/min}}{60 \text{ milliunits/ml}} = 0.06 \text{ ml/min} \times 60 \text{ min/hr} = 3.9 \text{ ml/hr or 4 ml/hr}$$

   $$\dfrac{5 \text{ milliunits/min}}{60 \text{ milliunits/ml}} = 0.08 \text{ ml/min} \times 60 \text{ min/hr} = 4.9 \text{ ml/hr or 5 ml/hr}$$

   Note: With this concentration of solution, there is a 1:1 relationship with milliunits/ml and ml/hr.

   b. Primary IV: $500 \text{ ml LR} \div \dfrac{\text{Minutes to administer}}{60 \text{ min/hr}} = 500 \text{ ml} \div \dfrac{30 \text{ minutes}}{60 \text{ min/hr}}$

   $$= 500 \times \dfrac{60}{30}$$
   $$= 1000 \text{ ml in 30 min}$$

Community

Although the metric system has become widespread in the clinical area, the home setting generally does not have the devices of metric measure. This becomes a problem when liquid medication is prescribed in metric measure for the home patient. The community nurse should be able to assist the patient in converting metric to household measure when necessary.

Preparation of solutions in the home setting may involve conversion between the metric and household systems. Solutions used in the home setting can be used for oral fluid replacement, topical application, irrigation, or disinfection. Although the majority of the solutions are commercially available, solutions that can be prepared in the home can be effective and less costly than the premixed items.

When commercially prepared drugs are too concentrated for the patient's use and must be diluted, it is necessary to calculate the strength of the solution to meet the therapeutic need as prescribed by the physician. Knowledge of solution preparation and metric–household conversion can be a useful skill for the community nurse.

METRIC TO HOUSEHOLD CONVERSION

When changing from metric to household measure, use the ounce from the apothecary system as an intermediary, because there is no clear conversion between the two systems.

The conversion factors for volume are:

Ounces to milliliters: multiply ounces × 29.57 or 30

Milliliters to ounces: multiply milliliters × 0.034

The conversion factors for weight are:

Ounces to grams: multiply ounces × 28.35

Grams to ounces: multiply grams × 0.035

Note that weight and volume measures differ in the metric system. The properties of crystals, powders, and other solids account for the differences more so than the liquids. Also, as liquid measures increase in volume, there are greater discrepancies between metric and standard household measure. Table 14-1 shows the current approximate equivalents. Deciliters and liters are also included with the volume measurements. These terms will be seen more commonly as the use of the metric system increases. Although conversion charts are helpful guides, a metric measuring device would be optimal for drug administration. Standard household measuring devices should be used instead of tableware if a metric device is not available.

| TABLE 14-1 | | | |

Household to Metric Conversions (Approximate)

Standard Household Measure	Apothecary	Metric Volume	Metric Weight
$^1/_8$ teaspoon	7-8 gtt/$^1/_{48}$ oz	0.6 ml	0.6 g
$^1/_4$ teaspoon	15 gtt/$^1/_{24}$ oz	1.25 ml	1.25 g
$^1/_2$ teaspoon	30 gtt/$^1/_{12}$ oz	2.5 ml	2.5 g
1 teaspoon	60 gtt/ $^1/_6$ oz	5 ml	5 g
1 tablespoon/3 teaspoons	$^1/_2$ oz	15 ml	15 g
2 tablespoons/6 teaspoons	1 oz	$^1/_4$ dl/30 ml	30 g
$^1/_4$ cup/4 tablespoons	2 oz	$^1/_2$ dl/60 ml	60 g
$^1/_3$ cup/5 tablespoons	2 $^1/_2$ oz	$^3/_4$ dl/75 ml	75 g
$^1/_2$ cup	4 oz	1 dl/120 ml	120 g
1 cup	8 oz	$^1/_4$ L/250 ml	230 g
1 pint	16 oz	$^1/_2$ L/480-500 ml	
1 quart	32 oz	1 L/1000 ml	
2 quarts/$^1/_2$ gallon	64 oz	2 L/2000 ml	
1 gallon	128 oz	$3^3/_4$ L/3840-4000 ml	

PRACTICE PROBLEMS: I Metric to Household Conversion

Answers can be found on page 357.

Use Table 14-1 to convert metric to household measure.

1. Bismuth subsalicylate 15 ml every hour up to 120 ml in 24 hr.

_____

2. Ceclor 5 ml four times per day.

_____

3. Tylenol elixir 1.25 ml every 6 hours as necessary for temperature greater than 102° F.

_____

4. Maalox 30 ml after meals and at bedtime.

_____

5. Neo-Calglucon 7.5 ml three times per day.

_____

6. Gani-Tuss NR liquid 10 ml, q6h, prn.

_____

7. Castor oil 60 ml at bedtime.

_____

Use Table 14-1 for conversions.

8. Metamucil 5 g in 1 glass of water every morning.

_____

9. Dilantin-30 pediatric suspension 10 ml twice per day.

_____

10. Homemade pediatric electrolyte solution:

H_2O 1 L, boiled _____

Sugar 30 g _____

Salt 1.5 g _____

Lite salt 2.5 g _____

Baking soda 2.5 g _____

11. A nonalcoholic mouthwash:

H_2O 500 ml boiled _____

Table salt 5 ml _____

Baking soda 5 ml _____

12. Magic mouthwash:

Benadryl 50 mg/10 ml _____

Maalox 10 ml _____

13. Gastrointestinal cocktail for gastric upset:

Belladonna/phenobarbital elixir, 10 ml _____

Maalox, 30 ml _____

Viscous lidocaine, 10 ml _____

PREPARING A SOLUTION OF A DESIRED CONCENTRATION

All solutions contain a solute (drug) and a solvent (liquid). Solutions can be mixed three different ways:

1. *Weight to weight:* Involves mixing the weight of a given solute with the weight of a given liquid.

Example: 5 g sugar with 100 g H_2O

This type of preparation is used in the pharmaceutical setting and is the *most accurate.* Scales for weight to weight preparation are not usually found in the home setting.

2. *Weight to volume:* Uses the weight of a given solute with the volume of an appropriate amount of solvent.

Example: 10 g of salt in 1 L of H_2O

or

$\frac{1}{3}$ oz of salt in 1 qt of H_2O

Again, a scale is needed for this preparation.

3. *Volume to volume:* Means that a given volume of solution is mixed with a given volume of solution.

Example: 10 ml of hydrogen peroxide 3% in 1 dl H_2O

or

2 T of hydrogen peroxide 3% in $1/_2$ c H_2O

Preparation of solutions volume to volume is commonly used in both clinical and home settings.

After a solution is prepared, the strength can be expressed numerically in three different ways:

1. A ratio—1:20 acetic acid
2. A fraction—5 g/100 ml acetic acid
3. A percentage—5% acetic acid

With a ratio, the first number is the solute and the second number is the solvent. In a fraction, the numerator is the solid and the denominator is the liquid. A solution labeled by percentage indicates the amount of solute in 100 ml of liquid. All pharmaceutically prepared solutions use the metric system, and the ratio, fraction, and percentages are interpreted in *grams per milliliter.*

Changing a Ratio to Fractions and Percentages

Change a ratio to a percentage or a fraction by setting up a proportion using the following variables:

Known drug : Known volume :: Desired drug : Desired volume

A proportion can also be set up like a fraction:

$$\frac{\text{Known drug}}{\text{Known volume}} = \frac{\text{Desired drug}}{\text{Desired volume}}$$

REMEMBER

Any variable in this formula can be found if the other three variables are known.

EXAMPLE

PROBLEM 1: Change acetic acid 1:20 to a percentage
1 g:20 ml = X g:100 ml
20 X = 100
X = 5 g
1 g:20 ml = 5 g:100 ml

Note: *In percentage, the volume of liquid is 100 ml.*

The ratio can be expressed as a fraction, 5 g/100 ml, or as a percentage, 5%. Another method of changing a ratio to a percentage involves finding a multiple of 100 for volume (denominator), then multiplying both terms by that multiple.

PRACTICE PROBLEMS: II Preparing a Solution of a Desired Concentration

Answers can be found on page 357.

Change the following ratios to fractions and percentages.

1. 4:1   **6.** 1:10,000

2. 2:1   **7.** 1:4

3. 1:50   **8.** 1:5000

4. 1:3   **9.** 1:200

5. 1:1000   **10.** 1:10

In the previous problems, grams per milliliter is the unit of measure used for preparing solutions. Scales for measuring grams are rarely found in the clinical area or the home environment. Volume (in milliliters) is the common measurement of drugs for administration. Drugs that are powders, crystals, or liquids are measured in graduated measuring cups with metric, apothecary, or household units. The milliliter, although a volume measure, can be substituted for a gram, a measure of mass, because at 4° C, 1 ml of water weighs 1 g. Mass and volume differ with the type of substance; thus grams and milliliters are not exact equivalents in all instances, but they can be accepted as approximate values for preparation of solutions.

Calculating a Solution From a Ratio

To obtain a solution from a ratio, use the proportion or fraction method.

EXAMPLES

PROBLEM 1: Prepare 500 ml of a 1:100 vinegar-water solution for a vaginal douche.

Known drug : Known volume :: Desired drug : Desired volume
1 ml   :   100 ml   ::   X ml   :   500 ml
100 X = 500
X = 5 ml

or

$$\frac{\text{Known drug}}{\text{Known volume}} = \frac{\text{Desired drug}}{\text{Desired volume}}$$

$$\frac{1\ \text{mL}}{100\ \text{ml}} = \frac{X}{500\ \text{ml}}$$

100 X = 500
X = 5 ml

Answer: 5 ml of vinegar added to 500 ml of water is a 1:100 vinegar-water solution.

Note: Five milliliters did not increase the volume of the solution by a large amount. When volume and volume solutions are mixed, the total amount of *desired volume* should not be exceeded. Therefore it is important to determine the volume of desired drug first, then remove that volume from the appropriate amount of solvent (solution). When mixing the solution, begin with the desired drug and add the premeasured solvent. This process ensures that the solution has an accurate concentration.

PROBLEM 2: Prepare 100 ml of a 1:4 hydrogen peroxide 3% and normal saline mouthwash.

Known drug:Known volume :: Desired drug:Desired volume

1 ml : 4 ml :: X ml : 100 ml

4 X = 100 ml

X = 25 ml

25 ml of hydrogen peroxide 3% is the amount of desired drug. To calculate the amount of normal saline, use the following formula:

Desired volume − Desired drug = Desired solvent

100 ml − 25 ml = 75 ml

Answer: 75 ml of saline and 25 ml of hydrogen peroxide 3% make 100 ml of a 1:4 mouthwash.

Calculating a Solution From a Percentage

To obtain a solution from a percentage, use the same formula with either the proportion or fraction method.

EXAMPLE

PROBLEM 1: Prepare 1000 ml of a 0.9% NaCl solution.

Known drug:Known volume :: Desired drug:Desired volume

0.9 g : 100 ml :: X g : 1000 ml

100 X = 900

X = 9 g or 9 ml

Answer: 9 g or 9 ml of NaCl in 1000 ml makes a 0.9% NaCl solution.

PREPARING A WEAKER SOLUTION FROM A STRONGER SOLUTION

When a situation requires the preparation of a weaker solution from a stronger solution, the amount of desired drug must be determined. The known variables are the desired solution, the available or on-hand solution, and the desired volume. The formula can be set up with the strength of the solutions expressed in either ratio or percentage. The proportion method or the fractional method can be used to solve the problem. The first ratio or fraction, the desired solution (weaker solution), is the numerator, and the available or on-hand solution (stronger solution) is the denominator.

Desired solution : Available solution :: Desired drug : Desired volume

or

$$\frac{\text{Desired solution}}{\text{Available solution}} = \frac{\text{Desired drug}}{\text{Desired volume}}$$

EXAMPLES

PROBLEM 1: Prepare 500 ml of a 2.5% aluminum acetate solution from a 5% aluminum acetate solution. Use water as the solvent.

2.5% : 5% :: X : 500 ml

2.5 ml : 5 ml :: X : 500 ml

5 X = 1250

X = 250 ml

Answer: Use 250 ml of 5% aluminum acetate to make 500 ml of 2.5% aluminum acetate solution.

Determine the amount of water needed.

Desired volume − Desired drug = Desired solvent

500 ml   −   250 ml   =   250 ml

or

Same problem using the fractional method:

$$\frac{2.5\%}{5\%} \times \frac{X}{500 \text{ ml}} =$$

5 X = 1250

X = 250 ml of 5% aluminum acetate

or

Same problem but stated as a ratio:

Prepare 500 ml of a 1:40 aluminum acetate solution from a 1:20 aluminum acetate solution with water as the solvent.

$$\frac{1}{40} : \frac{1}{20} :: X : 500 \text{ ml}$$

$$\frac{1}{20 \text{ X}} = \frac{500}{40}$$

$$X = \frac{500}{\overset{40}{\underset{2}{}}} \times \frac{\overset{1}{\cancel{20}}}{1} = \frac{500}{2}$$

X = 250 ml of 5% aluminum acetate solution

Guidelines for Home Solutions

For solutions prepared by patients in the home, directions need to be very specific and in written form, if possible. People often think that more is better. Teach the patient that solutions can be dangerous if they are too concentrated. Higher concentrations of solutions can irritate tissues and prevent the desired effect. Recommend that standard measuring spoons and cups be used rather than tableware. Level measures rather than heaping measures of dry solutes should be used. Utensils and containers for solution preparation should be *clean or sterilized by boiling* if used for infants. Mixing acidic solutions in aluminum containers should be avoided, especially if the solution is for oral use. Although there is no evidence of toxicity, a metallic taste is noticeable. Glass, enamel, or plastic containers can be used. Solutions should be made fresh daily or just before use. Oral solutions, especially for infants, require refrigeration; topical solutions do not.

When preparing the solution, start with the desired drug and then add the solvent. This helps to disperse the drug and ensures that the desired volume of solution is not exceeded. If the volume of solvent is several liters, then it is not always practical to subtract a small volume of solute.

Solution problems are best calculated within the metric system. Fractional and percentage dosages are difficult to determine within the household system.

PRACTICE PROBLEMS: III Preparing a Weaker Solution from a Stronger One

Answers can be found on page 358.

Identify the known variables and choose the appropriate formula. Perform calculations needed to obtain the following solutions using the metric system. Use Table 14–1 to obtain the household equivalent.

1. Prepare 250 ml of a 0.9% NaCl and sterile water solution for nose drops.

2. Prepare 250 ml of a 5% glucose and sterile water solution for an infant feeding.

3. Prepare 1000 ml of a 25% Betadine solution with sterile saline for a foot soak.

4. Prepare 2 L of a 2% Lysol solution for cleaning a changing area.

5. Prepare 20 L of a 2% sodium bicarbonate solution for a bath.

6. Prepare 100 ml of a 50% hydrogen peroxide 3% and water mouthwash.

7. Prepare 500 ml of a modified Dakin's solution 0.5% from a 5% sodium hypochlorite solution with sterile water as the solvent.

8. Prepare 1500 ml of a 0.9% NaCl solution for an enema.

_____

9. Prepare 2 L of a 1:1000 Neosporin bladder irrigation with sterile saline. (Omit the household conversion.)

_____

10. Determine how much alcohol is needed for a 3:1 alcohol and white vinegar solution for an external ear irrigation. Vinegar 30 ml is used. Solve using the proportion method.

_____

11. Prepare 1000 ml of a 1:10 sodium hypochlorite and water solution for cleaning.

_____

12. Prepare 1000 ml of a 3% sodium hypochlorite and water solution.

_____

13. Prepare 2000 L of a 1:9 Lysol solution to clean color-fast linens soiled with body fluids. (Omit the household conversion.)

_____

HYDRATION MANAGEMENT

Calculate Daily Fluid Intake for an Adult

Hydration problems normally increase with age as total body water is lost when muscle mass decreases. With aging, the sensation of thirst diminishes and the response to dehydration is not sufficient to meet metabolic needs. Kidney function begins to decline in middle age, slowly decreasing the ability of the kidney to concentrate urine, resulting in increasing water loss. Add health care problems, such as dementia and diabetes, along with commonly used medication that increases fluid loss, like diuretics and laxatives, and dehydration is a real risk.

Dehydration can exacerbate problems such as urinary tract and respiratory tract infections but can cause more subtle problems in the elderly, such as confusion, decreased cognitive function, incontinence, constipation, and falls. All elderly adults, especially those over 85 years old, should be assessed for dehydration on the basis of physical assessment, laboratory data, cognitive assessment, pattern of fluid intake, and medical condition. Once daily fluid intake is established, nursing measures can be taken to maintain an adequate hydration.

Standard Formula for Daily Fluid Intake*

100 ml/kg for the first 10 kg of weight
50 ml/kg for the next 10 kg of weight
15 ml/kg for the remaining kg

The standard formula includes fluid contained in foods. To determine how much liquid alone an adult needs to consume, multiply the daily fluid intake by 75%.

EXAMPLE

Adult weight is 94 kg

$$\underline{-10\ kg} \times 100\ ml = 1000\ ml$$
$$84\ kg$$
$$\underline{-10\ kg} \times\ \ 50\ ml =\ \ \ 500\ ml$$
$$74\ kg \times\ \ 15\ ml = \underline{1110\ ml}$$
$$2610\ ml$$

2610 ml × 75% = 2610 × 0.75 = 1957.5 or 1958 ml fluid/day.

Calculate Daily Fluid Intake for a Febrile Adult

When an adult is febrile, the need for fluids increases by 6% for each degree over normal temperature. For example, a 94-kg adult with an oral temperature of 100.8°, 2° above normal, needs a 12% increase in fluid. To find the increase, multiply the fluid/day, 1958 ml, by the percent increase, 12%, and add that to the total fluid/day.

1958 ml × 12% = 1958 × 0.12 = 234.9 or 235 ml
1958 ml + 235 ml = 2193 ml

PRACTICE PROBLEMS: IV Hydration Management

Answers can be found on page 360.

1. Calculate the standard formula, then the fluid need of an adult weighing 84 kg.
2. Calculate the standard formula, then the fluid need of an adult weighing 63 kg.
3. Calculate the standard formula, then the fluid need of an adult weighing 70 kg.
4. Calculate the standard formula, then the fluid need of an adult weighing 100 kg.
5. Calculate the standard formula, then the fluid need of an adult weighing 69 kg with a fever of 101°.

*Adapted from Skipper, A. (Ed.) (1993). *Dietitian's handbook of enteral and parenteral nutrition*. Rockville, Maryland: Aspen Publishers.

BODY MASS INDEX (BMI)

The importance of weight for the determination of overall health status and drug therapy must be emphasized. The current international standard is "body mass index" for adults and children as the criteria for healthy weight, overweight, and obese persons.

Body mass index (BMI) is a weight-for-height index that takes the place of previously used height and weight tables. BMI is a part of health assessments and is used as an indicator of risk factors for chronic diseases.

Calculate Body Mass Index Using Two Formulas

a. BMI pounds and inches formula:

$$\frac{\text{weight in pounds}}{(\text{height in inches})\,(\text{height in inches})} \times 703$$

EXAMPLE

A person who weighs 165 pounds and is 6 ft 1 inch (73 inches) has a BMI of

$$\frac{165}{73 \times 73} \times 703 = 21.8 \text{ BMI}$$

b. BMI metric formula:

$$\frac{\text{weight in kg}}{(\text{height in meters})\,(\text{height in meters})}$$

EXAMPLE

A person who weighs 165 pounds and is 6 ft 1 inch (73 inches) has a BMI of:

$$73 \text{ inches} \times 0.0254 \text{ meters} = 1.854 \text{ meters}$$
$$165 \text{ lbs} \div 2.2 \text{ kg} = 75 \text{ kg}$$
$$\frac{75}{(1.854)\,(1.854)} = \frac{75}{3.437} = 21.8 \text{ BMI}$$

 NOTE

Conversion factors from household to metric, see Chapter 2, Table 2-1. Formula is most accurate when rounded off to three decimal places.

PRACTICE PROBLEMS: V Body Mass Index

Answers can be found on page 361.

1. What is the BMI for a female weighing 208 lb and is 5'2"?

2. What is the BMI for a male weighing 198 lb and 5'11"?

3. What is the BMI for a female weighing 112 lb and is 5'4"?

4. What is the BMI for a male weighing 165 lb and is 6'1"?

5. What is the BMI for a male weighing 60 lb with a height of 3'10"?

ANSWERS

I Metric to Household Conversion
1. Bismuth subsalicylate 15 ml = 1 T. No more than 8 T in 24 hr
2. Ceclor 5 ml = 1 t
3. Tylenol elixir 1.25 ml = $^1/_4$ t
4. Maalox 30 ml = 2 T
5. Neo-Calglucon 7.5 ml = $1^1/_2$ t
6. Gani-Tuss NR, 10 ml = 2 t
7. Castor oil 60 ml = 4 T or $^1/_4$ c
8. Metamucil 5 g = 1 t
9. Dilantin-30 pediatric suspension 10 ml = 2 t
10. H_2O 1 L = 1 qt
    Sugar 30 g = 2 T
    Salt 1.25 g = $^1/_4$ t + $^1/_8$ t
    Lite salt 2.5 g = $^1/_2$ t
    Baking soda 2.5 g = $^1/_2$ t
11. H_2O 500 ml = 1 pt
    Table salt 5 ml = 1 t
    Baking soda 5 ml = 1 t
12. Benadryl 50 mg/10 ml = 2 t
    Maalox 10 ml = 2 t
13. Belladonna/phenobarbital elixir, 10 ml = 2 t
    Maalox 30 ml = 2 T
    Viscous lidocaine 10 ml = 2 t

II Preparing a Solution of a Desired Concentration
1. 4:1 = X:100
   X = 400
   $\frac{400}{100}$, 400%
2. 2:1 = X:100
   X = 200
   $\frac{200}{100}$, 200%
3. 1:50 = X:100
   50 X = 100
   X = 2
   $\frac{2}{100}$, 2%
4. 1:3 = X:100
   3 X = 100
   X = 33.3
   $\frac{33.3}{100}$, 33.3%

5. $1:100 = X:100$

$1000 X = 100$

$X = 0.1$

$\dfrac{0.1}{100}, 0.1\%$

6. $1:10,000 = X:100$

$10,000 X = 100$

$X = 0.01$

$\dfrac{1}{10,000}, 0.01\%$

7. $1:4 = X:100$

$4 X = 100$

$X = 25$

$\dfrac{25}{100}, 25\%$

8. $1:5000 = X:100$

$5000 X = 100$

$X = 0.02$

$\dfrac{0.02}{100}, 0.02\%$

9. $1:200 = X:100$

$200 X = 100$

$X = 0.5$

$\dfrac{0.5}{100}, 0.5\%$

10. $1:10 = X:100$

$10X = 100$

$X = 10$

$\dfrac{10}{100}, 10\%$

III Preparing a Weaker Solution from a Stronger One

1. Known drug: 0.6% NaCl $0.6:100 :: X:250$

Known volume: 100 ml $100 X = 150$

Desired drug: X $X = 1.5$ ml

Desired volume: 250 ml

1.5 ml of NaCl in 250 ml of water yields a 0.6% NaCl solution. Household equivalents are approximately $^1/_4$ teaspoon salt and 1 cup sterile water.

2. Known drug: 5% glucose (sugar) $5:100 :: X:250$

Known volume: 100 ml $100 X = 1250$

Desired drug: X $X = 12.5$ ml

Desired volume: 250 ml

12.5 ml of sugar in 250 ml of water yields a 5% glucose solution. Household equivalents are approximately 1 tablespoon in 1 cup of sterile water.

3. Known drug: 25% Betadine   25:100 :: X:1000
   Known volume: 100 ml   100 X = 25,000
   Desired drug: X   X = 250 ml
   Desired volume: 1000 ml   1000 ml − 250 ml = 750 ml

250 ml of Betadine in 750 ml saline yields a 25% Betadine solution. Household equivalents are 1 cup Betadine in 3 cups sterile saline.

4. Known drug: 2% Lysol   2:100 :: X:2000 ml
   Known volume: 100 ml   100 X = 4000
   Desired drug: X   X = 40 ml
   Desired volume: 2 L = 2000 ml

40 ml of Lysol in 2 L of water yields a 2% Lysol solution. Household equivalents are 2 tablespoons and 2 teaspoons (40 ml) of Lysol to 2 quarts or $^1/_2$ gallon of water.

5. Known drug: 2% sodium bicarbonate   2:100 :: X:20,000 ml
   Known volume: 100 ml   100 X = 40,000
   Desired drug: X   X = 400 ml or 400 g
   Desired volume: 20,000 ml

400 ml or 400 g of sodium bicarbonate (baking soda) in 20,000 ml of water yields a 2% sodium bicarbonate solution. Household equivalents are $1^1/_2$ cups and 2 tablespoons baking soda in 5 gallons of water.

6. Known drug: 50% hydrogen peroxide   50:100 :: X:100
   Known volume: 100 ml   100 X = 5000
   Desired drug: X   X = 50 ml
   Desired volume: 100 ml   100 ml − 50 ml = 50 ml

50 ml of hydrogen peroxide 3% in 50 ml water yields a 50% solution. Household equivalents are approximately 3 tablespoons of hydrogen peroxide 3% in 3 tablespoons of water.

7. Known drug: 0.5%   0.5:5 :: X:500
   Available solution: 5%   5 X = 250
   Desired drug: X   X = 50 ml
   Desired volume: 500 ml   500 ml − 50 ml = 450 ml

50 ml of sodium hypochlorite in 450 ml sterile water yields a 0.5% modified Dakin's solution. Household equivalents are 3 tablespoons and 1 teaspoon of Dakin's solution in 1 pint minus 3 tablespoons of water.

8. Known drug: 0.9%   0.9:100 :: X:1500
   Known volume: 100 ml   100 X = 1350
   Desired drug: X   X = 13.5 ml
   Desired volume: 1500 ml

13.5 ml of NaCl in 1500 ml water yields a 0.9% NaCl solution. Household equivalents are $2^1/_2$ teaspoons of salt in $1^1/_2$ quarts of water.

9. Known drug: 1 ml   1:1000 :: X:2000
   Known volume: 1000 ml   1000 X = 2000

Desired drug: X   X = 2 ml

Desired volume: 2000 ml

2 ml of Neosporin irrigant in 2000 ml of sterile saline yields a 1 : 1000 solution for continuous bladder irrigation. This treatment is done primarily in the clinical setting.

10. Use ratio and proportion to solve this problem.

    3 : 1 :: X : 30 ml

      X = 90 ml

Add 90 ml of alcohol to 30 ml of vinegar to yield a 3 : 1 solution for an external ear wash. Household equivalents are 6 tablespoons of alcohol and 2 tablespoons of vinegar.

11. Known drug: 1 ml   1 : 10 :: X : 1000

    Known volume: 10 ml   10 X = 1000

    Desired drug: X   X = 100 ml

    Desired volume: 1000 ml   1000 ml − 100 ml = 900 ml

100 ml of sodium hypochlorite (bleach) in 900 ml water yields a 1 : 10 sodium hypochlorite solution. Household equivalents are $^1/_3$ cup and 2 tablespoons sodium hypochlorite in approximately 1 quart minus $^1/_3$ cup and 2 tablespoons of water.

12. Known drug: 3 ml   3 : 100 :: X : 1000

    Known volume: 100 ml   100 X = 3000

    Desired drug: X   X = 30 ml

    Desired volume: 1000 ml   1000 ml − 30 ml = 970 ml

30 ml of sodium hypochlorite (bleach) in 970 ml water yields a 3% sodium hypochlorite solution. Household equivalents are 2 tablespoons in 1 quart minus 2 tablespoons of water.

13. Use ratio and proportion to solve this problem.

                  1 : 9 :: X : 2000 ml

                     9X = 2000 ml

                     X = 222 ml

Desired volume − Desired drug = Desired solvent

    2000 ml − 222 ml   = 1778 ml

222 ml of Lysol in 1778 ml of H_2O yields a 1:9 solution cleansing solution for colorfast linens soiled with body fluids.

IV Hydration Management:

1. Adult weight is 84 kg

    $\underline{-10 \text{ kg}} \times 100 \text{ ml} = 1000 \text{ ml}$

       74 kg

    $\underline{-10 \text{ kg}} \times 50 \text{ ml} = 500 \text{ ml}$

       64 kg × 15 ml = 960 ml

                     2460 ml

2460 ml × 75% = 2460 × 0.75 = 1845 ml

2. Adult weight is 63 kg

$\underline{-10 \text{ kg}} \times 100 \text{ ml} = 1000 \text{ ml}$
      53 kg
$\underline{-10 \text{ kg}} \times \; 50 \text{ ml} = \; 500 \text{ ml}$
      43 kg $\times \;\; 15 \text{ ml} = \;\; \underline{645 \text{ ml}}$
                              2145 ml

2145 ml $\times$ 75% = 2145 $\times$ 0.75 = 1608.75 or 1609 ml

3. Adult weight is 70 kg

$\underline{-10 \text{ kg}} \times 100 \text{ ml} = 1000 \text{ ml}$
      60 kg
$\underline{-10 \text{ kg}} \times \; 50 \text{ ml} = \; 500 \text{ ml}$
      50 kg $\times \;\; 15 \text{ ml} = \;\; \underline{750 \text{ ml}}$
                              2250 ml

2250 ml $\times$ 75% = 2250 $\times$ 0.75 = 1687.5 or 1688 ml

4. Adult weight is 100 kg

$\underline{-10 \text{ kg}} \times 100 \text{ ml} = 1000 \text{ ml}$
      90 kg
$\underline{-10 \text{ kg}} \times \; 50 \text{ ml} = \; 500 \text{ ml}$
      80 kg $\times \;\; 15 \text{ ml} = \underline{1200 \text{ ml}}$
                              2700 ml

2700 ml $\times$ 75% = 2700 $\times$ 0.75 = 2025

5. Adult weight is 69 kg

$\underline{-10 \text{ kg}} \times 100 \text{ ml} = 1000 \text{ ml}$
      59 kg
$\underline{-10 \text{ kg}} \times \; 50 \text{ ml} = \; 500 \text{ ml}$
      49 kg $\times \;\; 15 \text{ ml} = \;\; \underline{735 \text{ ml}}$
                              2235 ml

2235 ml $\times$ 75% = 2235 $\times$ 0.75 = 1676 ml

6% $\times$ 3° = 18% for increased temperature.

1676 ml $\times$ 18% = 1676 $\times$ 18 = 301.6 or 302 ml

1676 ml + 302 ml = 1978 ml fluid

V Body Mass Index (BMI)

1. 5 feet 2 inches = 62 inches (12 $\times$ 5 = 60 inches + 2 inches = 62 inches)

$$\frac{208}{(62) \;\; (62)} \times 703 = \frac{208}{3844} \times 703 =$$

$$0.054 \times 703 = 38 \text{ BMI}$$

2. 5 feet 11 inches = 71 inches

$$\frac{198}{(71) \;\; (71)} \times 703 = \frac{198}{5041} \times 703 =$$

$$0.039 \times 703 = 27.4 \text{ BMI}$$

3. 5 feet 4 inches = 64 inches

$$\frac{112}{(64)\ (64)} \times 703 = \frac{112}{4096} \times 703 =$$

$$0.027 \times 703 = 19\ \text{BMI}$$

4. 6 feet 1 inch = 73 inches

$$\frac{165}{(73)\ (73)} \times 703 = \frac{165}{5329} \times 703 =$$

$$0.31 \times 703 = 21.7\ \text{BMI}$$

5. 3 feet 10 inches = 46 inches

$$\frac{60}{(46)\ (46)} \times 703 = \frac{60}{2116} \times 703 =$$

$$0.028 \times 703 = 19.7\ \text{BMI}$$

PART V

POST-TEST: ORAL PREPARATIONS, INJECTABLES, INTRAVENOUS, AND PEDIATRICS

The post-test is for testing content of Part III, Orals, Injectables, Intravenous, and Chapter 10, Pediatrics. The test is divided into four sections. There are 60 drug problems, and the test should take 1 to 1½ hours to complete. You may use a conversion table as needed. Minimum passing score is 54 correct or 90%. If you get more than two drug problems wrong in a section of the test, return to the chapter in the book for that test section and rework the practice problems.

ORAL PREPARATIONS

1. Order: nifedipine (Adalat CC) 60 mg, po, daily for 1 wk; then 90 mg, po, daily.
   Drug available:

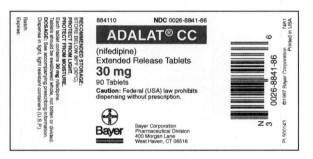
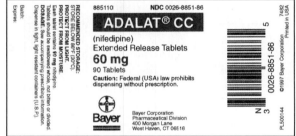

   a. Which Adalat CC container would you use for the first week? _____

   b. Explain how you would give 90 mg. _____

2. Order: Crestor (rosuvastatin calcium) 10 mg, po, daily at bedtime.
   Drug available:

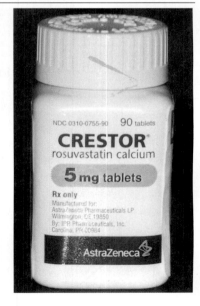

   a. How many tablet(s) would you give? _____

   b. When is/are the tablet(s) given? _____

3. Order: pravastatin sodium (Pravachol) 20 mg, po, at bedtime.

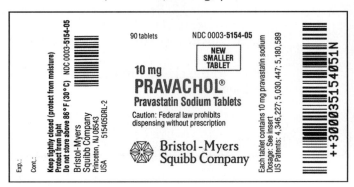

How many tablets of Pravachol should the patient receive? _____

4. Order: nitroglycerin (Nitrostat) gr 1/200, SL, STAT.
Drug available:

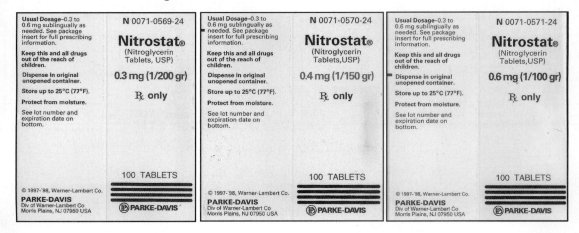

The drug is available in three different strengths. Which drug label would you

select? Why? _____

_____

5. Order: clorazepate sodium (Tranxene) gr 1/4/day, po, at bedtime.
Drug available:

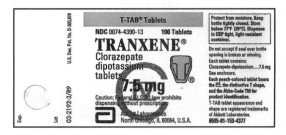

a. Change grain ¼ to milligrams. Use conversion table if needed. How many milligrams is equivalent to grain ¼? _____

b. How many tablets should the patient receive? _____

6. Order: clarithromycin (Biaxin) 0.5 g, bid × 10 days, po.
Drug available:

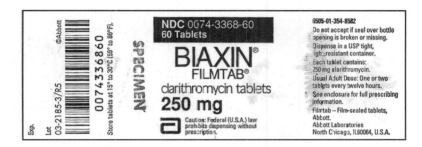

a. 0.5 gram is equivalent to _____ milligram.

b. How many tablets would you give? _____

7. Order: acetaminophen (Tylenol) gr x, po, prn, for headache.
Drug available:

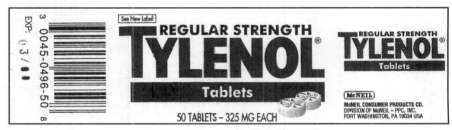

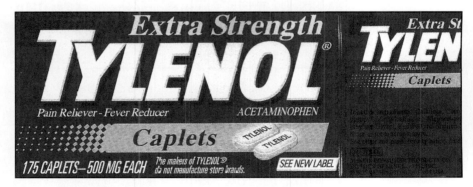

a. Grain x is equivalent to _____ milligrams.

b. Which Tylenol bottle would you select? _____

c. How many tablets or caplets should the patient receive? _____

8. Order: allopurinol (Zyloprim) 0.2 g, po, bid.
   Drug available:

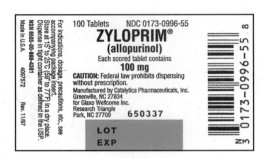

a. 0.2 g is equivalent to _____ milligrams.

b. The patient should receive how many tablets of allopurinol per dose?

   _____

9. Order: prochlorperazine (Compazine) 10 mg, po, tid.
   Drug available:

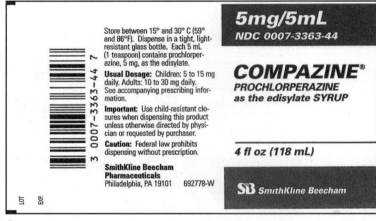

A

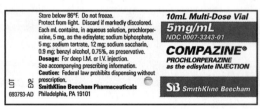

B

a. Which Compazine bottle would you select? Why? _____

b. How many milliliters would you give? _____

10. Order Synthroid (levothyroxine) 0.0375 mg, po, daily.
Drug available:

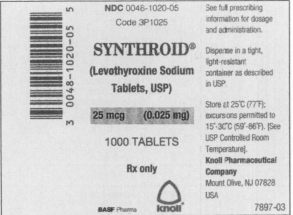
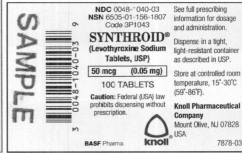

a. The micrograms for 0.0375 mg would be? _____

b. Which synthroid bottle would you select? _____

c. How many tablet(s) would you give per day? _____

11. Order: cefuroxime axetil (Ceftin) 500 mg, po, q12h.
Drug available:

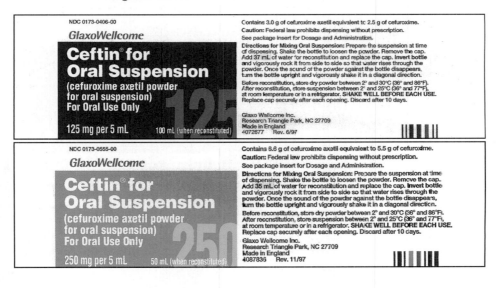

a. Which Ceftin bottle would you select? Explain. _____

b. The patient would receive how many grams _____ or

milligrams _____ of Ceftin per day?

c. How many milliliters should the client receive? _____

12. Order: cefaclor (Ceclor) 250 mg, po, q8h.
Drug available:

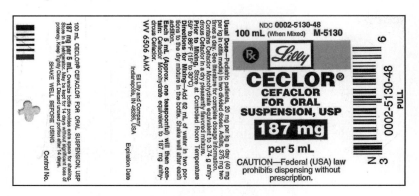

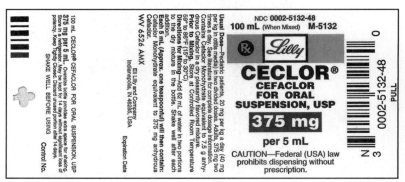

a. Which Ceclor bottle would you select? _____

b. How many milliliters should the client receive per dose? _____

c. Is there another solution to this drug problem? _____

13. Order: simvastatin (Zocor) 40 mg, po, daily.
Drug available:

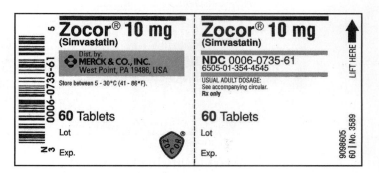

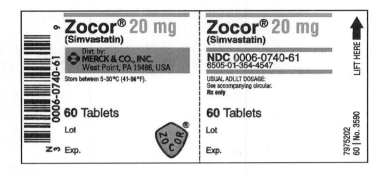

a. Which Zocor bottle would you select? Why? _____

b. How many tablets should the patient receive? _____

14. Order: Amoxil (amoxicillin) 0.4 g, po, q8h.
    Drug available:

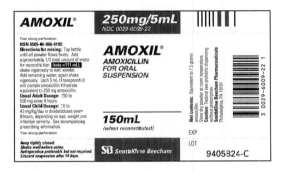

a. Change grams into milligrams: 0.4 grams = _____ mg.

b. How many milligrams should the patient receive per dose? _____

c. How many milliliters should the patient receive? _____

15. Order: Lamivudine (Epirvir) 150 mg, po, q12h.
    Drug available:

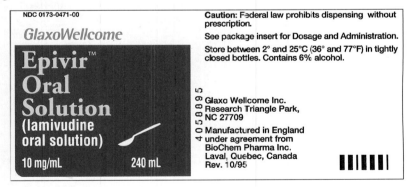

a. How many milligrams would you give per day? _____

b. How many milliliters would you give per dose? _____

16. Order: etretinate (Tegison) 0.75 mg/kg/day, po, in two divided doses. Patient weighs 150 pounds.
Drug available: Tegison 10-mg and 25-mg capsules.

    a. How many kilograms does the patient weigh? _____

    b. How many milligrams of Tegison should the patient receive per day?

    _____

    c. How many capsules of Tegison per dose? _____

17. Order: theophylline 5 mg/kg/LD (loading dose), po. Patient weighs 70 kg.
Drug available: Oral solution 80 mg/15 ml and 150 mg/15 ml.

    a. How milligrams should the patient receive? _____

    b. Which oral solution bottle would you select? _____

    c. How many milliliters of theophylline should the patient receive as a loading dose? _____

18. Order: docusate sodium (Colace) 100 mg, po, bid per NG (nasogastric) tube.
Drug available: Colace 50 mg/5 ml. Osmolality of docusate sodium is 3900 mOsm. The desired osmolality is 500 mOsm.

    a. How many milliliters of Colace should the client receive? _____

    b. How much water dilution is needed to obtain the desired osmolality?

    _____

INJECTABLES

19. Order: hydroxyzine (Vistaril) 25 mg, deep IM, STAT.
Drug available: (50 mg = 1 ml)

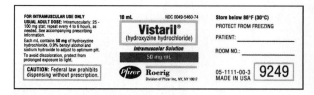

How many milliliters of Vistaril would you give? _____

20. Order: digoxin (Lanoxin) 0.25 mg, IM, daily.
Drug available:

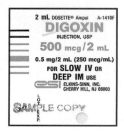

How many milliliters of digoxin would you give? _____

21. Order: meperidine (Demerol) 40 mg and atropine sulfate 0.5 mg, IM, STAT.
Drug available:

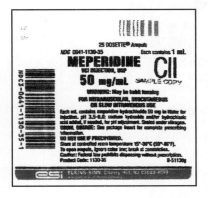 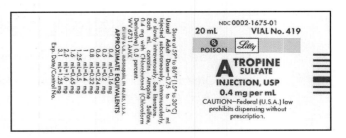

a. How many milliliters of meperidine and how many milliliters of atropine
would you administer? _____

b. Explain how the two drugs would be mixed. _____

22. Order: heparin 2500 units, SubQ, q6h.
Drug available:

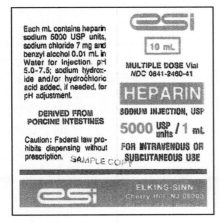 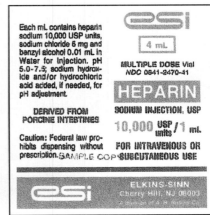

a. Which heparin would you use? _____

b. How many milliliters of heparin should the patient receive? _____

23. Order: Lovenox (enoxaparin Na) 20 mg, SubQ, q12h.
Drug available:

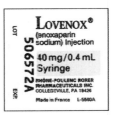

a. How many milliliters would you give?

24. Order: naloxone (Narcan) 0.5 mg, IM, STAT.
Drug available:

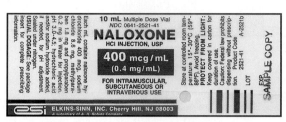

How many milliliters of naloxone should the patient receive? _____

25. Order: Humulin 70/30 insulin 35 units, SubQ, in AM.
Drug available:

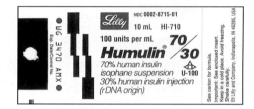

a. Indicate on the unit-100 insulin syringe how many units of 70/30 insulin should be given?

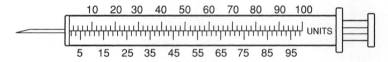

26. Order: Humulin N insulin 45 units and Humulin R (regular) 10 units.

a. Explain the method for mixing the two insulins.

_____

b. Mark on the units 100 insulin syringe how much regular insulin and NPH insulin should be withdrawn.

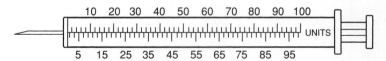

27. Order: vitamin B_{12} 500 mcg, IM, 3 × a week.
Drug available:

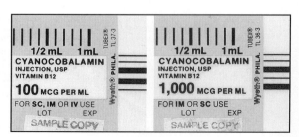

a. Which cyanocobalamin would you select? Why?

_____

b. How many milliliters would you give? _____

28. Order: morphine gr ⅙, IM, STAT.
    Drug available:

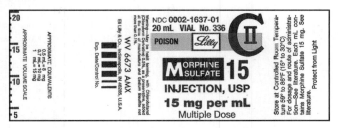

How many milliliters of morphine would you administer? _____

Note: Change grains to milligrams. Use conversion table if needed.

29. Order: phytonadione (AquaMEPHYTON) 5 mg, IM, STAT.
    Drug available:

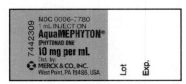

How many milliliters of AquaMEPHYTON would you administer? _____

30. Order: ranitidine HCl (Zantac) 35 mg, IM, q8h.
    Drug available:

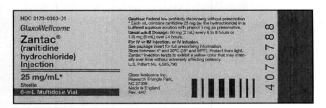

How many milliliters of Zantac should the patient receive? _____

31. Order: tobramycin (Nebcin) 3 mg/kg/day, IM, in three divided doses.
Patient weighs 145 pounds.
Drug available: (80 mg = 2 ml)

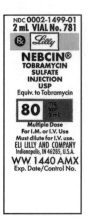

a. How many kilograms does the patient weigh? _____

b. How many milligrams of Nebcin should the patient receive per day?

_____

c. How many milligrams of Nebcin should the patient receive per dose?

_____

d. How many milliliters of Nebcin would you administer per dose?

_____

32. Order: bethanechol Cl (Urecholine) 2.5 mg, subQ, STAT and may repeat in
1 hour.
Drug available: (Note: 5.15 mg = 5 mg)

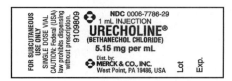

How many milliliters of Urecholine would you give? _____

33. Order: Tazidime (ceftazidime) 250 mg, IM, q8h.
Drug available:

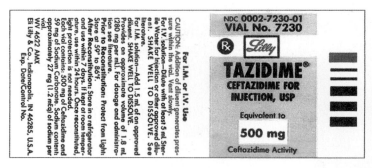

   a. How much diluent would you add to the Tazidime vial? (See label.)

   _____

   The diluent when mixed in the vial would equal _____.

   b. How many milligrams should the patient receive per day? _____

   c. How many milliliters would you give IM per dose? _____

   d. What type of syringe would you use? _____

34. Order: cefamandole (Mandol) 500 mg, IM, q12h.
    Drug available:

   a. How much diluent would you mix with the Mandol powder? (See label

   for mixing.) _____

   b. How many milliliters should be given? _____

35. Order: cefazolin (Ancef) 0.25 g, IM, q12h.
    Mixing: Add 2.0 ml of diluent = 2.2 ml drug solution.
    Drug available:

   a. Change grams to milligrams; drug label is in milligrams. _____

   b. How many milliliters of Ancef should the patient receive per dose?

   _____

36. Order: oxacillin sodium 150 mg, IM, q6h.
    Drug available:

   a. Label states to add _____ ml of diluent to equal _____ ml per
      250 mg.

b. How many milliliters of oxacillin should the patient receive per dose?

_____

37. Order: ceftazidime (Fortaz) 750 mg, IM, q12h.
Add 2.5 ml of diluent = 3 ml of drug solution.
Drug available:

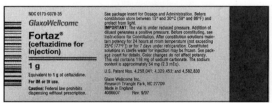

How many milliliters of ceftazidime would you administer per dose? _____

38. Order: gentamicin sulfate 4 mg/kg/day, IM, in three divided doses.
Patient weighs 165 pounds.
Drug available: gentamicin 10 mg/ml and 40 mg/ml.

a. How many kilograms does the patient weigh? _____

b. How many milligrams of gentamicin per day should the patient receive?

_____

c. How many milligrams of gentamicin per dose? _____

d. Which gentamicin bottle would you select? Explain.

_____

e. How many milliliters of gentamicin per dose should the patient receive?

_____

DIRECT IV ADMINISTRATION

39. Order: Furosemide (Lasix) 30 mg, IV direct, STAT.
Drug available:

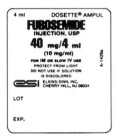

Instruction: Direct IV infusion not to exceed 10 mg/min.

a. How many milliliters should the patient receive? _____

b. Number of minutes to administer? _____

INTRAVENOUS

40. Order: 1000 ml of 5% dextrose/0.45% NaCl in 8 hours.
Available: 1 liter of 5% D/½ NSS; IV set labeled 10 gtt/ml.
How many drops per minute should the patient receive?

_____

41. Order: 500 ml of D_5W in 2 hours.
Available: 500 ml of D_5W; IV set labeled 15 gtt/ml.
How many drops per minute should the patient receive?

_____

42. Order: ticarcillin disodium (Ticar) 600 mg, IV q6h.
Available: Calibrated cyclinder (Buretrol) set with drop factor 60 gtt/ml;
500 ml D_5W.
Drug available: add 2 ml of diluent = 2.6 drug solution

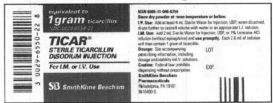

Instruction: Dilute drug in 60 ml of D_5W and infuse in 30 minutes.

a. _Drug calculation:_

_____

b. _Flow rate calculation:_

_____

43. Order: cefazolin (Kefzol) 500 mg, IV, q6h.
Available: Secondary set: drop factor 15 gtt/ml; 100 ml D_5W.
Add 2.5 ml of diluent to yield 3 ml of drug solution.
Drug available:

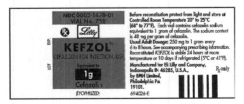

Instruction: Dilute drug in 100 ml D_5W and infuse in 45 minutes.

a. _Drug calculation:_

_____

b. _Flow rate calculation:_

_____

44. Order: chlorpromazine HCl (Thorazine) 50 mg, IV, to run for 4 hours.
Available: Secondary set: drop factor 15 gtt/ml; 500 ml of NSS (normal saline solution).
Drug available:

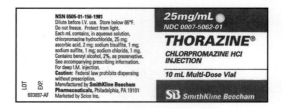

Instruction: Dilute Thorazine 50 mg in 500 ml of 0.9% NaCl (NSS) to run for 4 hours.

a. *Drug calculation:*

_____

b. *Flow rate calculation:*

_____

45. Order: Cefoxitin (Mefoxin) 1 g, IV, q6h.
Drug available: ADD-Vantage vial

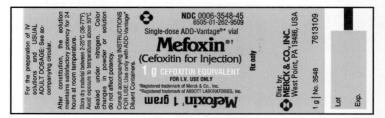

Set and solution: 50 ml of IV diluent bag for ADD-Vantage; Mefoxin 1 g vial for ADD-Vantage.
Instruction: Dilute Mefoxin in 50 ml of NaCl bag and infuse in 30 minutes.

a. How would you prepare Mefoxin 1 g powdered vial using the diluent

bag? (See page _____ as needed.)

b. Infusion pump rate (ml/hr): _____

46. Order: cefepime HCl (Maxipime) 0.5 g, IV, q12h.
Available: Infusion pump.
Add 2.0 ml diluent = 2.5 ml.
Drug available:

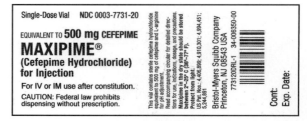

Instruction: Dilute in 50 ml of D_5W and infuse over 20 minutes.

a. *Drug calculation:*

_____

b. *Infusion pump rate:*

_____

47. Order: diltiazem (Cardizem) 10 mg/h, IV for 5 h.
    Available: Infusion pump; 500 ml of D$_5$W.
    Drug available:

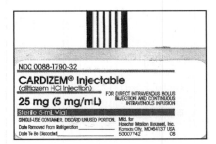

Instruction: Infuse diltiazem 10 mg/h over 5 hours.

a. *Drug calculation:*

_____

    (1) How many milligrams of Cardizem should the patient receive over

        5 hours? _____

    (2) How many milliliters of Cardizem should be mixed in the 500 ml of

        D$_5$W? _____

b. *Infusion pump rate:*

_____

48. Order: Ciprofloxacin (Cipro) 100 mg, IV, q6h.
    Drug available:

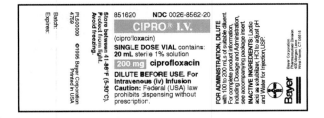

Set and solution: Secondary set with drop factor 15 gtt/ml; 100 ml of D$_5$W.
Instruction: Dilute drug in 100 ml of D$_5$W and infuse in 30 minutes; also calculate rate for infusion pump.

a. *Drug calculation:* _____

b. *Flow rate calculation* with secondary set (gtt/min): _____

c. *Infusion pump rate* (ml/hr): _____

49. Order: ifosfamide (Ifex) 1.2 g/m²/day for 5 consecutive days.
Patient: Weight: 150 pounds; Height: 70 inches = 1.98 m².
Available: Infusion pump; 5% dextrose solution.
Add 20 ml of diluent to 1 g of Ifex.
Drug available:

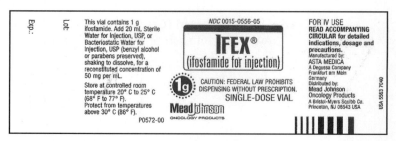

Instruction: Dilute Ifex in 50 ml of D₅W; infuse over 30 minutes.

a. *Drug calculation:*

_____

How many grams or milligrams of Ifex should the patient receive?

_____

b. How much diluent would you add to 2.4 g of Ifex?

_____

c. *Infusion pump rate:*

_____

PEDIATRICS

50. Child with cardiac disorder.
Order: Lanoxin pediatric elixir 0.5 mg, po, daily.
Drug available:

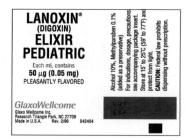

Child's age and weight: 3 years, 12 kg.
Pediatric dose range: 0.04–0.06 mg/kg.

a. Is this drug dose within the safe range? _____

b. How many milliliters would you administer? _____

51. Child with high fever.
Order: ibuprofen (Motrin) 0.1 g, prn temperature greater than 102°F.
Child's age and weight: 3 years, 15 kg.
Pediatric dose range: 100 mg, q6-8h, not to exceed 400 mg/day.
Drug available: (100 mg = 5 ml)

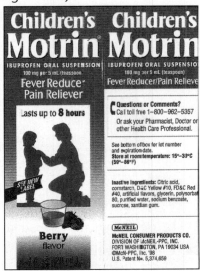

a. Is this drug dose within the safe range? _____

b. How many milliliters should the child receive per dose? _____

52. Child with strep throat.
Order: penicillin V potassium (Veetids) 400,000 units, po, q6h.
Child's age and weight: 8 years, 53 pounds.
Pediatric dose range: 25,000-90,000 units/kg/day in three to six divided doses.
Drug available:

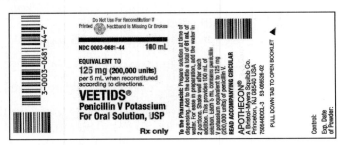

a. Is the drug dose within the safe range? _____

b. How many milliliters of penicillin V would you give? _____

53. Child with otitis media.
Order: amoxicillin (Amoxil) 250 mg, po, q6h.
Child's age and weight: 5 years, 19 kg.
Pediatric dose range: 20-40 mg/kg/day in three divided doses.

Drug available:

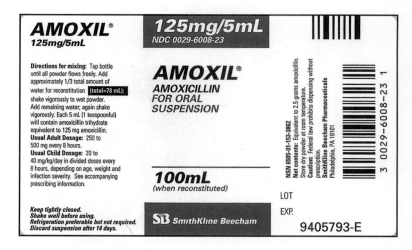

a. Is the drug dose within the safe range? _____

b. How many milliliters would you give? _____

54. Child with asthma.
Order: theophylline elixir 100 mg, po, q6h.
Child's age and weight: 7 years, 22 kg.
Pediatric dose: 400 mg/24 h in four doses.
Drug available: theophylline elixir 80 mg/15 ml.

a. Is the drug dose within the safe range? _____

b. How many milliliters would you give per dose? _____

55. Child with pruritus.
Order: diphenhydramine HCl (Benadryl) 25 mg, po, tid.
Child's age and weight: 2 years, 16 kg.
Pediatric dose: 5 mg/kg/day.
Drug available: Benadryl 12.5 mg/5 ml.

a. Is the drug dose within the safe range? _____

b. How many milliliters would you give? _____

56. Child with a lower respiratory tract infection.
Order: cefaclor (Ceclor) 100 mg, q8h.
Child's age and weight: 4 years, 44 pounds.
Pediatric dose range: 20-40 mg/kg/day in three divided doses.

Drug available:

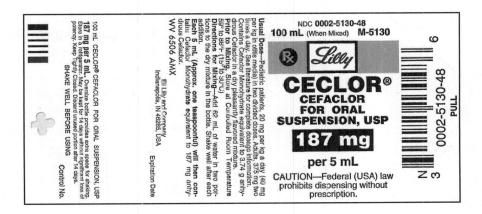

a. How many kilograms does the child weigh? _____

b. Is the drug dose within the safe range? _____

c. How many milliliters should the child receive? _____

57. Child with severe systemic infection.
    Order: tobramycin (Nebcin) 15 mg, IV, q8h.
    Child's age and weight: 18 months, 10 kg.
    Pediatric dose range: 3-5 mg/kg/day in three divided doses.
    Drug available:

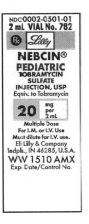

a. Is the drug dose within the safe range? _____

b. How many milliliters of tobramycin would you give? _____

58. Child with a severe central nervous system (CNS) infection.
Order: ceftazidime (Fortaz) 250 mg, IV, q6h.
Child's age and weight: 6 years, 27 kg.
Pediatric dose range: 30-50 mg/kg/day in three divided doses.
Add 2.0 ml of diluent = 2.4 ml of drug solution.
Drug available:

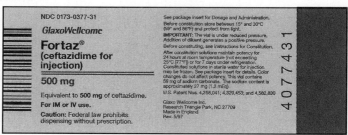

a. Is the drug dose within the safe range? _____

b. How many milliliters of Fortaz would be given? _____

59. Order: Cefazolin (Ancef) 400 mg, IV, q8h.
Child weight: 49 pounds.
Parameters: 50-100 mg/kg/day in 3 divided doses.
Drug available:

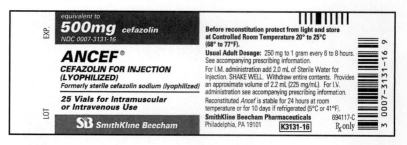

Instruction: Mix Ancef with 1.8 ml to equal 2.0 ml = 500 mg. Buretrol: Dilute drug in 50 mg of IV diluent; infuse in 30 minutes.

a. How many kg does the child weigh? _____

b. Is the drug dose within drug parameters? _____

c. How many ml of Ancef should be withdrawn from the vial? _____

d. Flow rate calculation (gtt/min): _____

60. Child with a severe respiratory tract infection.
Order: kanamycin (Kantrex) 60 mg, IV, q8h.
Child's age and weight: 1 year, 26 pounds.
Pediatric dose range: 15 mg/kg/day, q8-12h.

Drug available:

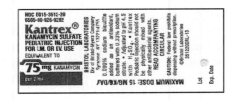

a. How many milligrams of kanamycin will the child receive per day? Per

dose? _____

b. How many milliliters of kanamycin will the child receive per dose?

_____

c. Is the drug dose within the safe range? _____

ANSWERS

Oral Preparations

1. **a.** The Adalat CC, 60 container.
   b. For 90 mg, remove 1 tablet from the 30-mg container and 1 tablet from the 60-mg container.
2. (a) 2 tablets; (b) in the evening or bedtime
3. 2 tablets of Pravachol.
4. Nitrostat 0.3 mg (use conversion table as needed)
5. **a.** grain $\frac{1}{4}$ = 15 mg
   b. 2 tablets
6. **a.** 0.5 gram = 500 mg
   b. 2 tablets
7. **a.** 600 to 650 mg = gr x
   b. 325-mg bottle
   c. 2 tablets from the 325-mg bottle
8. **a.** 0.2 g = 200 mg
   b. 2 tablets
9. **a.** Compazine 5 mg/5 ml; Compazine 5 mg/ml is for injection.
   b. 10 ml
10. **a.** 37.5 mcg = 0.0375 mg
    b. 0.025 mg or 25 mcg bottle
    c. BF: $\dfrac{D}{H} \times V = \dfrac{0.0375}{0.025} \times 1 =$

    $1\frac{1}{2}$ tablets

    or
    RP: $\quad$ H $\quad$: V :: $\quad$ D $\quad$: X
    $\quad$ 0.025 mg : 1 ml :: 0.0375 mg : X ml
    $\quad\quad$ 0.025X = 0.0375
    $\quad\quad\quad\quad$ X = $1\frac{1}{2}$ tablets

    or
    FE: $\dfrac{H}{V} = \dfrac{D}{X} = \dfrac{25 \text{ mcg}}{1 \text{ ml}} \times \dfrac{37.5 \text{ mcg}}{X} =$

    (Cross-multiply) 25 X = 37.5
    $\quad\quad\quad\quad$ X = $1\frac{1}{2}$ tablets

    or
    DA: ml = $\dfrac{1 \text{ ml} \times 0.0375 \text{ mg}}{0.025 \text{ mg} \times 1} = 1\frac{1}{2}$ tablets

11. **a.** Select 250 mg/5 ml bottle. However, either bottle could be used; 125 mg/5 ml = 20 ml.
   b. 1 gram; 1000 mg
   c. 500 mg = 10 ml

12. **a.** Either 187 mg/5 ml or 375 mg/5 ml.
   b. With (preferred) 187 mg/5 ml bottle:

$$\frac{250 \text{ mg}}{187 \text{ mg}} \times 5 \text{ ml} = \frac{1250}{187} = 6.67 \text{ or } 7 \text{ ml per dose}$$

   c. With the 375 mg/5 ml, 3.3 ml per dose.

13. **a.** Zocor 20 mg bottle. Either bottle; however, with the 10-mg Zocor bottle, more tablets would be taken (Zocor 10-mg bottle = 4 tablets).
   b. 2 tablets (Zocor 20-mg bottle)

14. **a.** Change 0.4 grams to milligrams = 400 mg
   b. 400 mg per dose.

   c. BF: $\dfrac{D}{H} \times V = \dfrac{400 \text{ mg}}{250 \text{ mg}} \times 5 \text{ ml} =$

   8 ml of amoxicillin

   or
   RP: H : V :: D : X
   250 mg : 5 ml :: 400 mg : X ml
   250X = 2000
   X = 8 ml

   or
   FE: $\dfrac{H}{V} = \dfrac{D}{X} = \dfrac{250}{5} \times \dfrac{400}{X} =$

   (Cross-multiply) 250X = 2000
   X = 8 ml of amoxicillin

   or
   DA: ml = $\dfrac{5 \text{ ml} = \overset{4}{\cancel{1000 \text{ mg}}} \times 0.4 \cancel{g}}{\underset{1}{\cancel{250 \text{ mg}}} = 1 \cancel{g} \times 1}$ = 8 ml of amoxicillin

15. **a.** 300 mg per day
   b. BF: $\dfrac{D}{H} \times V = \dfrac{150 \text{ mg}}{10 \text{ mg}} \times 1 \text{ ml} =$

   $\dfrac{150}{10} = 15 \text{ ml}$

   or
   DA: ml = $\dfrac{1 \text{ ml} \times \overset{15}{\cancel{150 \text{ mg}}}}{\cancel{10 \text{ mg}} \times 1} =$

   15 ml

16. **a.** 150 pounds = 68 kg
   b. $0.75 \times 68 = 51$ mg or 50 mg
   c. Select 25-mg capsule bottle. Two capsules.

17. **a.** 5 mg $\times$ 70 kg = 350-mg loading dose
   b. Select the 150 mg/15 ml bottle.
   c. 35 ml theophylline

18. **a.** 10 ml = 100 mg Colace
   b. $\dfrac{\textit{Known mOsm (3900)} \times \text{Volume of drug (10 ml)}}{\text{desired mOsm (500)}} = \dfrac{39,000}{500} = 78 \text{ ml drug solution and water}$

   78 ml of drug solution and water − 10 ml of drug solution =
   68 ml of water to dilute the osmolality of the drug

Injectables

19. ½ ml or 0.5 ml

BF: $\dfrac{D}{H} \times V = \dfrac{\overset{1}{\cancel{25}} \text{ mg}}{\underset{2}{\cancel{50}} \text{ mg}} \times 1 \text{ ml} = \frac{1}{2} \text{ ml}$

or

RP: H   : V ::   D   : X
       50 mg : 1 ml :: 25 mg : X

$$50 \text{ X} = 25$$
$$\text{X} = \frac{25}{50} = \frac{1}{2} \text{ ml}$$

or

DA: no conversion factor needed

$\text{ml} = \dfrac{1 \text{ ml} \times \overset{1}{\cancel{25 \text{ mg}}}}{\underset{2}{\cancel{50 \text{ mg}}} \times 1} = \frac{1}{2} \text{ ml or } 0.5 \text{ ml}$

20. 1 ml

21. a. Meperidine 0.8 ml; atropine 1.25 ml or 1.3 ml
  b. (1) draw 1.25 ml of air and insert into the atropine bottle
     (2) withdraw 1.25 ml of atropine and 0.8 ml of meperidine from the ampule.

22. a. Could use either vial, units 5000/ml or units 10,000/ml
  b. 0.5 ml from the units 5000 vial or 0.25 ml from the units 10,000 vial.

23. 0.2 ml of Lovenox

24. 1.25 ml of Naloxone.

25. Withdraw 35 units of Humulin 70/30.

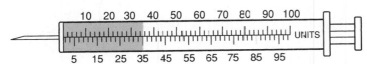

26. a. Withdraw the regular Humulin R insulin first and then the Humulin N insulin.

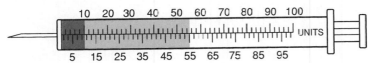

  b. Total of 55 units of Humulin R and Humulin N insulin (10 units regular, 45 units Humulin N).

27. a. Select 1000 mcg/ml. If you chose the 100 mcg/ml cartridge, you would need 5 cartridges to give 500 mcg.
  b. ½ ml or 0.5 ml

28. grain ⅙ = 10 mg (use conversion table as needed)
    0.66 ml or 0.7 ml

29. ½ ml or 0.5 ml

30. 1.4 ml

31. a. 145 ÷ 2.2 = 65.9 kg or 66 kg
  b. 3 mg × 66 kg = 198 mg/day
  c. 198 ÷ 3 = 66 mg per dose

   d. BF: $\dfrac{66 \text{ mg}}{80} \times 2 \text{ ml} = \dfrac{132}{80} = 1.65$ or 1.7 ml per dose **or**

   or
   DA: ml $= \dfrac{2 \text{ ml} \times 66 \text{ mg}}{80 \text{ mg} \times \quad 1} = \dfrac{132}{80} = 1.7$ ml per dose

32. 0.5 ml

33. a. Add 1.5 ml of diluent: 1.8 ml total
   b. 750 mg per day
   c. BF: $\dfrac{D}{H} \times V = \dfrac{250 \text{ mg}}{500 \text{ mg}} \times 1.8 \text{ ml} = 0.9$ ml of Tazidime

   or
   RP: H   :   V   ::   D   :   X
      500 mg : 1.8 ml :: 250 mg : X ml
            500X = 450
               X = 0.9 ml of Taxidime
   d. 3 ml syringe for mixing and administering; unable to mix the drug and diluent with a tuberculin syringe.

34. a. Add 3 ml diluent = 3.5 ml drug solution; 1 g = 1000 mg.

   b. $\dfrac{500 \text{ mg}}{1000 \text{ mg}} \times 3.5 \text{ ml} = \dfrac{1750}{1000} = 1.75$ ml or 1.8 ml per dose

35. a. 0.25 g = 250 mg

   b. BF: $\dfrac{250 \text{ mg}}{500} \times 2.2 \text{ ml} = \dfrac{550}{500} = 1.1$ ml per dose   **or** 1 ml
   or
   RP: H   :   V ::   D : X
      500 mg : 2.2 = 250 : X
            500 X = 550
               $X = \dfrac{550}{500} = 1.1$ ml or 1 ml

36. a. Add 5.7 ml diluent = 6.0 ml per 1 gram of oxacillin; 250 mg = 1.5 ml
   b. 0.9 ml per dose

37. 2.25 ml Fortaz

38. a. 165 lb ÷ 2.2 = 75 kg
   b. 4 mg × 75 kg = 300 mg/day
   c. 100 mg per dose
   d. Select 40 mg/ml bottle of gentamicin sulfate. (Normally less than 3 ml IM, should be given at one site.)
   e. 2.5 ml of gentamicin per dose

Direct IV Administration

39. a. 3 ml
   b. Known drug : Known minutes :: Desired drug : Desired minutes
         10 mg   :   1 minute   ::   30 mg   :   X
                              X = 3 minutes to administer 3 mg

Intravenous

40. 125 ml per hour

$$\frac{125 \text{ ml} \times 10 \text{ gtt/min}}{60 \text{ min/hr}} = \frac{1250}{60} = 20.8 \text{ gtt/min or } 21 \text{ gtt/min}$$

41. 62.5 to 63 gtt/min

42. Add 2.0 ml diluent = 2.6 ml drug solution; 1 g = 1000 mg.

a. $\dfrac{600 \text{ mg}}{1000 \text{ mg}} \times 2.6 \text{ ml} = \dfrac{15.6}{10} = 1.56 \text{ ml or } 1.6 \text{ ml Ticar per dose}$

b. $\dfrac{\text{Amount of solution} \times \text{gtt/ml}}{\text{Minutes}} = \dfrac{60 \text{ mg} \times \overset{2}{60} \text{ gtt/ml}}{\underset{1}{30} \text{ minutes}} = 120 \text{ gtt/min}$

43. a. 1.5 ml

b. $\dfrac{100 \text{ ml} \times \overset{1}{15} \text{ gtt/ml}}{\underset{3}{45} \text{ min}} = \dfrac{100}{3} = 33.3 \text{ or } 33 \text{ gtt/min}$

44. a. Add 2 ml Thorazine to 500 ml. For 4 hours: 500 ml ÷ 4 = 125 ml per hour.

b. $\dfrac{125 \text{ ml} \times \overset{1}{15} \text{ gtt/ml}}{\underset{4}{60} \text{ min/1 h}} = \dfrac{125}{4} = 31 \text{ gtt/min for 4 hours}$

45. a. Use the Mefoxin 1 g vial for ADD-Vantage and mix drug in the 50 ml IV bag for ADD-Vantage.

b. Amount of sol ÷ $\dfrac{\text{Minutes to admin}}{60 \text{ min/hr}}$ = ml/hr

50 ml ÷ $\dfrac{30 \text{ minutes}}{60 \text{ minutes}}$ = 50 ml × $\dfrac{\overset{2}{60} \text{ min}}{\underset{1}{30} \text{ min}}$ = 100 ml/hr

46. a. 0.5 g = 500 mg; add 2.0 ml of diluent = 2.5 ml of drug solution; 500 mg = 2.5 ml

b. Amount of solution ÷ $\dfrac{\text{Min to admin}}{60 \text{ min/h}}$ = ml/hr

2.5 ml drug + 50 ml ÷ $\dfrac{20 \text{ min}}{60 \text{ min/h}}$ = 52.5 ml × $\dfrac{\overset{3}{60}}{\underset{1}{20}}$ = 157.5 ml/hr or 158 ml/hr

Set pump to deliver in 20 minutes.

47. a. 10 mg/h × 5 h = 50 mg Cardizem

b. $\dfrac{50 \text{ mg}}{5} \times 1 \text{ ml} = 10 \text{ ml Cardizem to add to 500 m}$

c. 10 ml drug solution + 500 ml ÷ $\dfrac{300 \text{ min}}{60 \text{ min/hr}}$ = 510 ml × $\dfrac{\overset{1}{60} \text{ min}}{\underset{5}{300} \text{ min (5 h)}}$ = $\dfrac{510}{5}$ = 102 ml/hr

48. a. *Drug Calculation:*

BF: $\dfrac{D}{H} \times V = \dfrac{100 \text{ mg}}{200 \text{ mg}} \times 20 \text{ ml} = 10 \text{ ml}$ RP: H : V ::   D   : X

200 mg : 20 ml :: 100 mg : X ml

200 X = 2000

X = 10 ml

or

FE: $\dfrac{H}{V} = \dfrac{D}{X} = \dfrac{200}{20} \times \dfrac{100}{X} =$

(Cross multiply) 200X = 2000

$X = 10$ ml

or

DA: ml $= \dfrac{20 \text{ ml} \times \cancel{100}^{1} \text{ mg}}{\cancel{200}_{2} \text{ mg} \times 1} = 10$ ml

b. *Flow rate calculation* (secondary set):

$$\dfrac{110 \text{ ml } (100 + 10) \times \cancel{15}^{1} \text{ gtt/ml (set)}}{\cancel{30}_{2} \text{ minutes}} = 55 \text{ gtt/min}$$

c. *Infusion pump rate:*

$$110 \text{ ml} \div \dfrac{30 \text{ minutes to admin}}{60 \text{ min/hr}} = 110 \times \dfrac{\cancel{60}^{2}}{\cancel{30}_{1}} = 220 \text{ ml/hr}$$

49. a. 1.2 g × 1.98 m² = 2.37 g or 2.4 g or 2400 mg

    b. 2.4 g × 20 ml/1 g = 48 ml diluent added to Ifex vials to yield 54 ml of drug solution

    c. (54 ml of drug solution + 50 ml) $\div \dfrac{30 \text{ min}}{60 \text{ min}} = 104 \text{ ml} \times \dfrac{\cancel{60}^{2} \text{ min}}{\cancel{30}_{1} \text{ min}} = 208 \text{ ml/hr}$

    Set pump to deliver in 30 minutes.

Pediatrics

50. a. Drug dose is within safe range.

    b. 10 ml

51. a. Drug dose is within safe range.

    b. 5 ml

52. a. Drug dose is within safe range; 53 pounds ÷ 2.2 = 24 kg. 25,000 × 24 = 600,000 units; 90,000 × 24 = 2,160,000 units/day. Child receives 400,000 units × 4 (q6h) = 1,600,000 units/day.

    b. 400,000 units = 10 ml per dose

53. a. No; the drug dose is *NOT* within safe range. Do *NOT* give. Contact the physician or health care provider.

    Dosage parameters: 380 to 760 mg/day

    Order 250 mg × 4 (q6h) = 1000 mg/day; *not safe; exceeds parameters*

    b. Would not give medication.

54. a. Drug dose is within safe range.

    b. 18.75 ml or 19 ml theophylline elixir.

55. a. Drug dose is within safe range.

    5 mg × 16 kg = 80 mg; child receives 25 mg × 3 (tid) = 75 mg; *SAFE*

    b. 10 ml

56. a. 44 lb ÷ 2.2 = 20 kg

    b. Drug dose is less than pediatric drug range. Check with the health care provider.

    20 mg × 20 kg = 400 mg/day; 40 mg × 20 kg = 800 mg/day.

    Child to receive 100 mg × 3 (q8h) = 300 mg/day; less than 400-800 mg/day.

    c. 2.67 ml or 2.7 ml per dose = 100 mg

57. a. Drug dose is within safe range.

3 mg × 10 kg = 30 mg/day; 5 mg × 10 kg = 50 mg/day.

Child to receive 15 mg × 3 (q8h) = 45 mg/day.

   b. 1.5 ml per dose

58. a. Drug dose is within the safe range.

30 mg × 27 kg = 810 mg/day; 50 mg × 27 kg = 1350 mg/day.

Child to receive 250 mg × 4 (q6h) = 1000 mg/day.

   b. 1.2 ml per dose

59. a. 22 kg (child's weight in kg); 48 pounds ÷ 2.2 = 21.8 or 22 kg

   b. Yes, the daily dose is within the parameters; 50 × 22 = 1100 mg/day and 100 × 22 = 2200 mg/day

   c. *Drug calculation:* Child is to receive 400 mg × 3 = 1200 mg/day or 400 mg q8h

$$\text{BF: } \frac{D}{H} \times V = \frac{400 \text{ mg}}{500 \text{ mg}} \times 2 \text{ ml} = \frac{8}{5} = 1.6 \text{ ml}$$

or

$$\text{DA: ml} = \frac{2 \text{ ml} \times \overset{4}{\cancel{400 \text{ mg}}}}{\underset{5}{\cancel{500 \text{ mg}}} \times 1} = \frac{8}{5} = 1.6 \text{ ml}$$

   d. *Flow rate calculation:* $\dfrac{50 \text{ ml} \times \overset{2}{\cancel{60}} \text{ gtt/ml}}{\underset{1}{\cancel{30}} \text{ minutes}} = 100 \text{ gtt/min}$

60. a. 180 mg/day; 60 mg/dose

   b. $\dfrac{60}{75} \times 2 \text{ ml} = \dfrac{120}{75} = 1.6 \text{ ml per dose}$

   c. Drug dose is within safe range.

Child's weight: 26 lb ÷ 2.2 = 11.8 or 12 kg

15 mg × 12 kg = 180 mg/day; child to receive 180 mg/day or 60 mg per dose.

 Additional practice problems are available on the enclosed CD-ROM in the "Comprehensive Post-Test" section.

Guidelines for Administration of Medications

GENERAL DRUG ADMINISTRATION

1. Check medication order against doctor's orders, MAR (i.e., medication administration record), medicine card (if available), and/or other methods, such as computerized records.
2. Check label of drug container three times.
3. Check drug label for expiration date of *all* drugs. Return drugs that are outdated to the pharmacy.
4. Identify the patient by identification bracelet and by asking patient his or her name.
5. Stay with the patient until the medication is taken.
6. Give medications last to patients who need more assistance.
7. Report any drug error immediately to the head nurse and physician. An incident report must be made.
8. Record drug given, including the name of the drug, dosage, date, time, and your initials.
9. Record drugs soon after they are given, especially STAT medications. Also indicate on the drug sheet if the drug was not given.
10. Record the amount of fluid taken orally with medication if client's intake (I) and output (O) are being recorded.
11. Be aware that nurses have the right to question drug orders. Physicians are responsible for medication order, dosage, and route of drug administration. Nurses are responsible for administering medications.
12. Administer drug within 30 minutes of its prescribed time (30 minutes before or 30 minutes after prescribed time).
13. Do not guess when preparing medications. Check the order sheet if the drug order is not clear. Call the pharmacist, physician, and/or nursing supervisor if in doubt.
14. Do not give drugs poured by others.
15. Do not leave drug tray or cart out of your sight.
16. Know that patients have the right to refuse medication. If possible, ascertain why a patient refuses the medication. Report refusal to take medications.
17. Check if patient states that he or she has an allergy to a drug or a drug group.
18. Know the 6 *rights:* right drug, right dose, right route, right time, right patient, and right documentation.

ORAL MEDICATIONS

1. Wash hands before preparing oral medications.
2. Pour tablet or capsule into drug container's cap (top) and *not* into your hand. Drugs prepared for unit dose can be opened at the time of administration in the patient's room. Discard drugs that are dropped on the floor.
3. Pour liquids on a flat surface at eye level with your thumbnail at medicine cup line indicating the desired amount.
4. Do not mix liquids with tablets or liquids with liquids in the same container. Tablets and capsules can be put in the same container *except* for oral narcotics, digoxin, and PRN and STAT medications.

5. Do not pour drugs from containers with labels that are difficult to read.
6. Do not return poured medication to its container. Properly discard poured medication if not used.
7. Do not transfer medication from one container to another.
8. Pour liquid medications from the side opposite the bottle's label to avoid spilling medicine on the label.
9. Dilute liquid medications that irritate gastric mucosa, e.g., potassium products, or that could discolor or damage tooth enamel, e.g., SSKI (saturated solution of potassium iodide), or have client take the drug with meals.
10. Offer ice chips before administering bad-tasting medications in order to numb the client's taste buds.
11. Assist the patient into upright position when administering oral medications. Stay with the patient until medication is taken.
12. Give at least 50 to 100 ml of oral fluids with medications unless the patient has a fluid restriction. Doing so helps to ensure that medication reaches the stomach.
13. For patients having difficulty in swallowing or for patients receiving nutrients through a nasogastric or gastric tube, crush tablets (*not* capsules) and dissolve in juice or applesauce for oral ingestion or in water for tube administration. To maintain nasogastric and gastric tube patency, the tube should be flushed with specified amount of water; check with health care provider or the institution policy. Give oral medication in small amounts to prevent choking. For the patient who has difficulty swallowing, gently stroke the throat in a downward motion to enhance swallowing.
14. For drugs given by oral syringe, direct the syringe across the tongue and toward the side of the mouth.
15. If a patient or a child spits out *all* of the liquid medication, repeat the dose. If a patient or a child spits out more than one half of the liquid medication, repeat one half of the dose. If the patient or child spits out less than one half of the liquid medication or if there is a question regarding repeating the dose, the physician must be notified and another route of administration must be chosen.

INJECTABLE MEDICATIONS

1. Wash hands before preparing injectable medications.
2. Select the proper syringe and needle size for the type of medication to be administered.
3. Assess the amount of subcutaneous fat at the injection site before choosing the needle length for an intramuscular injection.
4. Select the injection site according to the drug.
5. Check for drug compatibility before mixing drugs in the same syringe.
6. Check the expiration date on the drug label before preparing medication. If in doubt, check with the pharmacist.
7. Check the label on the drug container to determine method(s) for drug administration, e.g., intravenous (IV), intramuscular (IM), subcutaneous (SubQ).
8. Do not give parenteral medications that are cloudy, are discolored, or have precipitated.

9. Aspirate the plunger before injecting medication. If blood returns, *stop*, withdraw the needle, and prepare a new solution. Check the policy of your institution. Aspiration does not apply to insulin, heparin, and lovenox.
10. Do not massage the injection site if using the Z-track method, intradermal injection, heparin, or any anticoagulant solution.
11. Do not administer injections into inflamed and edematous tissues or into lesion (moles, birthmarks, scar tissue) sites.
12. Recognize that individuals experiencing edema, shock, or poor circulation have a very slow tissue absorption rate with intramuscular injection.
13. Discard liquid drugs into the sink or toilet, *not* into the trash can.
14. Discard needles safely into the proper container.
15. Refrigerate unused reconstituted powdered medication in a vial. Write date, time, and your initials on the vial.
16. Discard unused solution in ampules. After they are opened, ampules cannot be used again.
17. Do not administer IM medications subcutaneously. Poor medication absorption and sloughing of the subcutaneous tissue could occur.

INTRAVENOUS FLUID AND MEDICATIONS

1. Wash hands before changing IV fluids and tubing and before preparing IV drugs.
2. Use aseptic technique when inserting IV catheters and changing IV tubing and bags. Be able to recognize symptoms of septicemia, such as chills, fever, and tachycardia.
3. Check for patency of the IV catheter (heparin lock) before administering drugs by injecting 2 ml of saline solution. Flush IV line with 15 ml of saline solution to empty the IV line of drug solution, if necessary.
4. Monitor all IV flow rates (conventional tubing or IV pumps) hourly as needed. IV flow rates can be altered by the patient's position or by a kink in the tubing.
5. Check for air bubbles in the IV tubing. Remove air from the tubing by clamping below the air bubbles and aspirating with a syringe, or use the method indicated by your institution.
6. Assess for allergic reactions to the IV drug. If reactions are seen, stop the flow of IV drug immediately.
7. Do not forcefully irrigate IV catheters. A clot could be dislodged from the catheter site and become an embolus.
8. Avoid using leg veins, elbow (antecubital) sites, and affected limbs for IV therapy.

9. Change the IV site daily or as indicated. Certain IV catheters, such as polyethylene catheters, can cause phlebitis.
10. Change IV tubing every 24 to 48 hours, and change IV bags every 24 hours.
11. Use the proper diluent to reconstitute a powdered drug. Follow institutional and pharmacy protocols for reconstituting and drug information inserts if available.
12. Vascular access sites should be labeled with the date and time of insertion.
13. When multiple catheters or multiple lumens are being used, all lines should be labeled with what medications and fluids are being infused through each line.
14. Assess infusion sites for signs of infiltration, which include coolness of skin around IV site, swelling, leakage, and pain. If these symptoms are present, discontinue IV. An infiltration scale should be used to grade the severity of the infiltration for accuracy of documentation.
15. For extravasation of vesicant medication or solution into the tissues around the IV site, the infusion should be discontinued immediately and the physician notified immediately so appropriate treatments can be instituted.
16. All IV sites should be monitored for signs of phlebitis, which is inflammation of the vein causing erythema, pain streaking noticeable along the vein, and a cord-like feeling along the vein. A phlebitis scale should be used for accuracy of documentation of symptoms.
17. All products and medications for IV infusion should be clearly labeled with the trade and generic names, along with the dosage and concentration of the drug or fluid, route of administration, expiration date, frequency, infusion rate, and sterility state.
18. All medications for IV infusion should be prepared in a clean environment.
19. When add-on devices are used, such as extension tubes, stopcocks, filters, access caps, and needleless systems, adhere to institutional policies and procedures, along with the manufacturer's directions.
20. Vascular access sites should be flushed at intervals according to institutional policies and procedures and manufacturer's policies and procedures.
21. Use an infusion pump for any medication with a narrow therapeutic range to prevent any error in dosage.
22. Every precaution should be taken to prevent a "free flow" incident of IV fluids.
23. Stabilize IV access sites to prevent the loss of site while maintaining the ability to monitor access.

Infiltration Scale

Grade	Clinical Criteria
0	No symptoms
1	Skin blanched
	Edema less than 1 inch in any direction
	Cool to touch
	With or without pain
2	Skin blanched
	Edema 1–6 inches in any direction
	Cool to touch
	With or without pain
3	Skin blanched, translucent
	Gross edema greater than 6 inches in any direction
	Cool to touch
	Mild to moderate pain
	Possible numbness
4	Skin blanched, translucent
	Skin tight, leaking
	Skin discolored, bruised, swollen
	Gross edema greater than 6 inches in any direction
	Deep pitting tissue edema
	Circulatory impairment
	Moderate to severe pain
	Infiltration of any amount of blood product, irritant, or vesicant

From *Infusion Nursing Standards of Practice.* (2006). New York: Infusion Nurses Society, p. S60.

Phlebitis Scale

Grade	Clinical Criteria
0	No symptoms
1	Erythema at access site with or without pain
2	Pain at access site with erythema and/or edema
3	Pain at access site with erythema and/or edema
	Streak formation
	Palpable venous cord
4	Pain at access site with erythema and/or edema
	Streak formation
	Palpable venous cord greater than 1 inch in length
	Purulent drainage

From *Infusion Nursing Standards of Practice.* (2006). New York: Infusion Nurses Society, p. S59.

Nomograms

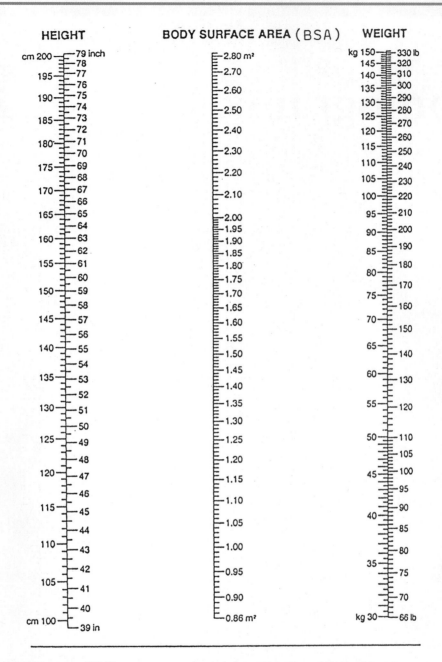

HEIGHT   BODY SURFACE AREA (BSA)   WEIGHT

Body surface area (BSA) nomogram for adults. *Directions:* (1) Find height; (2) find weight; (3) draw a straight line connecting the height and weight. Where the line intersects on the BSA column is the body surface area (m²). (From Deglin, J.H., Vallerand, A.H., & Russin, M.M. [1991]. *Davis's Drug Guide for Nurses* [2nd ed.]. Philadelphia: F.A. Davis, p. 1218. Used with permission from Lentner C. [ed.]. [1981]. *Geigy Scientific Tables.* [8th ed.] Vol. 1. Basel, Switzerland: Ciba-Geigy, pp. 226-227.)

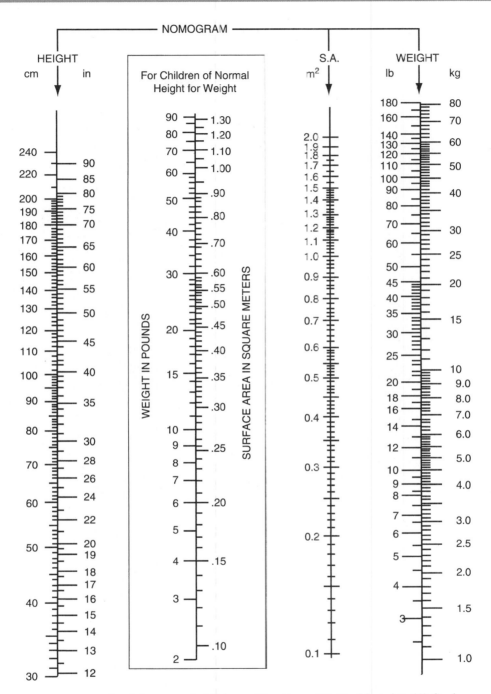

West nomogram for infants and children. *Directions:* (1) Find height; (2) find weight; (3) draw a straight line connecting the height and weight. Where the line intersects on the SA column is the body surface area (m²). (Modified from data of E. Boyd & C.D. West. In Behrman, R.E., Kliegman, R.M., & Jenson, H.B. [2000]. *Nelson Textbook of Pediatrics* [16th ed.]. Philadelphia: W.B. Saunders.)

References

Ambulatory infusion pump. (2001). Blackpool: McKinley Medical. From *www.mckinleymed.com*

Axton, S.E., & Fugate, T. (1987). A protocol for pediatric IV meds. *American Journal of Nursing, 7,* 943-945.

Barnhart, E.R. (1998). *Physician's desk reference* (52nd ed.). Oradell, NJ: Medical Economics.

Beckwith, C.M., Feddema, S.S., Barton, R.G., & Graves, C. (March, 2004). A guide to drug therapy in patients with enteral feeding tubes: dosage form selection and administration methods. *Hospital Pharmacy, 39,* 231.

Briars, G.L., & Bailey, B.J. (1994). Surface area estimation: pocket calculator vs. nomogram. *Archives of Disease in Childhood, 70,* 246-247.

Brown, B. (2000). *Calculating doses, flow rates, and administration of continuous intravenous infusion.* St. Louis: Elsevier Science.

Brown, M., & Mulholland, J.M. (2004). *Drug calculations: process and problems for clinical practice* (7th ed.). St. Louis: Elsevier/Mosby.

Burz, S. (2006). *Smart pumps get smarter.* From *www.nursezone.com/job/technologyreport.asp? article* ID=15520>

Conklin, S. (September 15, 2004). *UW Hospital and clinics install "smart" intravenous pumps.* From *www.wistechnology.com/article.php? id=1186>*

Conrad, M. (n.d.). *Infusion pumps.* From *www.rercami.org/ami/tech/tr-ami-mu-004_infusion-pumps/*

Crass, R. (2001). *Improving intravenous (IV) medication safety at the point of care.* Boston: ALARIS.

De Araujo, C.C., Dos Santos, M.V.D., & Barros, E. (1997). *A FPGA-based implementation of an intravenous infusion controller system,* p. 402. IEEE International Conference on Application-Specific Systems, Architectures and Processors.

Deglin, J.H., Vallerand, A.H., & Russin, M.M. (1991). *Davis's drug guide for nurses* (2nd ed.). Philadelphia: F.A. Davis.

Department of Veterans Affairs, Veterans Health Administration. (January 2002). *Bar code medication administration, version 2, training manual.* Washington, D.C.: Authors.

Dickerson, R.N., & Melnik, G. (April 1988). Osmolality of oral drug solutions and suspensions. *American Journal of Hospital Pharmacy, 45,* 832-834.

Estoup, M. (1994). Approaches and limitations to medication delivery in patients with enteral feeding tubes. *Critical Care Nurse, 14,* 68-79.

Foster, J. (2006). *Intravenous in-line filters for preventing morbidity and mortality in neonates.* From *www.nichd.nih.gov/cochrane/foster2 FOSTER.HTM*

Gahart, B., & Nazarento, A. (2003). *Intravenous medications* (19th ed.). St. Louis: Mosby.

Gin, T., Chan, M.T., Chan, K.L., & Yen, P.M. (2002). Prolonged neuromuscular block after rocuronium in postpartum patient. *Anesthesia-Analgesia, 94*(3), 686-689.

Green, B. (2004). *What is the best size descriptor to use for pharmacokinetic studies in the obese?* Brisbane: PubMed. From *www.ncbi.nlm.nih. gov/entrez/query.fegi?cmd*

Gurney, H. (1996). Dose calculation of anticancer drugs: a review of current practice and introduction of an alternative. *Journal of Clinical Oncology, 14*(9), 590-611.

Gurney, H.P., Ackland, S., Gebski, V., & Farrell, G. (1998). Factors affecting epirubicin pharmacokinetics and toxicity: evidence against using body-surface areas for dose calculation. *Journal of Clinical Oncology, 16,* 2299-2304.

Han, P.Y., Coombes, I.D., & Green, B. (October 4, 2004). *Factors predictive of intravenous fluid administration errors in Australian surgical care wards.* From *www.qhc.bmjjournals.com/cgi/ content/full/14/3/179*

Hardman, J. G., & Limbird, L.E. (2001). *Goodman & Gilman's the pharmacological basis of therapeutics* (10th ed.). New York: McGraw-Hill.

Hasler, R.A. (2004). *Administration of blood products.* San Diego: ALARIS. From *www.cardinalhealth.com/alaris/support/ clinical/pdfs/wp836.asp*

High tech IVs raise issues—intravenous infusion systems. (2001). Blackpool: McKinley Medical. From *www.mckinleymed.com*

Hodgson, B., & Kizior, R. (2006). *Mosby's 2006 drug consult for nurses.* St. Louis: Elsevier.

Husch, M., Sullivan, C., & Rooney, D. (2005). *Insights from the sharp end of intravenous medication errors: implications for infusion pump technology.* Chicago: BMJ Publishing Group, LTD. From *www.qhc.bmjjournals. com/content/full/14/2/80*

Infusion Nurses Society. (2006). *Infusion nursing: standards of practice,* Vol. 26. p. S 59, S 60. Philadelphia: Lippincott Williams & Wilkins. From *www.journalofinfusionnursing.com*

Infusion pumps. (n.d.). McKinley Medical. From *www.mckinleymed.com/infusion-pump-systems.shtml*

Intravenous therapy. (n.d.). McKinley Medical. From *www.mckinleymed.com/intravenous-therapy.shtml*

Kalyn, A., Blatz, S., & Pinelli, M. (2000). A comparison of continuous infusion and intermittent flushing methods in peripheral intravenous catheters in neonates. *Journal of Intravenous Nursing, 23*(3), 146-153.

Katzung, B.G. (1992). *Basic and clinical pharmacology* (5th ed.). Norwalk, CT: Appleton & Lange.

Kee, J.L., Hayes, E.R., & McCuistion, L. (2006). *Pharmacology: a nursing process approach* (5th ed.). Philadelphia: W.B. Saunders.

Kee, J.L., Paulanka, J.B., & Purnell, L. (2004). *Fluids and electrolytes with clinical applications* (7th ed.). Albany, NY: Delmar Publishers.

Krupp, K., & Heximer, B. (1998). The flow. *Nursing '98, 4,* 54-55.

Kuczmarski, R.J., & Flegal, K.M., (2000). Criteria for definition of overweight in transition: background and recommendations for the United States. *American Journal of Clinical Nutrition.* American Society for Clinical Nutrition, 72, 1074-1081.

Lack, J.A., & Stuart-Taylor, M.E. (1997). Calculation of drug dosage and body surface area of children. *British Journal of Anaesthesia, 78,* 601-605.

Lacy, C. (1990-2000). *Drug information handbook* (7th ed.). Cleveland: Lexi-Corp, Inc.

Lilley, L.L., & Guanci, R. (1994). Getting back to basics. *American Journal of Nursing, 9,* 15-16.

Loan, T., Magnuson, B., & Williams, S. (1998). Debunking six myths about enteral feeding. *Nursing '98, 8,* 43-48.

Macklin, D., Chernecky, C., & Infortuna, M.H. (2005). *Math for clinical practice.* St. Louis: Elsevier/Mosby.

Magnuson, V. (2005). Enteral nutrition and drug administration, interactions, and complications. *American Society for Parenteral and Enteral Nutrition, Vol. 20.* From *www.ncp. aspenjournals.org/cgi/content/full/20/6/618*

Maintaining oral hydration in older people. (2001). The Joanna Briggs Institute, Vol 5. From *www.joannabriggs.edu.au/ best_practice/BPIShyd.php*

Medscape. (2006). *ASHP National Survey of pharmacy practice.* From *www.medscape.com/ viewarticle/523005*

Mentes, J.C. (2004). *Hydration management evidence based-practice guidelines.* Iowa City: University of Iowa.

Mentes, J.C. (2006). Oral hydration in older adults. *American Journal of Nursing, 106*(6), 40-48.

Merenstein, G., & Gardner, S. (1998). *Handbook of neonatal intensive care* (4th ed.). St. Louis: Mosby.

MMWR. (2005). *Immunization management issues,* CDC. From *www.cdc.gov/mmwr/ preview/mmwrhtml/rr5416a3.htm*

Morris, D.G. (2006). *Calculate with confidence* (4th ed). St. Louis: Elsevier/Mosby.

Murray, M.D. (n.d.). *Chapter 10: unit-dose drug distribution systems.* From *www.ahrq.gov/clinic/ ptsafety/chap10.htm*

National Coordinating Council for Medication Error Reporting and Prevention. (2005). *Council recommendation.* From www.nccmerp. org/council/council1996-09-04.html

Niemi, K., Geary, S., Larrabee, M., & Brown, K.R. (2005). *Standardized vasactive medications: a unified system for every patient, everywhere.* Hospital Pharmacy. Vol. 40. Conshohocken, Pennsylvania: Wolters Kluwer Health, Inc.

National Institute of Health (NIH). (1998). *First federal obesity clinical guidelines released.* From *www.nhlbi.nih.gov/new/press/ober14f.htm*

Ogden, S.J. (2005). *Calculation of drug dosages* (7th ed.). St. Louis: Elsevier/Mosby.

Owen, D., Jew, R., Kaufman, D., & Balmer, D. (August, 1997). Osmolality of commonly used medications and formulas in the neonatal intensive care unit. *Nutrition Clinics, 12*(4).

Oyama, A. (2000). Intravenous line management and prevention of catheter-related infections in America. *Journal of Intravenous Nursing, 23*(3), 170-175.

Partners Healthcare System, Inc. (2003). *Project 4: safe intravenous infusion systems.* From *www.coesafety.bwh.harvard.edu/linkPages/ projectsPages/project4.htm*

Pediatrics. (1998). *Drugs for pediatric emergencies.* American Academy of Pediatrics. From *www.pediatrics.org/cgi/content/ full/101/1/e13*

Perinatal units: policy and procedural manual. (2005). Bryn Mawr, Pennsylvania: The Bryn Mawr Hospital.

Posidyne ELD intravenous filter set. (n.d.). East Hills, NY: PALL Medical. From *www.pall.com*

Prescribing in children. (n.d.). PatientPlus. From *www.patient.co/uk/showdoc/40024942*

Preventing magnesium toxicity in obstetrics. (2005). ISMP. From *www.ismp.org/ newsletters/acutecare/articles/20051020.asp*

Ratain, M.J. (1998). Body-surface area as a basis for dosing of anticancer agents: science, myth, or habit? *Journal of Clinical Oncology, 16*(7), 2297-2298.

Refurbished infusion pumps. (n.d.). CNA Medical. From *www.cnamedical.com/ infusionpumps.htm*

Rothschild, J.M. (2003). *Intelligent intravenous infusion pumps to improve medical administration safety.* AMIA Annual Symposium Process. From *www.pubmedcentral.nih.gov.articlerender. fegi?artid=1480207*

Savinetti-Rose, B., & Bolmer, L. (1997). Understanding continuous subcutaneous insulin infusion therapy. *American Journal of Nursing, 97,* 42-49.

Skokal, W. (1997). Infusion pump update. *RN, 60,* 35-38.

Spratto, G., & Woods, A. (2003). *PDR Nurse's drug handbook.* Albany, New York: Delmar Publishers.

Taxis, K. (2005). *Safety infusion devices.* Grogingen: BMJ Publishing Group. From *www.qhc.bmjjournals.com/cgi/content/ful/ 14/2/76*

Terry, J., Baranowski, L., Lonsway, R., & Hedrick, C. (1995). *Intravenous therapy: clinical principles and practice.* Philadelphia: W.B. Saunders.

Tessella Support Services. (2005). *Software that saves your life.* ALARIS. From *www.tessella. com/literature/articles/tessarchive/alaris.htm*

The Joint Commission (2000). *Infusion pumps: preventing future adverse effects* (15th ed.). From *www.jointcommission.org/ SentinalEvents/SentinalEventAlert/sea_15.htm*

Vanderveen, T. (2002). *Impact of intravenous (IV) infusion medication errors.* From *www.cardinalhealth.com/alaris/support/ clinical/pdfs/wpguardrails.asp*

Vanderveen, T. (2005). *Averting high risk errors is first priority.* PSQH. From *www.psqh.com/ mayjun05/averting.html*

Volumetric infusion pump manual. (1999). ALARIS Medical Systems, San Diego, California.

Wideman, M.V., Whittler, M.E., & Anderson, T.M. (n.d.). *Barcode medication administration: lessons learned from an intensive card unit implementation.* Columbia, Missouri: Agency for Healthcare Research and Quality.

Wong, D.L. (1995). *Nursing care of infants* (6th ed). St. Louis: Mosby.

Wyeth Laboratories. (1988). *Intramuscular injections.* Philadelphia: Wyeth Laboratories.

Zenk, K.E. (1987). Intravenous drug delivery in infants with limited IV access and fluid restriction. *American Journal of Hospital Pharmacy, 44,* 2542-2545.

Index

Note: Page numbers followed by "t" refer to tables.

NOTES

NOTES

NOTES

NOTES

NOTES

NOTES